Testimony and Trauma

At the Interface/Probing the Boundaries

VOLUME 118

The titles published in this series are listed at *brill.com/aipb*

Testimony and Trauma

Engaging Common Ground

Edited by

Cristina Santos, Adriana Spahr, and Tracy Crowe Morey

BRILL
RODOPI

LEIDEN | BOSTON

Cover illustration: Street graffiti Plazoleta de la Memoria, Buenos Aires. © 2015. Photographer Cristina Santos. Used with permission.

The Library of Congress Cataloging-in-Publication Data is available online at http://catalog.loc.gov
LC record available at http://lccn.loc.gov/2018968484

Typeface for the Latin, Greek, and Cyrillic scripts: "Brill". See and download: brill.com/brill-typeface.

ISSN 1570-7113
ISBN 978-90-04-37674-8 (paperback)
ISBN 978-90-04-39113-0 (e-book)

This book is printed on acid-free paper and produced in a sustainable manner.

Contents

PART 3
Scripts and Performances of Testimony

PART 4
Testimonial Embodiments

PART 5
The Curatorial Turn: Objects, Space, and Frames of Testimony

Illustrations

Notes on Contributors

Alison Atkinson-Phillips
is a research associate with the Newcastle University Oral History Unit and Collective. She completed her PhD in 2017 with the University of Technology, Sydney's Australian Centre for Public History.

Olga Bezhanova
is an Associate professor of Spanish Literature at Southern Illinois University, Edwardsville. She is the author the award-winning book *Growing Up in an Inhospitable World: Female Bildungsroman in Spain* and numerous articles.

Melissa Burchard
is Professor of Philosophy at the University of North Carolina, Asheville. Her research is on interpersonal and political violence, issues of sexuality and violence in identity, sexual ethics, and most recently on issues in trauma theory, including the parenting of traumatized children.

Mateusz Chaberski
graduated from Inter-faculty Individual Studies in Humanities at the Jagiellonian University in Cracow. He has an M.A degree in theatre studies and translation studies. He's now into his PhD programme in performance studies. His academic interests encompass memory studies, cyberculture, hybrid forms of contemporary art and drama translation. In 2015 he published his book *Doświadczenie (syn)estetyczne. Performatywne aspekty przedstawień site-specific.*

Candace Couse
was a 2012 finalist and winner from *The Primio Arte Laguna*, an international competition organized by the Cultural Association MoCA and Art Laguna, Couse's work has been exhibited across Canada, the USA, UK, Switzerland, Italy, Trinidad, Pakistan, Nepal and India.

Tracy Crowe Morey
Ph.D. (2007), University of Toronto, teaches Spanish at Ridley College and is a graduate student in Educational Studies at Brock University. She has published articles on women's testimonial literature and twentieth-century Latin American and Spanish film.

Marwa Sayed Hanafy
is an Assistant Professor in the Department of English Language and Literature, Faculty of Women for Arts, Sciences and Education, Ain Shams University. She received her PhD in Comparative Literature in 2014. She defended her second MA entitled: "Palestinian Rights: A Literary Multiple-Genre Approach" in the American University in Cairo in 2016.

Rachel Joy
is a sculptor, printmaker and PhD candidate based at the Centre For Ideas, Victorian College of the Arts at the University of Melbourne, Australia. Her work concerns relationships between identity, place, being and belonging.

Emma Kelly
is an independent researcher based in Belfast, Northern Ireland. Emma's research interests include Irish trauma narratives, contemporary Irish literature, women in 20th and 21st century Ireland, memory studies, and Irish cinema since 1970.

Timothy Long
is Head Curator of the MacKenzie Art Gallery in Regina, Saskatchewan, Canada and an Adjunct Professor of Visual Art at the University of Regina. His research interests include the application of mimetic theory to visual art and interdisciplinary approaches to film, dance, ceramics and performance art.

Elizabeth Matheson
is an independent curator, lecturer, and writer. Currently she is a co-curator of *Atom Egoyan and the Place of the Witness*, a multi-year research project on the film installation work of Atom Egoyan, funded by the Social Sciences and Humanities Research Council of Canada (SSHRC).

Antonio Prado del Santo
teaches Spanish language and literature at Knox College, Il., USA. He has worked on textual and visual representations of the Spanish Civil War and the post-2001 Argentine crisis.

Christine Ramsay
is Associate Professor of Film and Media Studies at the University of Regina. Her research, teaching and community service are in the areas of Canadian and Saskatchewan cinemas, masculinities in contemporary cultures, philosophies of identity, curating film installation art, and the culture of small cities.

Cristina Santos
teaches in Communication, Popular Culture and Film at Brock University. Her current research and scholarship reflect an interest in investigating the monstrous depictions of women as aberrations of feminine nature vis-à-vis the socio-culturally proscribed norm. She also investigates the construct of political and social deviance and trauma in life narratives as the construction of a personal and communal sense of identity that challenges official history and patriarchy. She is the author of *Unbecoming Female Monsters: Witches, Vampires, and Virgins* (2016).

Adriana Spahr
received her Ph.D. from the University of Toronto, Canada. At the present time she is an Associate Professor at MacEwan University in Edmonton, Canada. Her area of research focuses on political and social issues as reflected in works of literature. Part of her current research includes the role of testimony and the importance of human rights in our globalized world. On this topic she published articles and she is the co-author of the book *Madre de Mendoza/Mother of Mendoza* (Corregidor, 2013).

Introduction: Testimony and Trauma: Engaging Common Ground

Tracy Crowe Morey, Cristina Santos, and Adriana Spahr

1 Introduction

The turn to testimony in the twentieth century has given rise to our current state of reflection on how our societies bear witness to conditions of lives elsewhere. From political satires of North American apathy to organizational calls to act through giving to the most destitute among us, the beginnings of the current century can be marked as one of engagement. A cynic may agree with Mieke Bal's experience of bearing witness to images of suffering as she explains in her discussion of the photography exhibition *Beautiful Suffering* presented at the Williams College Museum of Art in 2006:

> Alone, I am not witnessing anyone's suffering. In all likelihood, the man is long dead, and he will never know that, in 2006, someone unknown to him felt an emotion for him that might approximate grief.[1]

Such spectacles of suffering and pain are questioned by many especially in terms of their possible engagement, if engaging at all. The overwhelming emotion affected through the proliferation of suffering from such images can actually render the witness unmoved.

Such complexities cannot be easily dismissed. However, the oversensitization of affect in the photography exhibition *Beautiful Suffering* provides a context for exploration regarding art's relationship with civic forms of engagement in the twenty-first century. Recent examples of political engagement include some of the more well-known grassroots movements coming from the youth such as Occupy Wall Street, Idle No More, the DREAMer movement, and the Arab Spring uprisings. As Henry Jenkins notes, these grassroots groups 'are actively recruiting and training young activists, helping them master basic practices that can support a lifetime of social change'.[2] Of interest

1 Mieke Bal, 'The Pain of Images', *Beautiful Suffering: Photography and the Traffic in Pain*, ed. Mark Reinhardt, Holly Edwards, & Erina Duganne (Chicago University Press, Chicago, 2007), 93.

2 Henry Jenkins, 'The New Political Commons', *Policy Options Politiques* November 1, 2012.

 | DOI:10.1163/9789004391130_002

to our study here is the fact that the youth are raising awareness through art-based forms of digital media and as a result they are self-actualizing their own participatory engagements in the public arena;[3]moreover, the public arena is being transformed and reactivated through the arts. For educational scholars and theorists, such as Henry Giroux, while much more work needs to be achieved, these grassroots movements are carving out 'new vocabularies and visions for clarifying our intellectual, ethical and political projects, especially as they work to reabsorb questions of agency, ethics, and meaning back into politics and public life'.[4]

Roger Simon's work on difficult knowledge and public pedagogy also attempts to construe and activate a newly transformed commons as a once again reclaimed democratic space of political alternatives. In *The Touch of the Past: Remembrance, Learning, and Ethics* (2005), Simon lays out what such a commons may look like:

> If there is to be an alternative to this stagnant horizon of community defined through usurpation and violence, what is needed is the reformulation of the prospect of a human solidarity that might reinvigorate new forms of relation within which one might conceive of a 'public life'.[5]

Such a public life 'must address questions as to what sets of relationships and social policies constitute a desirable society'.[6] Difficult knowledge is therefore a 'terrible gift' as Simon posits and such a gift represents, among many things, a legacy to future generations, a gift that demands reciprocity.[7] It is this reciprocity that we are still trying to figure out and it is here where we contextualize our discussions around the question of testimony as difficult knowledge.

From, a conceptual perspective, testimony is understood as an autobiographical narrative that presents evidence of first-person accounts of human

3 Ibid.

4 Henry Giroux, "Cultural Studies, Public Pedagogy and the Responsibility of Intellectuals", *Communication and Critical/Cultural Studies* 1.1 (2004): 75.

5 Roger Simon, *Touch of the Past: Remembrance, Learning and Ethics* (New York: Palgrave Macmillan, 2005), 5.

6 Roger Simon, 'Afterword: The Turn to Pedagogy: A Needed Conversation on the Practice of Curating Difficult Knowledge', *Curating Difficult Knowledge: Violent Pasts in Public Places*, ed. Erica Lehrer, Cynthia E. Milton, and Monica Eileen Patterson (Palgrave Macmillan, Basingstoke, 2011), 199.

7 Roger Simon, 'The Terrible Gift: Museums and the Possibility of Hope without Consolation', *Museum Management* 21 (2006): 187–204.

rights abuses, violence and war, and life under conditions of social oppression. Originally documenting claims of injustice and oppression that would otherwise have been erased or hidden from public recognition and unacknowledged in official histories, testimony has and continues to provoke controversy and debate surrounding issues of authenticity and accuracy. Yet, the continued use and evolution of testimony counters any claim that the genre has waned or lost audience appeal or interest.[8] Writers continue to use the genre as a source of information dissemination regarding human rights abuses and have begun to acknowledge testimony as an educational tool while also providing a means for solidarity and healing for its survivors and affected communities.

This collection of essays was initially motivated by one particular fascination shared by its editors. That is, we were interested in following the trajectory of testimony from its more traditional contexts of use in Latin America to how it was being used in the twenty-first century in ways that were becoming apparent to be much more diverse and inter-disciplinary.[9] However, we were becoming increasingly frustrated by the insular nature of the scholarship in this area. We wanted to bring together scholars and professionals on an international scale whose work on testimony would allow for discussions of the interdisciplinary nature of the phenomenon and also see if there was any common ground.

In the present collection, the contributing authors examine evolving forms and differing contexts of testimonial production. They do so with a critical eye to the ethical concerns that testimony brings to light for our present age. Some of the questions that are asked in this collection are the following: What are the methods and strategies used by these writers in their attempt to represent their own trauma or the witnessing of the trauma of others? What are the literary techniques and/or genres the writers make use of in their testimony? How do these testimonies relate to and/or challenge existing processes of restorative justice and healing, if at all? Can the promotion of restorative justice and/or healing be achieved and by what means? How are these testimonies received by members of their respective communities as well as by those outside their social/cultural networks? How does this form of testimonial creating constitute a means for political activism and/or social engagement?

8 Kimberly Nance, 'Something That Might Resemble a Call': Testimonial Theory and Practice in the Twenty-First Century', *Pushing the Boundaries of Latin American Testimony: Meta-Morphoses and Migrations*, ed. Louise Detwiler and Janice Breckenridge (New York: Palgrave Macmillan, 2012).

9 See Louise Detwiler and Janice Breckenridge for an updated analysis of twenty-first century *testimonio* scholarship: *Pushing the Boundaries* (New York: Palgrave Macmillan, 2012).

We hope that the current state of reflection and dialogue will challenge whether testimony in the twenty-first century is simply a new form of 'emotional tourism'[10] or can we take Simon's 'terrible gift' to imagine and construct alternative forms of solidarity? Can we reduce the state of affairs to mere apathy or does a socially engaging art-form like testimony offer up to a new generation a means of voice and agency in order to challenge 'the bankruptcy of old political languages and orthodoxies'?[11] Such an engaged public space is where we find many of the testimonies discussed in the following volume whose contents offer serious ponderings of these critically ethical concerns of our present age.

Organization of the Book

The present volume offers a series of papers first presented and expanded here for publication at one of two international conferences on *Testimony: Memory, Trauma, Truth, and Engagement* hosted at Oxford University, Oxford in July of 2014 and 2015. Initially the inaugural 2014 meeting aimed to bring together both researchers and practitioners engaged in the diverse forms of testimonial production in the twenty-first century. Many of the presentations reflected on the metamorphoses and hybrid forms of testimony especially production undertaken in the twenty-first century. A range of topics engaged with questions of genre, literary characteristics and modes of representation, reception, ethical concerns and the flaws and limitations of testimony. The papers selected for publication in the following volume reflect this broad range of testimonial production. Our second meeting continued the explorations and analyses of the multiple uses and contexts in which testimony finds a voice and receives a hearing. Again testimonial production showcased its diversity of expression and representation—from oral to written as well as nonfictional to fictional. The contexts of production were also diverse as examples covered clinical, pedagogical, religious, artistic, and performative environments, among others. Participants also began to reflect on questions pertaining to why testimony continues to thrive and evolve in the twenty-first century. It became clear that testimony encompassed a spectrum

10 Lisa Taylor, 'From Empathy to Estrangement, from Enlightenment to Implication: A Pedagogical Framework for (Re) Reading Literary Desire against the Slow Acculturation of Imperialism', *Muslim Women, Transnational Feminism, and the Ethics of Pedagogy: Contested Imaginaries in Post-9/11 Cultural Practice*, ed. Lisa K. Taylor and Jasmin Zine (Routledge, New York, 2014).

11 Giroux, 'Cultural Studies', 75.

of disciplines, conventions and practices, art forms, and embraced a broad range of geographical and historical contexts.

Throughout this volume, the reader will also notice the interactions and discussions taking place between the authors as they redrafted their chapters for expanded publication here. The authors from each conference were present to engage with all presenters for that particular conference as per the ethos of scholarship at Inter-disciplinary.net. In order to expand on this ethos for this collection, we asked the authors from both conferences to read the papers from the other contributors during the revision stage. We hoped that this process would ensure a much deeper level of engagement and discussion of the topic that could not be replicated in a stand-alone volume of individual papers on testimonial use and production. In this way, we were aiming to offer a common ground amongst the collection of culturally, disciplinary, and contextually divergent topics and essays. The fourteen chapters have been organized into five sections as follows:

Part 1. "Testimony, Time (In) Memorial" presents essays that examine testimony within the public sphere either as historical memorials or as official history. In Alison Atkinson-Phillips' "Material Testimony: Memorials Bearing Witness to Experiences of Loss and Trauma", memorials constitute an affirmation of the nation's previously hidden crimes revealed in national public inquiries into the forgotten and stolen children of Australia. In these public spaces, a narrative integrated with artistic and architectural form gives way to a commons that moves beyond the political debate of objectivity and rationality to actualize an affective space for mediation and thought. If nothing else, the commons holds out for a more inclusive space for those voices and stories previously disregarded or ignored.

In Antonio Prado del Santo's 'Spanish Republicans in the Holocaust: Historical Rights and Testimonial Literature', the importance of testimony is based on setting the historical record straight. Prado del Santo focuses on the experiences of Spanish Republicans imprisoned in the Nazi concentration camps after the end of the Spanish Civil War. It highlights the testimonies recently discussed in public forum attest to a historical solidarity based on class and political ideology amongst the Spanish Republican prisoners. The continuing debate on historical memory in Spain rests on testimonies such as those discussed by Prado del Santo in order to challenge the national amnesia surrounding Spain's Republican history and to re-politicize the commons.

Olga Bezhanova's 'Writing Spain's Fraught History: Testimony or Fiction?' also deals with the Spanish Civil War and public forms of memory that address Spain's history of national amnesia. However, the narrative here plays on fiction and history to include innovative uses of both novelistic and autobiographic forms of second hand witnessing. Similar to the other papers in this section, the importance of telling the story, in this case a private one, becomes a public form of unsettling of the amnesic or apathetic commons.

Part 2. "Suffer the Children" contains essays that deal with the consequences of inter-generational trauma and the implications of suffering and violence on children. In the case of Cristina Santos' 'When the Personal Becomes Collective: A Mother's Re-membering of a Disappeared Daughter in *Madre de Mendoza*', keeping the memory alive of the political and social activism of a politicized youth and its effects on an older generation is to ensure that these stories become part of a national remembering of the victims of Argentina's military dictatorship of 1976 to 1983. In this case, Santos' discussion of testimony reflects the life story of an Argentine mother whose personal story of trauma becomes an example of an entire society affected by the brutal disappearances of Argentina's children.

Adriana Spahr's 'Growing Up in Pain: Children of the Victims of the Argentinean Dictatorship' is an essay that discusses the author's collection of oral testimonies aimed at providing a medium for healing in a society that suffered a horrific state violence and human rights abuses. The healing in this case is of the children living in Argentina and abroad whose parents were victims of the state violence of the military dictatorship of 1976 to 1983. Spahr speaks to the inter-generational effects of political persecution especially on the growth and attitudes of the youth toward life and civic participation in Argentina and in Canada.

Melissa Burchard's 'Non-Standard Witness: Lessons from Working with/for Traumatized Children' examines recent cases of testimony with traumatized children to argue that current requirements and rigid conceptualizations of testimony work against the aims for healing of these survivors. Burchard speaks within a framework of care ethics over a justice-oriented one that must be considered when dealing with traumatized children's testimonies. In this way, Burchard offers an alternate and ethically-informed application of testimony's juridical use for healing from trauma.

Part 3. "Scripts and Performances of Testimony" brings together examples of the diversity of the literary nature of recent testimonial production from contexts like cinema and theatre to novelistic forms of writing such as autobiography and scriptotherapy.

Marwa Sayed Hanafy's 'Trauma and Healing in Izzeldin Abuelaish's *I Shall Not Hate*' examines the Palestinian novel as a form of narrative therapy as well as communal healing. Hanafy's examination of the testimony of a Palestinian survivor and doctor attests to the themes of memorialization as peace-making as a major drive of Abuelaish's testimony.

Emma Kelly's 'The 'piercing breach of a border': Irish Cinema as a Mediator of Modern Trauma' turns to recent cinematic representations of the Irish state's abuse of 'abjected' and 'othered' women placed in reformatories such as the Magdalene Laundries during the twentieth century. Kelly offers an analysis of the importance of cinema as an educational tool, one that endeavours to uncover the political and social reasons behind the institutionalization and abuses of Ireland's so-called 'fallen' women.

Mateusz Chaberski's 'Performing Witnesses: Frameworks of Memory in Contemporary Performing Arts' looks at the contemporary performances of Rimini Protokoll's *Mnemopark* (2008) and Jan Klata's *Transfer!* (2006) in order to examine concepts of theatrical techniques as frameworks of memory. Engagement at this level crosses over between audience member and stage performer to actualize a means for collective and credible witnessing within an ever-changing time and space permitted within the art of performance.

Part 4. "Testimonial Embodiments" contains essays that are both academic and autoethnographic; that is, the authors showcased here use their scholarly research and craft—whether through text or image—as a form of testimonial witnessing. Two of the selections offer testimonies of witnessing to the authors' body pain and suffering and a third paper offers an account of the artist's unsettling narrative crafted as a second hand witnessing to acts of genocide. These papers also offer insight into not only the reception of testimonial text/art, but also, into the production or process of bearing witness in testimony.

Candace Couse's 'Sick: Negotiating Body Trauma through Visual Art Practice' examines the social contexts of aberrance of the sick body as a form of trauma in a number of recent art exhibitions by the artist. As a feminist practitioner of the arts, Couse offers an autobiographical reading of the sick female body to conceptualize trauma as defined within existing normalized confines of Western science and medicine. The affect produced by Couse's embodied artwork offers an opening for a more humane and less estranged configuration or reorientation of relations between bodies.

The final piece in this section is Rachel Joy's 'Very Becoming: Transforming Our Settler Selves in Occupied Australia'. Here the author explores ways of unsettling through art practices within the context of settler/non-settler relations. The artist works to challenge Australia's ontological position of the Occupier as well as the nation's amnesic memory by engaging in artistic forms that look to unsettle the self or the object in relation to others. Again, the importance of process over product becomes manifest in such testimonial works. In essence, all of the essays presented here highlight how effective the affective forms of art can be as a means for engagement.

Part 5. "The Curatorial Turn: Objects, Space, and Frames of Testimony" is the last section in this collection and centres on the collaborative curatorial project of the Canadian-Armenian art filmmaker Atom Egoyan. The project called *Atom Egoyan and the Place of the Witness* fittingly finds a home here for scholarly discussion concerning questions of testimony and acts of witnessing through diverse mediums. The papers in this section address the medium of film installation art and speak to the importance of the immersive space, objects and frames of testimonial witnessing.

Christine Ramsay's 'Haunted Geographies in Atom Egoyan's *Calendar* and *Return to the Flock*' is the first paper in the curatorial series which offers a comparative analysis of the Armenian Genocide in his feature film *Calendar* (1993) and his installation *Return to the Flock* (1996–1997). In such a comparison, Ramsay highlights the symbolic power of cultural objects such as the church, the sheep, and the Armenian countryside as a way in which to bring to light Egoyan's use of artefacts from both the cinema and the gallery space as a means for engagement of testimonial witnessing.

Timothy Long's 'Atom Egoyan's *Auroras: A Chorus of Witnesses*' deals with the lens-based installation *Auroras* (2007) that presents the tragic story of Aurora Mardiganian, a survivor of the Armenian genocide who becomes a celebrity phenomenon due to the publication and filming of her story in the United States. Long explains the use of what he terms 'theatroclasm' or 'breaking the place of the viewer' as an example of Egoyan's strategy to engage with and unsettle the act of witnessing. Long's analysis of this particular lens-based installation also delves into Egoyan's unmaking of an often too simplistic polarity between victim and victimizer thereby offering a much more complex engagement with accounts of genocide.

Elizabeth Matheson's 'Immersive Spaces and the Place of the Witness' considers the space of testimony in Egoyan's filmic installation *Steenbeckett* (2002). As important as objects and frames are to testimony as discussed in the previous two essays, Matheson's analysis looks to space itself and the act of witnessing and non-witnessing in order to field questions related to our engagement and non-engagement with a most existential being: the self. It is no wonder that this highly immersive and impressionistic experience is fittingly achieved through a remembered-life on celluloid as represented in *Krapp's Last Tape*. This final paper in the collection in essence brings us back home to the question of how, as individuals within our own private space, will respond and engage with the world around us.

3 Furthering Explorations of a Common Ground

The editors' hope that this collection not only reveal the 'common ground' of the wide range of testimonial production but that it also initiate further discussions and examinations of the 'sources' of testimonial production. That is, the social injustices and human rights infractions suffered by both individuals and the collective through varying historical, geographic, political, and socio-cultural contexts. It is a desire to recover what has been lost; to unveil that which has been hidden; to uncover what has been repressed; to seek meaning in what has been unexplainable by telling one's story. James Dawes in his essay 'Human Rights in Literary Studies' makes this point very clear:

> We make sense of ourselves and our lives, individually and collectively, by telling stories. Basic work in social psychology supports this idea: some key studies on altruism, for instance, argue that our choices about whether or not to help in certain circumstances are dependent upon a 'self-concept' we develop based on the stories we have learned to tell ourselves to explain our sometimes arbitrary past actions. ... This means that when considering basic issues about the 'self' that are fundamental to the work of human rights and humanitarianism—sympathy, community building and activism, trauma and recovery (to name a few)—we need to be highly sensitive to the structure of narrative and the role of storytelling.[12]

This collection aspires to engage with a broader and inter-disciplinary dialogue of testimonial production and reception that surpasses questions of genre and geography (to name a few) to focus on the human story—to seek to make sense of human suffering with the prospect of 'making sense' of these lived experiences. The editors believe this is but a small contribution to the life stories that embody realities not always part of official histories.

Bibliography

Bal, Mieke. 'The Pain of Images'. *Beautiful Suffering: Photography and the Traffic in Pain*, edited by Mark Reinhardt, Holly Edwards, and Erina Duganne, 93–115. Chicago University Press, Chicago, 2007.

12 James Dawes, 'Human Rights in Literary Studies', *Human Rights Quarterly* 31.2 (2009): 395.

Dawes, James. 'Human Rights in Literary Studies'. *Human Rights Quarterly* 31.2 (2009): 394–409.

Detwiler, Louise and Janice Breckenridge, eds. *Pushing the Boundaries of Latin American Testimony: Meta-Morphoses and Migrations.* New York: Palgrave Macmillan, 2012.

Giroux, Henry. "Cultural Studies, Public Pedagogy and the Responsibility of Intellectuals". *Communication and Critical/Cultural Studies* 1.1 (2004): 59–79.

Jenkins, Henry. 'The New Political Commons'. *Policy Options Politiques,* November 1, 2012. Viewed on 8 September, 2016. http://policyoptions.irpp.org/magazines/come-together/jenkins.

Nance, Kimberly. '"Something That Might Resemble a Call": Testimonial Theory and Practice in the Twenty-First Century'. *Pushing the Boundaries of Latin American Testimony: Meta-Morphoses and Migrations,* edited by Louise Detwiler and Janice Breckenridge, 239–247. New York: Palgrave Macmillan, 2012.

Simon, Roger. 'Afterword: The Turn to Pedagogy: A Needed Conversation on the Practice of Curating Difficult Knowledge'. *Curating Difficult Knowledge: Violent Pasts in Public Places,* edited by Erica Lehrer, Cynthia E. Milton, & Monica Eileen Patterson, 193–209. Palgrave Macmillan, Basingstoke, 2011.

Simon, Roger. *Touch of the Past: Remembrance, Learning and Ethics.* New York: Palgrave Macmillan, 2005.

Simon, Roger. 'The Terrible Gift: Museums and the Possibility of Hope without Consolation'. *Museum Management* 21 (2006): 187–204.

Taylor, Lisa K. 'From Empathy to Estrangement, from Enlightenment to Implication: A Pedagogical Framework for (Re) Reading Literary Desire against the Slow Acculturation of Imperialism'. *Muslim Women, Transnational Feminism, and the Ethics of Pedagogy: Contested Imaginaries in Post-9/11 Cultural Practice,* edited by Lisa K. Taylor and Jasmin Zine, 218–243. Routledge, New York, 2014.

PART 1

Testimony, Time (In)Memorial

CHAPTER 1

Material Testimony: Memorials Bearing Witness to Experiences of Loss and Trauma

Alison Atkinson-Phillips

Abstract

Public memorials play an increasing role in the repertoire of commemorative practices through which societies attempt to come to terms with difficult or uncomfortable pasts. Increasingly, memorials are also used to acknowledge lived experiences of loss and trauma. This represents a shift in the kinds of experiences memorials can be expected to acknowledge and challenges ideas of what a memorial is and what it does. This chapter draws on research conducted within Australia, and considers three examples of memorials that are influenced by transitional justice approaches to truth-telling, and which are used to bring difficult stories of child abuse, forced separation of families and loss of land into the public sphere. Using a narrative therapy approach, this chapter considers the relationships of power that allow such stories to be told in particular ways. These examples offer insights into the strategies survivors of human rights abuses and their supporters use to claim the right to speak and to have their stories heard, and the ways such testimony is constrained. At their best, memorials to lived experience are part of an arsenal of tools available to survivors and their supporters to bear witness to difficult pasts. The materiality of the memorial form can be helpful in assisting such histories to be absorbed into mainstream narratives.

Keywords

memorial – trauma – witness – testimony – post-colonial – Australia

Introduction

In a busy pedestrian thoroughfare in the centre of Perth, the state capital of Western Australia, stands a human-scale sculpture of a chatterbox – a child's toy usually made of paper that is folded and unfolded to reveal stories and

 | DOI:10.1163/9789004391130_003

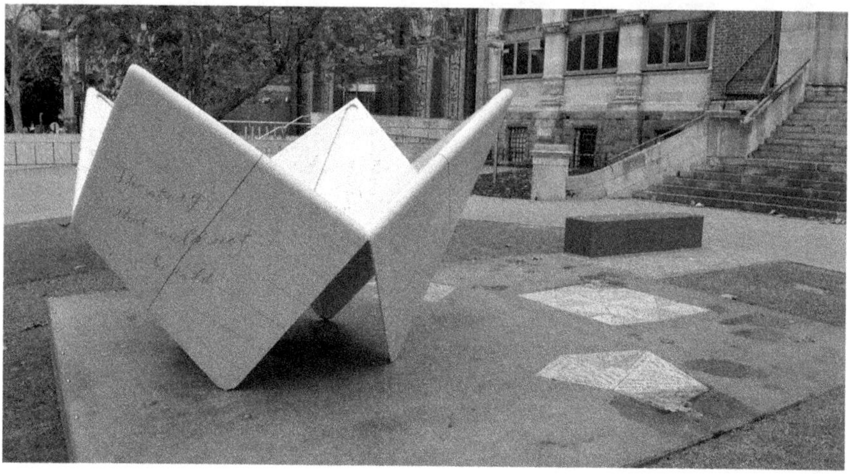

FIGURE 1.1 *Unfolding Lives* by Judith Forest
© 2014. PHOTOGRAPHER ALISON ATKINSON-PHILLIPS. USED WITH PERMISSION.

secrets. This chatterbox, made of fibreglass, is just the right height for an adult to lean over to read inside; also a good height for children to climb. The outside of the chatterbox offers fragments of text, clues about the secrets within. The side closest to the path reads, 'The story that could not be told'. But the very existence of this sculpture bears witness to the fact its story is no longer a secret, no longer unspeakable. This is a government-funded memorial that remembers the experiences of children who were in Australian out-of-home care during the 20th century—children who suffered the effects of institutionalisation and were often neglected and abused. It is a story that emerged slowly into the public sphere in a variety of ways, including through a national Australian Senate inquiry in the mid 2000s. This sculpture, named 'Unfolding Lives', takes the story that could not be told and places it upon the land, in one of the most public places of the city.

'Unfolding Lives' is just one example of an emerging genre of memorials that commemorate lived experiences of loss and trauma. They represent a shift in the kinds of experiences memorials can be expected to acknowledge, and challenge ideas of what a memorial is and what it does. These commemorative objects physically entered public spaces in the 1990s, at around the same time as the emergence of trauma studies as an academic discourse.[1] Like

1 Andreas Huyssen, 'Trauma and Memory: A New Imaginary of Temporality', *World Memory: Personal Trajectories in Global Time*, edited by Jill Bennett and Rosanne Kennedy, (London: Palgrave Macmillan, 2003), 16–29.

'Unfolding Lives', other memorials to lived experience commemorate stories that have been slow to be told publicly. In Australia, where my research is focussed, these are the stories of (post)settler-colonisation that include child abuse, rape, forced separation of families and loss of land. International examples can include retrospective commemoration of collective traumas such as the trans-Atlantic slave trade, as well as experiences with living survivors, such as the World War 2 'comfort women'.[2] Indeed, there is increasing recognition of the continuity between the stories of colonial trauma and these 20th century experiences.[3] I have found Deborah Britzman's term 'difficult knowledge' to be a useful way to describe these stories. Difficult knowledge is 'knowledge that does not fit'; knowledge that disrupts our sense of the world as we expect it to be.[4] Because of this, it is knowledge that is difficult to speak and difficult to receive. Margaret Smith does not use the term, but offers an example of the barriers that are created when those in positions of power are not ready to receive difficult knowledge.[5] The term draws attention to the experience of receiving such knowledge, and the need to pay attention to the conditions under which survivors' stories are able to be told and be heard. Whereas within trauma discourse, silence is most often interpreted as the inability of the victim to assimilate their experience, the concept of difficult knowledge points to the possibility of other reasons for silence, including the lack of a public discourse into which it is possible to speak.[6]

---

2 Carole Gluck, 'Operations of Memory: "Comfort Women" and the World', *Ruptured Histories: War, Memory, and the Post-Cold War in Asia*, edited by Sheila Myoshi Jager and Rana Mitter, (Cambridge, Massachusetts: Harvard University Press, 2007), 27–57.

3 See, for example, the exploration of the Parramatta Female Factory heritage site edited by Paul Ashton and Jacqueline Z. Wilson, *Silent System: Forgotten Australians and the Institutionalisation of Women and Children* (Melbourne: Australian Scholarly Publishing 2014).

4 Erica T. Lehrer and Cynthia E. Milton, 'Introduction', *Curating Difficult Knowledge: Violent Pasts in Public Places,* edited by Erica T. Lehrer, Cynthia E. Milton and Monica Eileen Patterson, (New York: Palgrave Macmillan, 2011), 1–18. See also Deborah P. Britzman, 'If the Story Cannot End: Deferred Action, Ambivalence, and Difficult Knowledge', *Between Hope and Despair: Pedagogy and the Remembrance of Historical Trauma,* edited by Roger I. Simon, Sharon Rosenberg and Claudia Eppert (Oxford: Rowman and Littlefield Publishers Inc, 2000), 27–57.

5 See 'Testimony in Northern Ireland: Abandoning the Past as a Source of Societal Healing?' (Paper presented at the *2nd Global Meeting of Testimony: Memory, Trauma, Truth, Engagement* July 2015).

6 Rosanne Kennedy and Jan Tikka Wilson, 'Constructing Shared Histories: Stolen Generations Testimony, Narrative Therapy and Address', *World Memory: Personal Trajectories in Global Time,* edited by Jill Bennett and Rosanne Kennedy (New York: Palgrave Macmillan, 2003), 124.

When memorials are created to acknowledge the painful experience of people who are *still* living, this creates both practical and theoretical challenges. Not only must these memorials engage in a different way with the ongoing experience of survivors, but they themselves confront the idea contained in much theoretical trauma writing of the absent (dead) 'ideal witness'. A common assumption is that all survivor-testimonies are grounded in the experience that cannot be spoken, that of the non-survivor'.[7] This statement suggests a hierarchy of trauma, with death at the top, which non-death memorials disrupt. In fact, such memorials draw attention to a crucial paradox at the heart of trauma theory, that trauma is fundamentally an experience of the living, not the dead. As Rothberg bluntly states, 'the dead are not traumatised, they are dead'.[8] An alternative way of approaching the work of bearing witness is offered by Rosanne Kennedy and Tikka Jan Wilson in their essay on Stolen Generations' testimony included in *World Memory*, edited by Kennedy and Jill Bennett. Kennedy and Wilson suggest a reading strategy based on the narrative therapy model as a possible approach to thinking about testimony as 'an address and appeal to community'.[9] This approach has helpfully informed discussion of literary testimony in Stef Craps' *Postcolonial Witnessing*[10] and I propose to use it here to consider the ways memorials to lived experiences of loss and trauma constitute an act of witnessing that allows difficult knowledge to be assimilated into publicly shared story or 'imagined community'.[11]

Narrative therapy is grounded in an understanding that 'no-one is a passive recipient of trauma' that: within the limited circumstances in which they find themselves, people will take action to preserve what is of value to them.[12] The aim of its therapeutic approach is to assist the traumatised person to re-build a 'sense of self' by assisting them to recognise their own agency. This is done

7 I am grateful to Steven Rita-Procter for drawing my attention to this through his unpublished paper at the *1st Global Meeting of Testimony: Memory, Trauma, Truth, Engagement.*

8 Michael Rothberg, *Multidirectional Memory: Remembering the Holocaust in the Age of Decolonization* (Stanford: Stanford University Press, 2009), 90.

9 Kennedy and Wilson, 'Constructing Shared Histories', 127.

10 Stef Craps, *Postcolonial Witnessing: Trauma Out of Bounds* (Basingstoke: Palgrave Macmillan, 2013).

11 Benedict Anderson, *Imagined Communities: Reflections on the Origin and Spread of Nationalism* 2nd ed. (London: Verso, 1991).

12 Michael White, 'Working with People Who Are Suffering the Consequences of Multiple Trauma: A Narrative Perspective', *International Journal of Narrative Therapy and Community Work* 1 (2004): 45.

through active listening, by the therapist and also through the involvement of an 'outsider-witness', whose job is to reflect back to the trauma survivor their story. A crucial difference between this model and a traditional psychoanalytic approach is that it frames the trauma survivor as the owner of the story. The outsider-witness partners in their witnessing by listening and reflecting back. Their role is not so much to empathise with the survivor-witness, but to hear and reflect back the story that is told, 'interweaving it with their own life stories' in a social act.[13] Importantly, the 'story' does not have to be the story of the traumatic event itself; rather the survivor-witness is encouraged to 'map the areas of their lives that have been invaded or are not always taken over by the problem'.[14] The point made by Kennedy and Wilson is that testimony in a narrative therapy model is 'an inherently social process, requiring a community that shares and participates in the discourse—both retrospectively and prospectively'.[15] The point of the participation of the outsider-witness is not the witnessing as such, but what comes next. As Craps argues, when testimony comes out of experiences that are ongoing or have continuing repercussions, it often contains the need for a response.[16] Craps offers a list of trauma literature coming out of or addressing traumatic African history which 'denounce and fight the indifference of a privileged and empowered Western public to the suffering of the racial, ethnic or cultural other'.[17] Many examples from around the world can be found in the chapters that make up the rest of this volume. Although memorials might inspire an empathic response, viewed through the lens of narrative therapy, they can be understood as an appeal to 'enter into the story' in solidarity, not sympathy. While memorials to lived experience, in common with traditional memorials, often serve a mourning or recovery role for survivors, this chapter is focussed on what Viebach calls their 'outside' role as truth telling or testimony[18] that is aimed at gaining entry into a shared, public story.

In teasing out the idea of public memorial as testimony, this chapter will consider three examples with a specific connection to testimony as it is usually understood; that is, testimony as narrative. These are memorials that

13 Kennedy and Wilson, 'Constructing Shared Histories', 132.

14 Ibid., 131.

15 Ibid., 132.

16 Stef Craps, *Postcolonial Witnessing*, 42.

17 Ibid., 42.

18 Julia Viebach, '"Alétheia" and the Making of the World: Inner and Outer Dimensions of Memorials in Rwanda', *Memorials in Times of Transition*, edited by Susanne Buckley-Zistel and Stefanie Schafer (Cambridge, Antwerp, Portland: Intersentia, 2014), 69–94.

commemorate experiences that have come to public consciousness through the oral and written testimony given as part of national public inquiries. My first and third examples are state-funded memorials constructed in response to the Australian Senate Community Affairs Reference Committee's *Forgotten Australians: A Report on Australians who experienced Institutional or Out of Home Care as Children.*[19] The second memorial acknowledges the experiences of the Stolen Generations, a name given to Aboriginal children removed from their families as a result of government assimilationist policies. This history came to be widely recognized following an earlier Australian inquiry by the Human Rights and Equal Opportunities Commission, with findings published as *Bringing Them Home: Report of the National Inquiry into the Separation of Aboriginal and Torres Strait Islander Children from Their Families.*[20] *Forgotten Australians* references this other inquiry as the first of a 'trilogy' that includes, as a middle instalment, an Australian Senate report on child migrants.[21] Child migrants in this context are children who were transported to Australia from the UK during the 20th century and raised in Australian orphanages. Although the memorials considered in this chapter do not specifically refer to child migrants, it is important to understand these histories as interrelated and part of Australia's history as a settler-colonial nation. All three of the inquiries drew heavily on personal testimony, and all three of their final reports quote directly and extensively from oral and written testimony. The narrative testimonies included in the reports, along with an increasing body of oral history and memoir, therefore inform these memorials.

1 Going Public

The memorials explored in this chapter are those described by Hamilton as 'material, three dimensional memorials, that can be touched, scratched,

19 Parliament of Australia, *Forgotten Australians: A Report on Australians Who Experienced Institutional or Out of Home Care as Children*, 30 August 2004, viewed on 18 May 2014, http://www.aph.gov.au/~/media/wopapub/senate/committee/clac_ctte/completed_inquiries/2004_07/inst_care/report/report_pdf.ashx.

20 Australian Human Rights Commission, *Bringing Them Home: Report of the National Inquiry into the Separation of Aboriginal and Torres Strait Islander Children from Their Families*, 1997, viewed on 18 May 2014, http://www.humanrights.gov.au/sites/default/files/content/pdf/social_justice/bringing_them_home_report.pdf.

21 Parliament of Australia, *Forgotten Australians*, 2.

venerated, visited, photographed or defaced—that have a visibility in a public place'.[22] In other words, two of their important characteristics are their materiality and their publicness. These two qualities are intertwined, in part through the tradition of public art and the monument. There is some slippage between the terms monument, memorial and public art, and they are often used interchangeably. All refer to material, symbolic objects placed in public space, but the terms of their publicness are contested.[23] Public memorials are not public by definition of the land on which they are situated, or how they are funded, but because of the way they function to allow the co-production of meaning. Approaching memorials with this understanding of publicness, I consider them as art objects; that is, as aesthetic objects that are encountered physically and affectively.[24] Whereas for Habermas and later for Warner, the public sphere is defined by rational debate,[25] I understand the public sphere as an imaginary space where various publics negotiate their shared meanings and ideas. This sharing and negotiation is not limited to either speech or textual acts, but includes visual and other forms of communication. Memorials arise out of stories that must be negotiated and, to some extent, shared in order to make it to the construction phase; as aesthetic objects, they are encountered and made meaning of by memorial participants. Such meanings also circulate within a broader public sphere through images and text *about* the memorials and the histories they represent. So, memorials can be understood as interventions into the public sphere that not only serve as an 'address and appeal to community'[26] but also expand that community and in doing so constitute a public.

---

22 Paula Hamilton, 'Material Memories and the Australian Memorial Imagination', *Melbourne Historical Journal* 39 (2011): 11–12.

23 Miles argues that both traditional monuments and contemporary public artworks 'make visible the values of the public sphere'; however, Deutsche contends that public art should be understood as 'a practice that constitutes a public'. Malcolm Miles, *Art, Space and the City: Public Art and Urban Futures* (London: Routledge, 1997); Rosalyn Deutsche, *Evictions: Art and Spatial Politics* (Cambridge: MIT Press, 1996), 288.

24 Jill Bennett, *Practical Aesthetics: Events, Affects and Art after 9/11* (London: I B Tauris, 2012), 14–15.

25 Craig Calhoun, 'Introduction', *Habermas and the Public Sphere,* edited by Craig Calhoun (Cambridge: MIT Press, 1992), 1–48; Michael Warner, *Publics and Counterpublics* (New York: Zone Books, 2002).

26 Kennedy and Wilson, 'Constructing Shared Histories', 124.

2 Unfolding Lives, Perth

The various components of 'Unfolding Lives' cover a flattened concrete space on a small grassy knoll, edged by a low, red concrete wall on which the artwork's title is embossed and on which a memorial plaque rests. The memorial is located in the Perth cultural centre, to the right of the Western Australian (WA) Museum entrance. On the other side of the museum entrance is a children's play space. For the casual passer-by, the four outside 'folds' of the sculpture offer only clues about the story within. To find out more, the visitor must move closer, almost like the action of drawing near to hear a secret whispered in the children's game the sculpture represents. Some of the information contained within is indeed difficult knowledge: 'They told me my parents were dead. They were not'. 'My name was once a number'. This is taken from testimony directly from survivors whose identity was either purposefully removed or simply not valued by the adults responsible for them.[27] Similarly confronting phrases are on two diagrams embedded into the red concrete surface. Alongside these are more redemptive snippets: 'someone is listening to my story'; 'regaining our identity'. A third tile names the institutions where children lived.

The process through which 'Unfolding Lives' came to be constructed offers an insight into the complex challenges of bringing difficult knowledge into the public sphere through the memorial form. Its construction was not driven directly by care leavers (people previously in out-of-home 'care' as children),[28] and in this sense it differs from a usual understanding of testimony as the address of a victim or witness. Nonetheless, the memorial came about as a result of Recommendation 32 of *Forgotten Australians*, which in turn was a response to the submission of the Care Leavers Australia Network (CLAN).[29] Appearing before the Senate Inquiry in February 2004, Dr. Joanna Penglase, then president of CLAN, made it clear that she saw the public inquiry and the idea of a memorial as connected, and as both being about making 'history visible'. Penglase, a care leaver and memory activist who has published on the topic of the

27 These stories of lost or stolen identity have echoes of the policies of the Franco dictatorship, as discussed by Olga Bezhanova in this volume. The use of numbers rather than names to address people in institutions is a practice continued in Australia's immigration detention system.

28 Not all of those who spent time in state care as children identify as Forgotten Australians. The term 'care leavers' is an alternative name that implies a greater sense of agency.

29 Parliament of Australia, *Forgotten Australians*, 325.

children in care, was a founding member of CLAN. She appeared before both the 2004 inquiry into children in care and the earlier inquiry into child migration. She advocated for widespread public acknowledgement of the suffering twentieth century child welfare practices caused.[30] The Senate Committee, drawing on the advice of CLAN, suggested that memorial forms should include gardens, plaques placed on the site of institutions, and heritage centres, again on the site of former institutions. The Federal Government accepted the recommendations to the extent that it recognised memorials as 'an appropriate way to acknowledge past injustices'[31] and responded by making $AU100,000 available for memorial projects. This, divided up equally between the six Australian states, meant each received a total of $16,666. The Government did not take into account the different numbers of children in care in each state, even though, if memorials were to be located at specific sites, it would seem logical that there may be more demand for memorials in states where there had been more institutions. In every state but Queensland, the funding was used instead to create a single state memorial.

In Western Australia, the Forgotten Australians memorial project was part of a program known as Redress WA, a scheme based on a transitional justice framework and designed to provide some restitution to people who experienced abuse or neglect in state care when they were children. This fits in with a broader international trend for memorials to be considered 'symbolic reparation' within transitional justice mechanisms.[32] The Federal Government funds covered the costs of landscaping at the memorial site, and the State Government provided an additional $100,000, plus consultancy and project management costs, towards the memorial. So, while the Senate inquiry and its recommendations provided the impetus for the memorial, there is not a straightforward line between the Federal Government response and the finished Perth memorial.

30 Senate of Australia, Community Affairs Reference Committee *Official Committee Hansard*, 4 February 2004, viewed on 18 May 2014, http://parlinfo.aph.gov.au/parlinfo/download/committees/commsen/721/toc_pdf/3131-2.pdf.

31 Senate of Australia, Community Affairs Reference Committee, *Australian Government Response to Forgotten Australians: A Report on Australians Who Experienced Institutional or Out-of-Home Care as Children*, 2005, viewed 19 January 2016, http://www.aph.gov.au/~/media/wopapub/senate/committee/clac_ctte/completed_inquiries/2004_07/inst_care/gov_response/gov_response_pdf.ashx.

32 Susanne Buckley-Zistel and Stefanie Schaefer, 'Introduction', *Memorials in Times of Transition*, eds. Susanne Buckley-Zistel and Stefanie Schafer (Cambridge: Intersentia, 2014), 1–24.

The WA Department for Child Protection (DCP) had overall responsibility for the project, and one particular worker played an important role as a liaison between various stakeholders. It is not clear who made the decision to locate the memorial in its particular spot outside the WA Museum, and on the edge of the Perth Cultural Centre. However, the choice led to the involvement of a number of high-level stakeholders, some of whom were driven by concerns about the artistic or aesthetic 'quality' of the finished product, as much as by a desire to fulfil the spirit of the Senate's recommendations. It was this group of stakeholders, representatives of various state government departments and agencies, that selected the artist and approved the final design. A Forgotten Australians Committee was involved in the project, offering advice to the DCP worker which fed through into the development of the project brief. This Committee was consulted during the design development phase through a series of informal workshops. These structures clearly restricted the involvement of the survivors of the state care system in the project; only those who were able to participate in the particularly structured 'consultation' process could have a say, and only then in a very limited way.

Nonetheless, considered in terms of the narrative therapy model, the memorial can be understood as a form of state listening and acknowledging, despite the fact that the 'reflecting back' of the stories was always mediated through available discursive and institutional structures. One care leaver I interviewed about the memorial connected it with the Federal Government's formal apology to the Forgotten Australians, which he had attended. It was not the apology that was important to him, but the moment when Opposition Leader Malcolm Turnbull said, 'We believe you'. For some survivors, the memorial is seen as a way the state says, 'We believe you'. For survivors who have had to work hard to have the difficult knowledge of state-sanctioned child abuse accepted by the community, this is a powerful message.

The role individuals play in the development of public memorials is often under-acknowledged. Despite the clear power imbalance between those whose experience the memorial sought to represent (the care leavers/Forgotten Australians) and the design selection committee, previous memory work meant key actors in the project were able to 'hear' the story and to reflect it back respectfully. Both artist Judith Forrest and writer Terri-ann White drew on existing testimony, including *Forgotten Australians*, public submissions to the Inquiry, and autobiographical texts, to inform their approach. The 'chatterbox' form of the final memorial developed out of Forrest's research. Her initial written proposal had suggested the sculpture would make use of 'the sort of soft rounded forms and tactile surfaces that evoke comfort and security' but she soon realised that forms which might suggest 'comfort' to one person, may have more sinister resonance when associated with stories of abuse, particularly

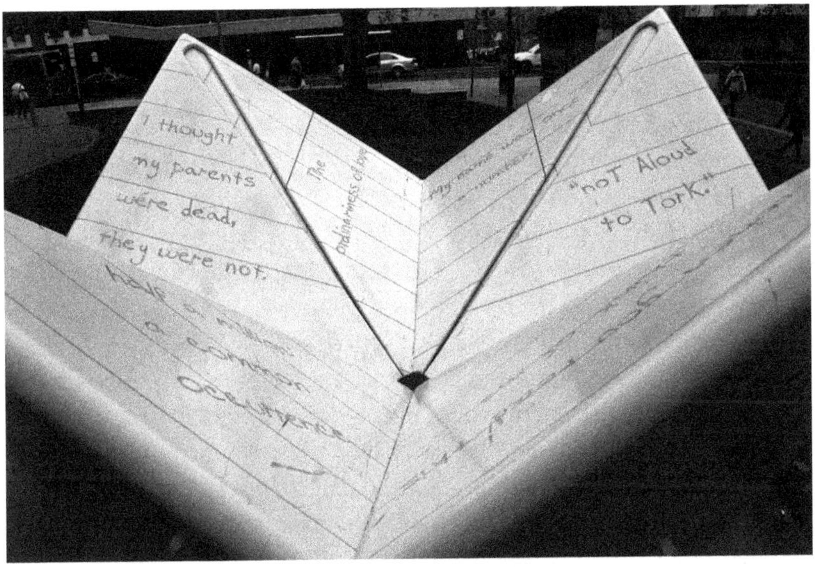
I thought
my parents
were dead,
they were not.
"noT Aloud
to Tork."

FIGURE 1.2 *Unfolding Lives*, view inside the chatterbox
© 2014. PHOTOGRAPHER ALISON ATKINSON-PHILLIPS. USED WITH PERMISSION.

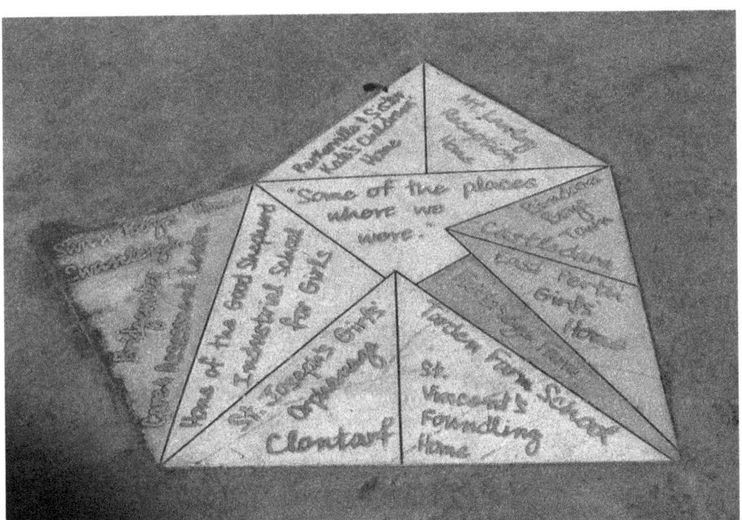

FIGURE 1.3 *Unfolding Lives*, floor detail
© 2014. PHOTOGRAPHER ALISON ATKINSON-PHILLIPS. USED WITH PERMISSION.

sexual abuse. After playing with the idea of a shelf holding a trio of toys, she settled on the idea of the chatterbox. In part, this was because her research suggested it was a toy that had been played with by children around the world in different ways, and because it was a toy that could be made 'even when the kids had nothing else'. Its use as a 'fortune teller' also suggested the variability of children's fortunes, and the element of luck. The tiled areas emerged from the artist's fascination with diagrams, and provided further space for text.

The writer involved in the project, Terri-ann White, is director of University of Western Australia (UWA) Press and has a well-developed theoretical background in memory and history. She brought to this work her own understanding of the role of the memorial and the work it had to do in the public sphere. In particular, White was keen to avoid a didactic approach, and the chatterbox form allowed her to avoid a simplistic, closed narrative approach. White said her aim was to encourage visitors to 'ask the questions and put them into an empathic space'.[33] However, her understanding of empathy is not based on a passive victim. For example, even one of the most confronting statements, 'Not aloud to Tork', which is very deliberately misspelt as a direct quote, contains within it a sense of the agency of the speaker, in the very fact that they are speaking now. Drafts of the text were presented to the Forgotten Australians Committee during the design process and feedback was listened to, leading to a collaborative outcome. For example, the initial design included only a few names of institutions, but responses of care leavers allowed both White and Forrest to understand that having all the institutions publicly named was important for ex-residents. Forrest renegotiated production deadlines to allow for more names to be added. By giving voice the care leavers and avoiding locking down their story, 'Unfolding Lives' creates a sense of empathic unsettlement which acknowledges the impossibility of inhabiting another's experience.[34]

3 Stolen Generations Memorial, Mt. Annan

As Kennedy and Wilson argue, the healing power of testimony lies not necessarily in 'speaking per se, but rather in challenging the particular historical

33 'Chatterbox Speaks of Childhood Pain', *Stirling Times*, 21 December 2010, viewed on 18 May 2014, http://stirling.inmycommunity.com.au/news-and-views/local-news/chatterbox-speaks-of-childhood-pain/7579913/.

34 Jill Bennett, *Empathic Vision: Affect, Trauma, and Contemporary Art* (Stanford: Stanford University Press, 2005), 8.

relationship of speaking and listening'.[35] In (post)settler-colonial Australia, Aboriginal peoples' right to speak and be heard is by no means settled. The very use of the title 'Aboriginal' masks the complexity of the vast network of language and kinship systems that cover the continent and associated islands of Australia, as well as the very different experiences of colonisation these distinct peoples have had. For example, whereas Aboriginality is often characterised as being defined by a particular spiritual connection to country, many Stolen Generations people have experienced dislocation from their family and their country that has not been resolved. For some, this means working out what it might mean to be Aboriginal but without any specific place of belonging.

The particular history of site of the Stolen Generations memorial at the Mt. Annan Royal Botanical Gardens has implications for the way it is able to be understood. Mt. Annan was a traditional meeting place for clans of the Tharawal/Dharawal people before being taken over as farm lands by Europeans. In the mid-1980s, the land was designated a 'botanical gardens' by the New South Wales (NSW) Government as a Bicentennial project. That is, as a part of the celebration of British arrival in Australia, an event remembered as 'invasion' by many Aboriginal and non-Aboriginal Australians, and as 'settlement' by others. The memorial is constructed in an area that retained some of the native bushland and has been extensively replanted. It should be noted that this return to a pre-colonial bush setting has not included a return of ownership of the land to the traditional owners, now represented by the Tharawal Local Aboriginal Land Council. However, for the purpose of having the land set aside as a memorial to the Stolen Generations, this creates in some sense a neutral territory where the experiences of all those affected by the assimilation policies of child removal can be acknowledged. In contrast to the highly bureaucratic processes followed in the development of 'Unfolding Lives', this memorial was created as a result of direct advocacy by Aboriginal people. One thing it does have in common is the significant role played by certain individuals, in this case Carol Kendall, an Aboriginal woman who was taken from her family and adopted by a non-Aboriginal family. Kendal became a well-known Stolen Generations campaigner and the memorial's signage acknowledges the important advocacy role she played in bringing it into being. The memorial was developed as a partnership project of the Botanical Gardens Trust, Link-Up NSW (a community organisation committed to reconnecting Aboriginal families) and the NSW Stolen Generations Committee.

Tabled in the Australian parliament in May 1997, at about the same time as the South African Truth and Reconciliation Commission process was

35 Kennedy and Wilson, 'Constructing Shared Histories', 129.

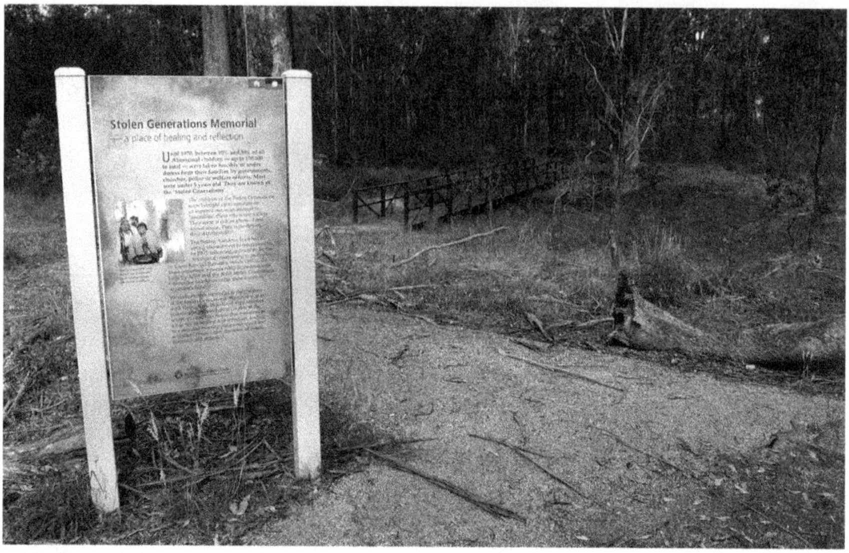

FIGURE 1.4 Mt Annan Stolen Generations Memorial, entrance

underway, *Bringing Them Home* drew on a similar philosophical belief in the power of truth telling.[36] It was both acclaimed and criticised for its extensive use of first person testimony within the body of the report, including testimony given individually and some that had been collated as part of submissions by groups such as Link-Up NSW. This commitment to testimony as truth telling carries through to the interpretive signs of the memorial, which include information and statistics about the removal of Aboriginal children from their families. However, as Kennedy and Wilson point out, within this broad 'truth telling' approach, other discursive frames can operate.[37] The main signage is written in the 'voice' of the Trust, and is addressed to a non-Stolen audience. It gives factual and historical background about the Stolen Generations, and makes clear the important role of Link-Up and the Stolen Generations Committee. It especially recognises the agency of Kendall, who was deceased by the time construction was completed. As Kennedy and Wilson point out, Link Up, and other groups like it, first 'provided a discursive community' in which

36 Bernadette Brennan, 'Bringing Them Home: The Power of Story as Public Discourse', *Journal of the Association for the Study of Australian Literature* (2013): 27.

37 Kennedy and Wilson, 'Constructing Shared Histories', 122.

Aboriginal people were able to speak as a 'valued and authentic Aboriginal subject'.[38] In the case of this particular memorial site, they then lobbied and negotiated to provide a physical and symbolic space in which the story of the Stolen Generations could be acknowledged. The interpretive signage at the entry and central points of the memorial include advice on how to approach it, and leave the memorial participant in no doubt that this is a solemn place. The memorial takes the form of a circular journey along a wheelchair-accessible boardwalk through the bush, leading to a central clearing with a sculpture, water feature and bench seat. The path then leads back out to the main road, not far from a picnic area. This gives visitors the option of walking the path alone and returning to their companions when they are ready. The journey is punctuated by plaques containing short first-person narratives, some of which are taken from *Bringing Them Home* and may have been taken from the Link-Up NSW submission. These story fragments directly address the memorial participant, and offer a sense of the multi-layered experiences of separation and assimilation masked by the Stolen Generations label.

At the central point of the walkway is a clearing. The large sandstone sculpture there was carved on site by Badger Bates, a Paakantji artist from rural New South Wales. One side, facing the entry from the boardwalk, is a relief sculpture depicting a nuclear family of a man, woman, baby and small child in a circular composition, framed by gum branches above. The inclusion of a nuclear family is surprising, given that one of the factors leading to the removal of children was a rigid understanding of family which refused to acknowledge Aboriginal kinship networks. So, for example, a baby whose Aboriginal mother died in childbirth could be taken without regard to the wishes of their extended family. However, the use of the nuclear family taps into western notions of what 'family' looks like, and in doing so it assists westernised memorial participants to consider the pain of having a family unit torn apart.

Between the man and boy on one side and the woman and baby on the other is a niche into which two small bowls are nested. Visitors are invited to fill the bowls with water from the small pond at the foot of the sculpture and pour them out as a symbol of their tears. From the boardwalk, concrete slabs imprinted with a child's footprints lead to the sculpture, with more concrete slabs, this time showing adult footprints, leading away. Footprints are a common motif used in Stolen Generations memorials. In this case, there is a sense that only through undertaking a 'journey of healing' can the Stolen child emerge fully as an adult. The other side of the sculpture is more abstract,

38 Ibid., 137.

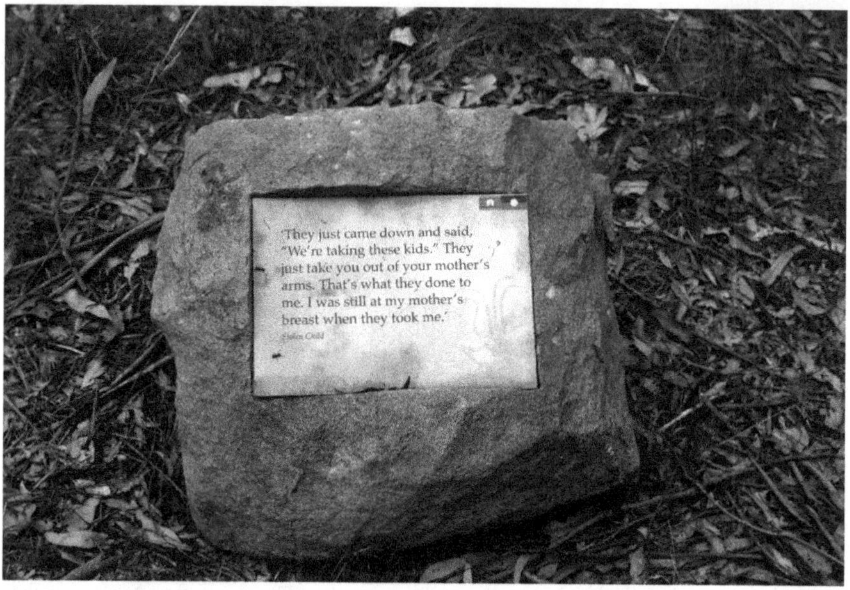

FIGURE 1.5 Mt Annan Stolen Generations Memorial, testimony plaque

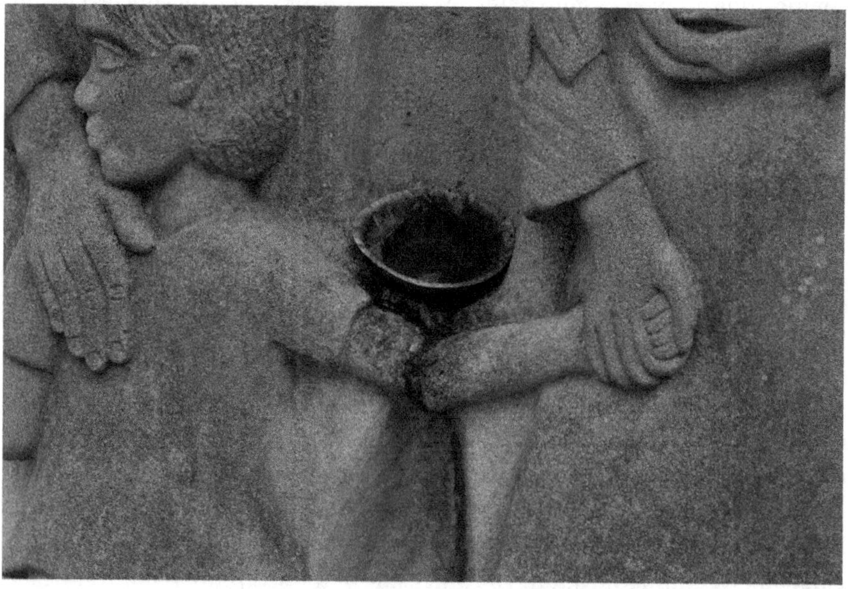

FIGURE 1.6 Mt Annan Stolen Generations Memorial, central sculpture

and interpretive signage at the site explains that it represents the anger and sadness of the Ngatyi or Rainbow Serpent, 'over the hurt done to his people who were taken away from their Country'.[39] While the circular journey of the memorial offers a healing ritual for Stolen Generations people, the interpretive signage is directed at a 'non-Stolen' public, who are asked to take part in the ritual pouring out of tears and to put themselves 'in the place' of the families who were, and often continue to be, separated. In this way, the memorial itself claims the right of the Stolen Generations to tell their story, and challenges the wider public to bridge the gap between Aboriginal and non-Aboriginal history by attempting to enter into that story.

4 World Within, World Without, Melbourne

Finally, and very briefly, I want to consider 'World Within, World Without' by Helen Bodycomb, a memorial in central Melbourne, Victoria, which differs from the other two examples in its minimal use of text. Like 'Unfolding Lives', this state memorial to care leavers was created in response to *Forgotten Australians* and the Senate Committee's recommendations. It was unveiled in October 2010, just over a month before 'Unfolding Lives', and the plaque references the national apology to care leavers given by Australian Prime Minister Kevin Rudd in November 2009. Comparing this memorial to the previous two examples helps to demonstrate how the form and location, as well as the process of memorialisation are important. Standing about two feet off the ground, 'World Within, World Without' is a mosaic artwork embedded within a stone slab. In common with other forms of testimony, memorials can only enter the public sphere when survivors are able to gain access to the discursive space in which to tell their story. As my discussion of the Perth memorial to the Forgotten Australians shows, the creation of physical memorials involves multiple negotiations and is mediated by mechanisms of power.

An important issue of memorials, like other testimony, is the way the story is able to be received. For public memorials, a key aspect of this is their physical location. The Victorian memorial to the Forgotten Australians is lacking the access to symbolic space available to the other examples in this chapter. The Stolen Generations Memorial is given a level of symbolic status through its location within the botanical gardens site, and its physical design requires a bodily performance that makes visiting the memorial a kind of pilgrimage.

39 Badger Bates, *Stolen Generations Memorial*, Mount Annan Botanical Gardens (2007). Artist statement on plaque.

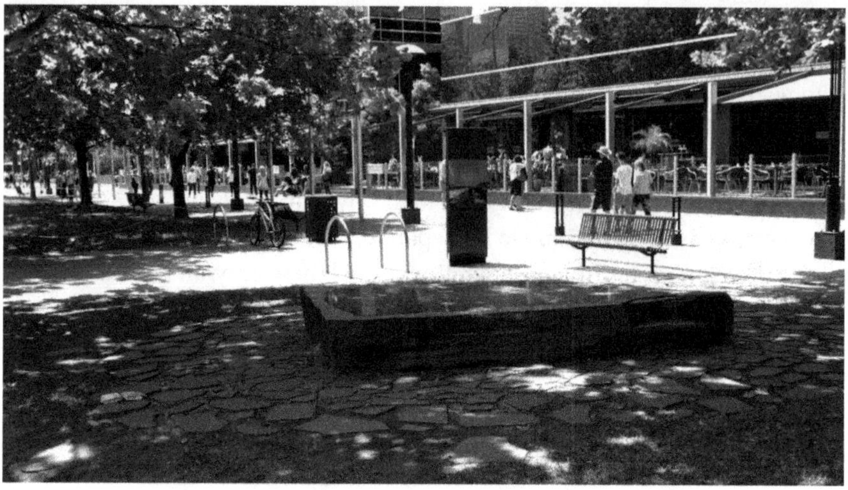

FIGURE 1.7 *World Within, World Without*

This is an integral part of the memorial's testimonial power of claiming the right to speak. 'Unfolding Lives' and 'World Within, World Without' are both located in pedestrian areas, but whereas the Perth memorial is on a raised platform, close to a number of other Western Australian cultural institutions, the Melbourne memorial is located in the Southbank precinct most closely associated with shopping and entertainment. The patch of grass on which it sits is bordered by the river on one side, and a café strip on the other, leading into the Southbank shopping mall. Apart from the scattering of stone slabs around the mosaic itself, there are no clues for visitors that distinguish it from the numerous other public artworks in the surrounding area. If 'Unfolding Lives' is usually experienced in fleeting encounters, at least its slightly elevated site and close proximity to the WA Museum gives it some sense of status. 'World Within, World Without' enjoys no such visual cues to separate it from the wider leisure context in which it finds itself.

The polished black granite surface of the mosaic visually references the famous Vietnam Veteran's Memorial (VVM) in which visitors are able to see themselves reflected. The design set into this surface is a scattering of coloured circles and flower-like motifs in a pallet of yellows and greens. A brief plaque explains that the design reflects the constellations in the sky above Victoria at the time and date of the Australian Prime Minister's formal apology to the Forgotten Australians in 2009. 'Wattle blossoms represent the one thousand most visible stars and planets, one for every one hundred children who were in

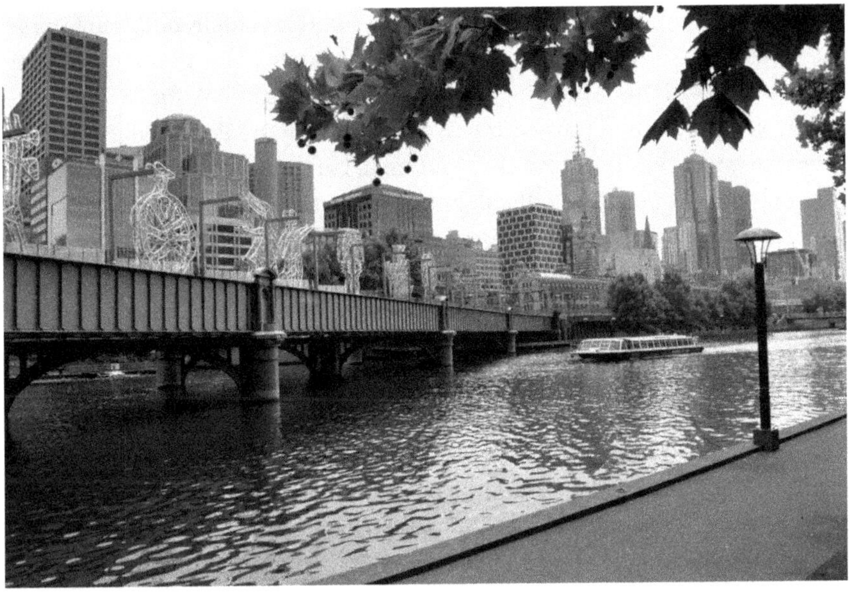

FIGURE 1.8 View across Yarra River from Southbank

Victorian state care'.[40] Architect Russell Rodrigo argues that memorial designers following in the tradition of VVM designer Maya Lin have failed to grasp the complexity of her minimalist approach. Rodrigo suggested that Lin used a mix of abstract and 'figurative' elements in the form of the names engraved in the memorial, which act on a symbolic level as 'linking objects' that allow visitors to engage empathically with the memorial.[41] In the case of 'World Within, World Without', the imagery of the stars attempts to provide the figurative element. The idea of the star connects to ideas of wishing and dreaming, and hints that these were children denied the opportunity to dream dreams. By connecting the stars with the very Australian motif of wattle blossoms, the artist makes the children 'ours' and asks this particularly located community to both acknowledge the vastness of the problem and to situate themselves within that story. In doing so it carefully draws the visitor as witness into the national community of Australia, and the more localised community of the state of Victoria.

40 Helen Bodycomb, *World Within, World Without*, Southbank (2010). Artist statement on plaque.

41 Russell Rodrigo, 'Mediating Memory: Minimalist Aesthetics and the Memorialization of Cultural Trauma' (PhD diss., University of Syndey, 2009).

However, by connecting each star with a hundred children, the memorial loses the sense of individuality and instead can only point to the magnitude of the problem. Both 'Unfolding Lives' and 'World Within, World Without' are playful sculptures, and prove attractive to children. The Perth sculpture is located close to a children's play area, and small children can often be seen using it as a climbing frame. The difficult knowledge written onto the interior of the sculpture means that adults coming closer are confronted with this story and with the choice of whether or not to discuss it with their children. 'World Within, World Without' is similarly attractive to small people. It is a good height for toddlers to climb and for slightly older children to jump from. However, whereas 'Unfolding Lives' makes creative use of the contrast between the playfulness of the sculptural form and the difficult knowledge contained in the text, the full meaning of 'World Within, World Without' is only available through reading the plaque. And while the wording of the plaque draws the reader into the story, the imagery of the memorial itself is focussed on the moment of apology, rather than the ongoing experience of care leavers. Even if memorial participants can get past the many symbolic barriers that limit access to the artwork, the moment of empathy they may experience is unlikely to lead to the kind of unsettlement the Perth memorial aims at.

5 Conclusion

By ending with that brief example, I want to draw attention to twin questions that must be considered when approaching memorials as testimony. The first is about the relationships of power and the mechanisms by which the story is allowed to be told in the first place. The second is about the discursive and spatial framing that affects the way the story is received. Difficult knowledge enters the public sphere through particular pathways, and through the agency of specific individuals and groups. Memorials have come to be understood as part of a transitional justice framework, and memorials to lived experience tend to be built when they are able to connect with ideas of truth telling and as a means to 'heal' social division. Discursive framing constantly draws memorials into a way of speaking about the past as finished business, and when memorials acknowledge experiences with ongoing effects, they must work hard to break through such frames. Careful attention should be paid to the power relationships at play, and the ways certain voices may be missing.

Considering memorials to lived experience through the lens of narrative therapy means paying attention to the way shared meaning is developed, respecting the voices of survivor-witnesses and resisting the desire to make

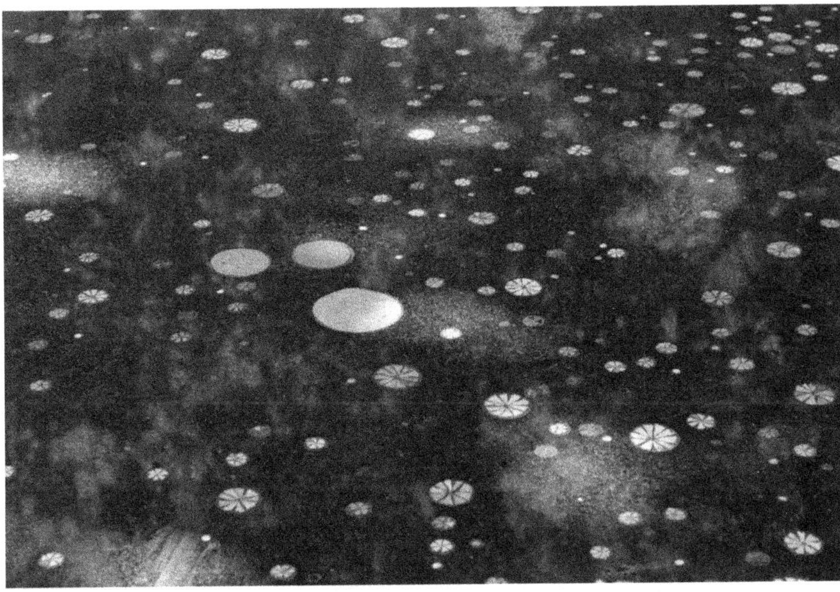

FIGURE 1.9 *World Within, World Without*, detail
© 2014. PHOTOGRAPHER ALISON ATKINSON-PHILLIPS. USED WITH PERMISSION.

difficult knowledge comfortable. There is always a risk that the very fact of the acknowledgement means painful stories become a kind of melancholic entertainment for the wider public, who are not, of course, able to truly 'enter into' that experience and who may be implicated in the acts that generated the initial trauma. One the other hand, like many other memorials, memorials to lived experience can become absorbed into the landscape, to be easily ignored or taken for granted. Yet this may not be such a bad thing. From being denied a discursive space in which to be heard, the materiality of the memorial form is one way difficult knowledge can be absorbed as part of the collective history. At their best, memorials to lived experience are a part of the arsenal of tools available to survivors and their supporters to bear witness to difficult knowledge. The materiality of the memorial form can be helpful in assisting painful histories to be absorbed into the mainstream narrative of the nation or another public as 'imagined community'.[42] There is no such thing as the perfect memorial, but designs that avoid a didactic approach have a chance of negotiating this ethical minefield and, creating space for dialogue, become truly public.

42 Anderson, *Imagined Communities*, 200–201.

Bibliography

Anderson, Benedict. *Imagined Communities: Reflections on the Origin and Spread of Nationalism*, 2nd edition. London: Verso, 1991.

Ashton, Paul and Jacqueline Z. Wilson, editors. *Silent System: Forgotten Australians and the Institutionalisation of Women and Children.* Melbourne: Australian Scholarly Publishing, 2014.

Australian Human Rights Commission. *Bringing Them Home: Report of the National Inquiry into the Separation of Aboriginal and Torres Strait Islander Children from Their Families,* 1997. Viewed on 18 May 2014. http://www.humanrights.gov.au/sites/default/files/content/pdf/social_justice/bringing_them_home_report.pdf.

Bennett, Jill. *Practical Aesthetics: Events, Affects and Art after 9/11.* London: I. B. Tauris. 2012.

Bennett, Jill. *Empathic Vision: Affect, Trauma, and Contemporary Art.* Stanford: Stanford University Press, 2005.

Brennan, Bernadette. 'Bringing them Home The Power of Story as Public Discourse.' *Journal of the Association for the Study of Australian Literature* (2013): 23–32.

Britzman, Deborah P. 'If the Story Cannot End: Deferred Action, Ambivalence, and Difficult Knowledge'. *Between Hope and Despair: Pedagogy and the Remembrance of Historical Trauma*, edited by Roger I. Simon, Sharon Rosenberg and Claudia Eppert, 27–57. Oxford: Rowman and Littlefield Publishers Inc., 2000.

Buckley-Zistel, Susanne and Stefanie Schaefer. 'Introduction'. *Memorials in Times of Transition*, edited by Susanne Buckley-Zistel and Stefanie Schafer, 1–24. Cambridge: Intersentia, 2014.

Calhoun, Craig. 'Introduction'. *Habermas and the Public Sphere,* edited by Craig Calhoun, 1–48. Cambridge: MIT Press, 1992.

'Chatterbox Speaks of Childhood Pain'. *Stirling Times*, 21 December 2010. Viewed on 18 May 2014. http://stirling.inmycommunity.com.au/news-and-views/local-news/chatterbox-speaks-of-childhood-pain/7579913/.

Craps, Stef. *Postcolonial Witnessing: Trauma Out of Bounds.* Basingstoke: Palgrave Macmillan, 2013.

Deutsche, Rosalyn. *Evictions: Art and Spatial Politics.* Cambridge: MIT Press, 1996.

Gluck, Carole. 'Operations of Memory: "Comfort Women" and the World'. *Ruptured Histories: War, Memory, and the Post-Cold War in Asia*, edited by Sheila Myoshi Jager and Rana Mitter, 44–47. Cambridge, Massachusetts: Harvard University Press, 2007.

Hamilton, Paula. 'Material Memories and the Australian Memorial Imagination'. *Melbourne Historical Journal* 39 (2011): 11–23.

Huyssen, Andreas. 'Trauma and Memory: A New Imaginary of Temporality'. *World Memory: Personal Trajectories in Global Time*, edited by Jill Bennett and Rosanne Kennedy-, 16–29. New York: Palgrave Macmillan, 2003.

Kennedy, Rosanne and Jan Tikka Wilson. 'Constructing Shared Histories: Stolen Generations Testimony, Narrative Therapy and Address'. *World Memory: Personal Trajectories in Global Time*, edited by Jill Bennett and Rosanne Kennedy, 119–40. New York: Palgrave Macmillan, 2003.

Lehrer, Erica T., Cynthia E. Milton and Monica Eileen Patterson. *Curating Difficult Knowledge: Violent Pasts in Public Places*. New York: Palgrave Macmillan, 2011.

Miles, Malcolm. *Art, Space and the City: Public Art and Urban Futures*. London: Routledge, 1997.

Parliament of Australia. *Forgotten Australians: A Report on Australians Who Experienced Institutional or Out of Home Care as Children*, 2004. Viewed on 18 May 2014. http://www.aph.gov.au/~/media/wopapub/senate/committee/clac_ctte/completed_inquiries/2004_07/inst_care/report/report_pdf.ashx.

Rodrigo, Russell. 'Mediating Memory: Minimalist Aesthetics and the Memorialization of Cultural Trauma'. PhD Dissertation, University of Sydney, 2009.

Rothberg, Michael. *Multidirectional Memory: Remembering the Holocaust in the Age of Decolonization*. Stanford: Stanford University Press, 2009.

Senate Community Affairs Reference Committee, Australia. *Official Committee Hansard*. 4 February 2004. Viewed 18 May 2014. http://parlinfo.aph.gov.au/parlinfo/download/committees/commsen/721/toc_pdf/3131-2.pdf.

Senate of Australia, Community Affairs Reference Committee, *Australian Government Response to Forgotten Australians: A Report on Australians Who Experienced Institutional or Out-of-Home Care as Children*, 2005. Viewed 19 January 2016. http://www.aph.gov.au/~/media/wopapub/senate/committee/clac_ctte/completed_inquiries/2004_07/inst_care/gov_response/gov_response_pdf.ashx.

Smith, Margaret. 'Testimony in Northern Ireland: Abandoning the Past as a Source of Societal Healing?' Paper presented at the *2nd Global Meeting of Testimony: Memory, Trauma, Truth, Engagement* July 2015. http://www.inter-disciplinary.net/probing-the-boundaries/wp-content/uploads/2015/06/MESmith-testimony2-wpaper.pdf

Viebach, Julia. '"Alétheia" and the Making of the World: Inner and Outer Dimensions of Memorials in Rwanda'. *Memorials in Times of Transition*, edited by Susanne Buckley-Zistel and Stefanie Schafer, 69–94. Cambridge: Intersentia, 2014.

Warner, Michael. *Publics and Counterpublics*. New York: Zone Books, 2002.

White, Michael. 'Working with People Who Are Suffering the Consequences of Multiple Trauma: A Narrative Perspective'. *International Journal of Narrative Therapy and Community Work* 1 (2004): 45.

CHAPTER 2

Spanish Republicans in the Holocaust: Historical Rights and Testimonial Literature

Antonio Prado del Santo

Abstract

This chapter analyses the testimonial literature of Spanish Republicans who suffered the experience of the Nazi concentration camps. I argue against the universalist interpretation of the Holocaust testimonies as exemplified in Tzvetan Todorov's approach. In his classical *Facing the Extreme* Todorov understands the survival in the Nazi camps from an exclusive humanist perspective of universal virtues and the rights of men above any other manifestation of humanity, including the desire for political subjectivity and solidarity. However, when reading the testimonies of the Spanish Republicans, we find that their motivation for survival in the Nazi camps was that which gave *political* meaning to their existence. Survival was the continuation of the political resistance initiated in Spain against Franco, and his allies Hitler and Mussolini. In contrast to the universalist position of Todorov, I rely on perspectives like those of Slavoj Žižek, Giorgio Agamben and Hannah Arendt, who contend that the defence of universal human rights above human particularism contradicts the very premise of such universalism. Ironically, this universal position negates the elemental contextual connections from which every human being is related, such as language, collectively, and political subjectivity. By analysing the partisan component of the Spanish Republican survivors, I seek to show the limits of the universal imaginary regarding the Holocaust, through which the Nazi genocide is interpreted, *solely*, as one of the most historical attempts against human rights. The case studied here reveals another dimension of the Nazi perversion: an extermination project of the political condition of the human being, and according to the non-universalist dimension of these testimonies, the total annihilation of the political body and memory of the antifascist European left resistance, initiated in 1936 in Spain by Spanish Republicans and International brigadiers, and succumbed in the Nazi camps 1945 by world-wide anti-fascist combatants.[1]

1 Chapter translated by Rod Brookes.

 | DOI:10.1163/9789004391130_004

Keywords

Holocaust – Spanish Civil War – Spanish – Republicans – Mauthausen – political rights – human rights

1 Historical Anomaly or Official Amnesia? Spaniards in Nazi Camps

The current official history of Spanish democracy still fails to assimilate the important body of historical work demonstrating an intimate relationship between the Spanish Civil War and World War II. Hence the presence of Spanish Republicans in the Holocaust still does not register in the popular imaginary of the Spanish nation. Significantly, this 'national amnesia' is replicated throughout other Western democratic nations in which a hegemonic narrative represents World War II as a war waged by liberal democracy against global fascism, marginalising other ideological positions from which fascism was also fought at an international level, such as socialism, communism and anarchism. Within this narrative, Nazism is an ideology predominantly focused on anti-Semitism. The Holocaust becomes a synonym for Nazi genocide, but a definition of Nazi genocide limited to the extermination of six million Jews which excludes the other eleven million non-Jewish people who also succumbed in Nazi camps.[2] Based on this logic we should not be surprised that the particular ideological dimension of the Spanish Civil War connecting anti-fascist struggle with class war, is, nevertheless, usually disconnected from the European crisis which triggered World War II. And yet, when Hitler and Mussolini decided to support Franco militarily, Spain became the first European democracy attacked by the Nazi regime. The main response against such an aggression included, not only the participation of communists, socialists and anarchists in the Republican government, but also a working class revolution, which collectivized the land and industry in most parts of the Republican zone and also declared that the anti-fascist war was going to be a "revolutionary war". The enemies of Nazism in Spain were not the Jews, but rather the armed working class who was defending a democratically elected Republic against a military *coup d'état*.

Recent historical studies claim that more than 30,000 Spaniards interned as refugees in France after the Spanish Civil War were deported to Germany.

2 Donald Niewyk and Francis Nicosia, *The Columbia Guide to the Holocaust* (New York: Columbia University Press, 2000), 45.

Of these, around 15,000 were imprisoned in Nazi camps.[3] These figures do not seem to alter the official versions of history which still minimise or ignore the connection between the Spanish Civil War and World War II. According to these versions, Spain closed its borders to the rest of Europe in 1939, the same year the war finished in Spain and the war in the rest of Europe began. It follows that the Fascist government which won in Spain did not participate in World War II in support of Hitler, and therefore in that war there was no resistance of anti-Fascist Spaniards fighting against Hitler, i.e. the Spanish war was not 'continued' beyond Spanish borders. However, the Spanish Civil War did continue in the context of World War II in some form. It is estimated that more than 100,000 Spanish citizens participated militarily in World War II, approximately half on each side: republicans fought for the Allies and nationalists for the Axis. Hence, despite the official positions of Franco's Spain from initial neutrality to non-belligerence in 1940, it is worth noting that Franco's regime collaborated with the Axis by participating in the siege of Leningrad through the formation of the 250th Division of the Wehrmacht, better known as the Blue Division, composed of 47,000 Spanish soldiers a fifth of whom would lose their lives. Another of the consequences of Franco's alliance with Hitler was to permit Germany to refuse prisoner of war status and Spanish citizenship to all Spanish Republicans captured by Germany in its occupied territories and especially France, thus permitting the transfer of prisoners of war from the *stalags* to the Nazi death camps.[4] Regarding the participation of Spaniards on the side of the Allies, it is estimated that out of approximately 500,000 Republicans exiled to France after the end of the Spanish Civil War and interned in refugee camps, around 60,000 left the internment camps to enlist in the French marching battalions or the semi-militarised companies of workers fortifying the Maginot line. These Spanish Republicans fought against the German invasion from these positions. Thousands of them were imprisoned by the Nazis while thousands more of them joined the French resistance forces on the retreat. Furthermore, of the 2,000 Spanish combatants exiled to the Soviet Union, it is estimated that 700 fought in Stalingrad against the Nazi invasion, of whom half would lose their lives. In total, it is estimated that some 10,000 Spanish Republicans died in

3 David Wingeate Pike, *Spaniards in the Holocaust: Mauthausen, the Horror on the Danube* (London: Routledge, 2014), 9.

4 Helen Graham, *The Spanish Civil War: A Very Short Introduction* (New York: Oxford University Press, 2005), 126.

the Nazi camps, a figure which is equivalent to if not higher than the number of Republicans who died fighting in World War II.[5]

Nevertheless, the figures on Spanish Republicans in Nazi camps are reduced to a kind of historic accident, either ignored as part of the general state of amnesia or at best incorporated into yet another vision of a depoliticised Holocaust. However, these figures point straight to a historical dimension which is very significant politically.

In the light of this apparent lapse in the official history, the existing testimonial literature written by Spanish Republicans in Nazi camps has greater potential significance. In many of these writings the logic of the vital resistance in the Nazi camps is explicitly ideological: it is the same logic that propelled Spanish Republicans to resist the fascist coup in Spain for three years, to survive the following months in the French refugee camps, and finally to fight the German army on the side of the allies. Therefore, these sources demonstrate that the resistance of Spanish Republicans in the Nazi camps was linked to political resistance, the aim of which was an end to fascism in Europe and above all liberation from fascism in Spain. However, the primary national imaginary responsible for this monumental amnesia and historical depoliticisation is significantly the current Spanish democratic state. During the Spanish democratic transition the decision to grant *amnesty* for crimes against humanity committed by Franco's regime effectively led to *amnesia* regarding Spain's republican past and an interminable wait for a true process of national reconciliation leading right up to the present.

2 From Spanish Republicans to Spain's Enemies: from Undesirable Aliens to Europe's Stateless

The Spanish Republicans crossing the French border *en masse* after defeat in the Spanish Civil War to Franco's fascist forces, could not have found a worse time to seek the political refuge they expected there. During the 1920s France was a country of refuge to numerous citizens fleeing European authoritarian regimes. However, during the 1930s, the European economic crisis and the rise of totalitarianism led to an increase in the number of refugees from the rest of Europe, with alarm and xenophobia gripping the more conservative sections of French society who saw the mass of refugees as a threat to national security. Hence, from April 1938 the Daladier government created a body of

5 Ibid., 120–126.

legislation to limit the right to asylum at the same time as the number of Spaniards fleeing the Spanish Civil War to France spectacularly increased. These legal measures were passed on the 12 of November in the form of a decree aimed at 'undesirable aliens' who could no longer find in France a country of refuge, only 'special centres' intended to intern them. According to Geneviève Dreyfus-Armand, the adjective 'undesirable' used to designate foreigners for some years became official after this legal measure was passed.[6] From the date of this decree to February 1939, the month of the great exodus following the retreat of the Republican forces, France opened its borders to 500,000 Spanish Republicans, thus respecting their traditional right to asylum but with an important legal contradiction. Spanish Republicans were no longer political refugees. Rather they were undesirable aliens who were dangerous to French national security, interned in concentration camps intended to control, guard and even repress them.[7]

After months of surviving these camps, a large number of Spanish Republicans enlisted in the Foreign Legion, the Marching Battalions of Foreign Volunteers and the military branch of the Companies of Foreign Workers. Enlistment was voluntarily or, according to some testimonies, the result of coercion by the authorities in camps like Septfonds.[8] Once Germany's occupation of France began, thousands of Republicans still managed to escape and join the French Resistance. After Republicans of these three fronts were captured by the Nazis, they were taken to Nazi camps as political prisoners. From that moment on, Franco ceased to recognise the prisoners' Spanish nationality. Therefore, Germany considered them to be stateless and as such they were treated as political prisoners and sent to the Nazi concentration camps. This policy was officially disclosed to Ramón Serrano Suñer, Spanish Foreign Minister and Head of the Spanish Fascist Party, in October 1940. In light of the Spanish state's approval and Vichy France's disavowal of any responsibility, Nazi Germany considered the Spanish Republicans to be stateless, refusing to apply to them the Geneva Convention on political prisoners, and deporting them straight to the Nazi camps branded with a blue triangle.[9]

After the end of World War II, France amended its laws to permit Spanish Republicans who survived the war to take up residence and citizenship. As a

---

6 Geneviève Dreyfus-Armand, 'L'exili republicà i la seva significació dins del segle de les catàstrofes', *Reflexionant l'exili. Aproximació a l'exili republicà: entre la història, l'art i el testimoniatge*, edited by Jordi Font Agulló (Barcelona: Catarroja, 2019), 33.

7 Ibid., 32.

8 Ibid., 24, 34.

9 Graham, *The Spanish Civil War*, 126.

result, the great majority chose to settle in France instead of returning to Franco's Spain where, for obvious reasons, the republican status of these Spaniards was still not recognised. When Franco's regime finally came to an end after three long decades of republican exile, one of the foundations of the Spanish transition to democracy (1975–1982) was to be the Amnesty Law of 1977. This law considered that for the good of a democratic and peaceful transition in Spain it was necessary to grant an amnesty for political crimes committed before 1976, including Spanish fascism's crimes against humanity from the Civil War up to that date. Ironically, the statute of limitation on fascist crimes in the democratic era ended up denying the legitimacy of the democratic history of Spanish Republicans in their fight against international fascism. It marked the continuation of the suppression of the historical and political rights of Spanish Republicans initiated when they were 'enemies of the Fatherland' (under Franco's victorious Spain), 'undesirable aliens' (both in democratic France prior to the occupation and in Petain's collaborationist France) and 'stateless reds' (in Germany of the Third Reich).

Hence the Spanish democratic transition perpetuated Franco's regime of amnesia regarding the republican, anti-fascist and revolutionary memory of the Spanish Civil War which had been maintained for forty years. And this state of affairs continued until very recently, when the Spanish Historical Memory Law was passed on the 26 December 2006. This event happened 67 years after the end of the Spanish Civil War, 31 years after Franco's death and 24 years after the consolidation of the democratic transition. This law was the Spanish democratic state's first legal measure established to recognise and extend the rights of the victims of Franco's repression during the Civil War and the dictatorship. From the date it was passed the first measures aimed at fulfilling its objectives were initiated. However, numerous Spanish historical memory groups have complained that the measures are minimal and insufficient. The most aggressive official initiative was launched in 2008 by the judge Baltasar Garzón with the opening of cases of crimes against humanity committed by Franco's regime. One year later the ultra-right group Manos Limpias filed a law suit against Garzón alleging that he had abused his legal authority by infringing the Spanish transition's amnesty laws. In April 2010 Garzón was stripped of his legal powers and it became impossible to proceed with the cases against Franco's repression. From 2011 to the present, the Argentinian courts have pursued the cases against Franco's regime under the principle of 'universal justice'. In Spain, this measure was broadly denounced by countless groups, and on the international level, Spanish justice has been denounced by numerous organisations including Amnesty International and Human Rights Watch. Moreover, United Nations recently denounced the impunity of the 1977 law for blocking the investigation of genocide and enforced disappearances during the Civil War and Franco's regime.[10] In turn, since the first decade of the century, dozens of historical memory organisations have sprung up echoing the demands of relatives of the victims of Franco's repression, which historians such as Paul Preston have begun to call the Spanish Holocaust.[11]

3 Towards a Theorisation of Historical Rights: from Human Rights to Political Rights

Therefore, the Spanish state's current position regarding the historical memory of the Spanish Civil War seems to be an apolitical position consistent with the theory of the two demons defence: that the two sides in the civil war share equal responsibility for its tragedies. This is the reconciliatory position of the Spanish transition's policy of amnesia, the prime component of which was the 1977 Amnesty Law. This official 'egalitarian' vision finds its logical parallel in the treatment of the participation of Spaniards in World War II. Some cases of state commemorative ceremonies denounced by historical memory associations serve as examples. The Spanish government is the only government in Europe whose citizens perished in the Mauthausen Nazi concentration camp that does not participate in their memory in the annual international commemoration of the liberation of the camp.[12] By contrast, ceremonies have been held such as the controversial official tribute to Spanish ex-combatants for the Third Reich, the Blue Division, which was staged by a government's regional office in Catalonia in 2013. The ceremony was justified by the Ministry

10 On 10 February 2012 Navanathem Pillay, the United Nations' High Commissioner for Human Rights, asked Spain to repeal the law as it does not comply with international human rights legislation. However, the Spanish Constitution of 1978 which established the amnesty law prevents its repeal due to the legal principle of non-retroactivity.

11 Paul Preston, *The Spanish Holocaust: Inquisition and Extermination in the Twentieth-Century Spain* (New York: N.W. Norton & Co., 2012).

12 For examples of detailed descriptions of this ceremony denouncing the absence of Spanish officialdom see Archivo, Guerra y Exilio, 'Actos del memorial de Mauthausen - 2013: El vergonzoso caso de la delegación española', (*Sociología crítica*, 20 May 2013), viewed on 29 May 2015, https://dedona.wordpress.com/2013/05/20/actos-del-memorial-de-mauthausen-austria-2013-el-vergonzoso-caso-de-la-delegacion-oficial-espanola-age-y-rps-cantabria/; and Pedro A. García Bilbao, 'Mauthausen, 12 de mayo de 2013: España ya no puede caer más bajo', (*Sociología crítica*, May 20 2013), viewed on 29 May 2015, http://dedona.wordpress.com/2013/05/20/mauthausen-12-de-mayo-de-2013-espana-ya-no-puede-caer-mas-bajo-pedro-a-garcia-bilbao/.

of the Interior as one of a number of acts promoting 'historical reconciliation'. Also, during the Armed Forces Day parade on 12 October 2004, an ex-member of the Blue Division marched alongside a volunteer republican who fought for the Free French Forces. Protests from republican historical memory associations were not long in coming, epitomised by the following quote from Florén Dimas of the *Foro por la Memoria* (*The Memory Forum*):

> The presence in the 12 October parade of a Blue Division representative alongside an ex-republican combatant enlisted in the Free French Forces who disembarked in Normandy, helped liberate Paris, and reached Hitler's alpine refuge in Berchtesgaden in April 1945, is a travesty of monumental proportions, as it aims to depict harmony between parties directly opposed after the Civil War spread to the Second World War, honouring brave Spanish Republicans fighting for freedom in Europe while paying tribute to those who tried to subjugate freedom by swearing allegiance to Hitler. This association roundly condemns the presence in Madrid's 12 October parade of a representative of a unit established by history to be an icon of the support provided by Franco's regime to its Nazi equivalent, and believes that the commission of a ceremony disgracing the historical memory of Spaniards who died fighting such ideologies on the battlefields is unworthy of the Spanish government.[13]

Hence, it is logical that in addressing the hardships suffered by exiled republicans, first in the French internment camps and then in the Nazi death camps, this reconciliatory position applies the universalist stance on the defence of human rights to all voices. However, this position also ignores one of the key reasons for the very existence of Spanish Republicans in Nazi camps: the exercise of their political and historical rights. Above all, the story is about Spaniards in these camps, not Spanish *Republicans*. These 'Spaniards' are discussed as if they were a historical anomaly, contradicting the common sense view that Spain did not (*officially*) participate in World War II. However, the reality is that these testimonies demonstrate beyond dispute the connection between the Spanish Civil War and World War II. Time and time again, these testimonies insist that not only were these wars connected but rather they were part of the same war. For official Spanish culture to recognise this reality would be to

13 Florén Dimas, 'La division azul en el desfile del 12 de octubre en Madrid. Una Equidistancia histórica, anacrónica e inmoral', *Foro por la Memoria*, 11 October 2015, viewed on 29 May 2015, http://foroporlamemoria.info/documentos/2004/fdimas_11122004.htm.

shoot itself in the foot regarding the alleged miracle of the Spanish transition, which was based on making a pact with Francoism to forget the republican cause. But if Spanish fascists and anti-fascists continued fighting in World War II on their respective sides, can it seriously be said that the allies were as evil as the Nazis? And by the same logic regarding this historical connection, would it make sense for Europe behind the Pyrenees to treat the Holocaust's crime against humanity with a Pact of Forgetting similar to that adopted by Spanish law? Faced with these slippery issues, Spanish officialdom agrees to ignore these connections, thus reaching a historical impasse.

The case of the deportation of some 15,000 Spanish citizens to Nazi concentration camps has received barely any attention in studies of the Holocaust. However, the existing body of written testimonies by survivors of this significant episode makes a vitally important historical contribution. The study of these testimonies obliges us to revise our interpretation of the intimate connections between the Spanish Civil War, World War II and the Holocaust from the present perspective of the historical memory of Western democratic nations, especially Spain.

Above all, analysing these texts raises the limitation of approaches to the Holocaust based exclusively on the discourse of human rights and moral universalism which ignore political and ideological dimensions. The classic example of this type of approach is the study by Tzvetan Todorov, who from a universalist perspective questions the possible reasons why millions of people in the Nazi and Soviet Concentration camps survived.[14] The common denominator found by Todorov is the presence of three main virtues he calls ordinary: dignity, caring closely for someone enduring the same suffering and the stimulus of the life of the mind. Other possible reasons for survival foreign to the moral individualist perspective, such as political sacrifice or group solidarity, are dismissed. For Todorov, the violence and suffering in these camps is too real for political, ideological and abstract subtleties. The key to survival seems to have been these ordinary and universal virtues. However, having read the Spanish testimonies, I am obliged to rethink the moral framework of this type of approach. In these testimonies, besides the appearance of non-politicised virtues, we also find one impulse repeated over and over again: resistance in the camp is a quintessential version of the political resistance begun in the fight against Fascism in Spain. Therefore, in opposing Todorov's narrative, I find myself more in agreement with the position of critics such as Slavoj

14 Tzvetan Todorov, *Facing the Extreme. Moral Life in the Concentration Camps* (New York: Henry Hold and Company, 1996).

Žižek, Giorgio Agamben and Hannah Arendt regarding 'the depoliticised politics of human rights as ideology'.[15] These critics set out to invert the order of the opposition between universal pre-political human rights and the specific rights of the citizen, arguing that 'man is made by citizenship and not citizenship by man'.[16] This reflection seems more evident in the cases of people who have been stripped of every human quality except that they are still human. This relates to Giorgio Agamben's notion of *homo sacer* as a human being reduced to 'bare life': a concept inherited from Roman law according to which a human being excluded from all forms of community as a citizen loses his socio-political identity and can be killed by anyone without it constituting a crime, since he has lost all value and cannot even be sacrificed to the gods. That is to say, he has regressed from a being recognised as a citizen (inhabitant and participant in the *polis*) to a being recognised *solely* as human.[17]

In turn, Hannah Arendt raises an interesting paradox in her study of the status of the human rights of all those people who lost their nationality after the emergence of the new political map following World War I. The paradigm case of new stateless masses within Europe was Jews living in Nazi Germany. For Arendt, the Nuremberg laws of 1935 synthesised the situation of this new stateless group as it distinguished between the Reich's full citizens and citizens of 'alien blood'. The latter would be declared second class citizens without political rights who could lose their citizenship by decree. In this case, national laws could no longer apply to them and they lost their right to have rights. That is to say, the end of national rights is the end of political rights, the end of the right to the 'polity', the right to history, and consequently the end of human rights. Therefore, for Arendt, there are no human rights without political rights, and any human rights policy which forgets this principle is in itself a policy which denies those same rights:

> The paradox involved in the loss of human rights is that such loss coincides with the instant when a person becomes a human being in general – without a profession, without a citizenship, without an opinion, without a deed by which to identify and specify himself – and different in general, representing nothing but his own absolute unique individuality

15 Slavoj Žižek, 'Against Human Rights', *New Left Review* 34 (2005): 126, viewed on 29 May 2015, http://newleftreview.org/II/34/slavoj-zizek-against-human-rights.

16 Ibid., 127.

17 Giorgio Agamben, *Homo Sacer: Sovereign Power and Bare Life* (Stanford: Stanford University Press, 1998), 73.

> which, deprived of expression within and action upon a common world loses all significance.[18]

It follows from Arendt's paradox that the only existing right in the life of the Nazi camps was precisely the *right to be human* in strictly biological terms as proposed by Agamben, suppressing all the other social, political and historical rights which distinguish human beings from animals. It is precisely from the perspective of the violation of the Spanish Republicans' political rights and Žižek's suspicion of the apolitical universalisation of human rights 'in general' that I wish to discuss the historical treatment of the experience of Spanish republicans in Nazi camps after the Spanish Civil War was lost. This was a moment when those internees became citizens without citizenship and republicans without a Republic, an essential prerequisite to the Nazis imprisoning all stateless persons in a no-place, no-history limbo: the Nazi concentration camp.

4 Testimonial Literature by Spanish Republicans in Nazi Camps

In his rigorous historiographical study of Franco's repressive policies towards republican exiles in France from 1937 to 1951, Jordi Guixé Coromines demonstrates the collaboration between Franco's government and successive French governments during three wars: the Spanish Civil War, World War II and the Cold War. He notes that the obsessive persecution of republican exiles by Franco's dictatorship during these witch hunts was not accidental:

> … it formed part of an objective and a policy of the State: to *annihilate the history* of the Second Republic and those who made it possible within and beyond Spain. (emphasis mine)[19]

The imposition of Francoist history as official Spanish history would therefore be proportionate to the effectiveness of its revisionist anti-republican mechanisms. These mechanisms were no other than those comprising the monumental and all-powerful repressive and ideological fascist state apparatus over four decades (1939–1975). The imbalance with the discursive weaponry possessed by republican exiles is absolute. The paradigm of this attempt to reduce

18 Hannah Arendt, *The Origins of Totalitarianism* (New York: Houghton Mifflin Hartcourt, 1951), 302.

19 Jordi Guixé Coromines, *La república perseguida: Exilio y represión de la Francia de Franco, 1937–1951* (València: Universitat de València, 2012), 25.

republican historical subjectivity to nothing can be found specifically in the context of World War II, where the legal status of republicans as 'undesirable aliens' in France or 'stateless reds' under the Nazi regime gave the green light to their imprisonment in the Nazi concentration camps. Therefore, the attempt to eliminate these Spanish Republicans reduced solely to the 'bare life' of the human species (whether through indifferent neglect of the camp regime, through forced labour or through the explicit intention to exterminate) was also an attempt to suppress Spanish republican history.

It is against the background of this complete obliteration of the political and historical rights of Spanish Republicans in Nazi camps that all the political and historical potential of the testimonial literature stands out. However, as we can see in the canonical case of Todorov, the premise of testimony as the bridge between individual memory and a political and historical memory running counter to official accounts cannot be found in the canonical tradition of the testimonial studies of the Holocaust. However, there are other critical traditions within testimonial literature which do openly recognise the historical and political dimension of the texts, including post-colonial theory and Latin American subaltern studies focussing on testimony.

Studies of Latin American testimony such as the testimony by Rigoberta Menchú recording the complaints of the victims of the Guatemalan genocide lend themselves to comparisons with other testimonies at a global level also acting as resistance through denouncing abuses of historical rights. One example is the literary testimony by Radwa Ashour on the 1948 Arab-Israeli War, denouncing the war not as a war of independence (the official Israeli historical version) but rather as a 'Nakba' (catastrophe) for Palestine. Whether in Latin America or the Middle East, the common denominator in the abuse of human rights is the same one indicated by Arendt in the case of World War II Europe: the prior elimination of the national, political and historical rights of stateless groups. The case of the testimonies of Spanish Republicans in Nazi camps is not substantially different. As we can see, they testify to the act of resistance involved in recording the history that officialdom tries to eliminate, the concentration camp being the place designed for this disappearance.

Testimonial literature written by Spanish Republicans deported to Nazi camps is in this sense important, since we systematically find in their writings a battle between the *homo sacer* destined to be obliterated by the official history and the collective scream of a partisan memory which clings to its own combative version of history. The testimonies of the Nazi camp survivors under study here all record their experiences of torment in these camps within a historical narrative uniting all Republican combatants in the Spanish Civil War. The common axis of this narrative is the fight against and resistance to

European Fascism. For these survivors, World War II was the logical continuation of the Spanish Civil War. Furthermore, these testimonies tell us that World War II began in Spain, since it was in Spain that the Hitler/Mussolini/Franco Fascist axis was established when the three armies intervened against the democratic Spanish Republic. So for example, in *El largo viaje* (*The Long Voyage*), Jorge Semprún (1923–2011), who was exiled to France while still a boy before much later becoming a Resistance fighter and then a Buchenwald camp survivor, writes the following fictional account of a dialogue between a German soldier and the novel's protagonist, who is arrested in France by the German army for collaboration with the French Resistance. The conversation is slanted by the soldier's assumption that the prisoner is French:

> -France is not my country.
> -That doesn't make sense -he says, disconcerted.
> -Yes it does. Anyway, I defend my country in defending France, which is not my country.
> -Which is your country?
> -Spain.
> -But Spain is our friend -he says.
> -You think? Before starting this war, you started the war in Spain, and Spain was not your friend.[20]

Later, the narrator feels indignant that the majority's reaction of 'absolute shock' at the horrific tactics employed by the Nazi army only comes after the beginning of World War II, when for three years the Spanish Civil War had already been a testing ground for Nazism and fascism:

> Perhaps, because I didn't see anything else after July 1936 ... Perhaps, because I saw the German and Italian fighters flying over the roads at low altitude and calmly machine-gunning the crowds along my country's roads.[21]

After arriving in France, Semprún's narrator discovers to his surprise how the Spanish Civil War is seen beyond the Spanish/French border. He is amazed that he is called 'Red' while Franco's faction is called 'Nationalist':

---

20 Jorge Semprún, *El largo viaje* (Barcelona: Tusquets, 2011), 45.
21 Ibid., 68.

> When I read in the newspaper that there were Reds on one side and Nationalists on the other, it took me by surprise. It was not easy to understand how they could be called Nationalists when they fought the war with Moroccan troops, the Foreign Legion, German planes and Italian infantry divisions.[22]

But above all it is after being captured by the Nazis that the interpellation 'Spanish Red' carries most weight with him, as an internal process of appropriation followed:

> Afterwards, I never ceased to be a Spanish red. It is a way to be valid everywhere. Hence, in the concentration camp I was a *rotspanier*. I looked at the trees and I was happy to be a Spanish Red. As the years passed, I became more happy to be one.[23]

A connection can be gleaned here between the Nazi Germany that participated in the Spanish Civil War against the 'Reds' and the France that signed the Non-Intervention Agreement because it did not want to assist the 'Reds'. We can see the connection on one of the occasions when the convoy taking the protagonist to Germany stops and he sees the contemptuous stares of curious Germans. At that moment his memory takes him back to when he arrived in the French port of Bayonne on his return from Spain and a mob of curious bathers crowded round to see the Spanish exiles disembark. He realises that the way the French once stared at the 'Spanish Reds' was the same as the way the Germans now stare at the prisoners of the convoy, now seen as 'delinquents or terrorists'.[24]

Therefore, for the Spanish Republicans, the fight against Franco was also a fight against Hitler. They believe the Spanish Civil War to be in reality a European Civil War confined to a single country thanks to the containing effect of the Non-Intervention Committee established by the democratic nations of France and England in August 1936. They see the Non-Intervention Agreement signed by these nations in response to the Spanish Civil War as a pact to appease Hitler and allow Germany to occupy and annex Austria and part of Czechoslovakia in 1938. For example, Semprún's protagonist decides to distract himself from the agony of his long journey to Buchenwald by fondly remembering the

22 Ibid., 106.
23 Ibid., 106.
24 Ibid., 133.

library where he grew up, which was itself a refuge against the news about the outcome of the Spanish Civil War and the progress of Nazism in Europe. He remembers it as a ...

> ... child's universe bombarded from everywhere by deafening rumours about the world, by the howling of the radio which during the Anschluss of Vienna and the sad, stupid stupor of September 1938 confirmed the defeat of my country, vanquished everywhere, beaten like the dykes of Scheveningen ...[25]

The second historical process the Spanish Republicans record as connecting with their experience in the Nazi concentration camps is the mass crossing of the French border in February 1939 by half a million people and the subsequent internment in improvised camps on French beaches. Here they suffered as the result of being mistrustfully treated as 'Spanish Reds', enduring shortages, the militarisation of their camps, punishments, and insalubrious living conditions and food. The Spanish Republicans do not hesitate to call them concentration camps, considering them to be simple precursors of the Nazi camps.[26] This abandonment by the French government of the Republican exiles who hoped to find a warm welcome and asylum in a democratic and friendly country is interpreted as an abandonment of the European anti-Fascist cause. It is another reason to keep reflecting that the French Government who signed the Non-Intervention Agreement in response to the Spanish Civil War was a government allied with Nazism, as Mariano Constante, survivor of the Mauthausen camp, states:

> It was not possible for us to forget that the government who subjugated us had abandoned Austria, Czechoslovakia and the Spanish Republic to the power of Fascism. If when we arrived in France we had seen in this government a clear determination to fight Nazism, we would all have volunteered to resume the fight against our enemy. But from its attitude towards us, the way it repressed us, we had decided that this was a capitulating government.[27]

25 Ibid., 206.

26 Mariano Constante and Manuel Razola, *Triángulo azul* (Zaragoza: Gobierno de Aragón. Departamento de Educación, cultura y deporte, 2008), 23.

27 Ibid., 24.

Responsibility for internment in the Nazi camps is shared between the Nazi government and the Spanish pro-Franco government. For example, regarding the famous meeting between Hitler and Franco in Hendaye, Manuel Razola, Mauthausen survivor, writes:

> Franco's meeting with Hitler on the French border on 23 October increased the number of those shipments. The Francoists preferred to leave us in the hands of the Nazis. They probably thought it was the way to ensure that nobody would know how thousands of Spanish anti-Fascists disappeared or where they went.[28]

Hence, the testimonies tell us that the crossing of the border into France, survival in the French camps, enrolment in the militarised companies of workers and marching battalions of volunteers, participation in the French resistance, detention in German *stalags* and now survival in Nazi concentration camps, were all part of the same act of resistance which led Spanish Republicans to take up arms against Fascism in Spain for 32 months in the first place. Esteban Balogh, a Hungarian volunteer in the International Brigades during the Spanish Civil War and prisoner in the Mauthausen Nazi camp, convinced that he was going to die there, wrote: 'We did not fall in Spain but it will probably be here where we perish. This is the same fight against the same enemy'.[29] Or as the French Mauthausen survivor Pierre Daix wrote about the Spanish Republicans, 'the honor of being a revolutionary was the very reason to live'.[30]

According to Eduardo Pons Prades, there were 15 main camps in which Spanish Republican men and women were imprisoned by the Nazi government, but the great majority, around 7,000, were found in the Mauthausen camp, the only concentration camp classified as Category III and the most extreme.[31] Although it was not technically classified as an extermination camp, more than half its prisoners died there in a planned way. The testimonies of these survivors revolve around a high level of political awareness as the necessary basis of resistance and survival. This awareness has been noted by Francie Cate-Arries in her study of Spanish Republicans in French concentration camps, in which she argues that these texts insist on positioning resistance in the camps as a republican national identity in exile. Nevertheless, although living conditions

28 Ibid., 30.

29 Ibid., 76.

30 Ibid., 17.

31 Eduardo Pons Prades, *Morir por la libertad: Españoles en los campos de exterminio nazis* (Madrid: VOSA SL, 1995), 14.

in the French camps were very hard, they are still a separate paradigm compared to the Nazi holocaust camps. For example, in Todorov's study we find much more present when we analyse the testimonies of republicans in Nazi camps. Even so, I maintain that in these testimonies premises for survival can be found that are as important as Todorov's moral conditions. Above all, after Franco's coup of 1936 the political identity of Spanish Republicans continues to be that of anti-fascist combatants. According to Todorov, these premises for survival would be too abstract and fragile as pillars on which to sustain oneself in the Nazi camps.

However, in opposition to individualist interpretations of the Holocaust, we find that the logic of anti-Fascist resistance amassed in these testimonies during previous years of fighting persisted in these camps across a whole range of possibilities: from individual survival understood as an act of political conscience to individual and isolated acts of sabotage; from acts of solidarity between anti-Fascist comrades to the astonishing creation, in the case of the aforementioned Mauthausen camp, of an authentic solidarity network transformed into a truly political resistance organisation in the camp. Neus Català, captured from the French Resistance and deported to the Ravensbrück women's concentration camp, discusses several ways that she, together with other prisoners, were able to sabotage the construction of armaments in a military factory close to the camp, risking execution for treason:

> Although we were consumed by hunger we weren't capable of stealing a piece of bread, but when it came to the fight we were the perfect thieves: sabotage, sabotage, sabotage. It took all our effort, it was all we cared about. We were risking our lives … but it had to be done.[32]

She tells us about her conviction that she should take this type of risk by connecting the anti-Fascist resistance in Spain to the French Resistance of World War II: 'I left Spain having lost the war, but I was not defeated and here, locked up, I am fighting to win it back'.[33] Later she writes: 'At the same time we managed to continue the Resistance: by not producing Nazi weapons or by sabotaging them by any means necessary'.[34]

Regarding the organisation of resistance among Spanish Republicans in the Mauthausen camp, according to the testimonies and the historical studies, a

32 Neus Català, *De la resistencia y la deportación: 50 testimonios de mujeres españolas* (Barcelona: Península, 2000), 58.

33 Ibid., 57.

34 Ibid., 58.

clandestine solidarity network was formed among the Spanish Republicans which managed to infiltrate all the most important *komandos*, giving access to valuable information. Through this infiltration missions were organised which consisted of seizing material and important Nazi documents both to reduce the level of extermination in the camp and to achieve political ends. One of the most successful results of this clandestine network was the confiscation of photographic material by Antonio García and Francesc Boix, the Spanish Republicans working in the photographic laboratories. Through working together they managed to get a very valuable photographic archive out of the camp to the village of Mauthausen, which would later be used in the Nuremberg trials as testimony against the Nazi horror.[35] It is revealing that this solidarity group was precisely composed of all the political factions in the Spanish Republic's Popular Front government during the war, including as it did Anarcho-Syndicalists, Socialists, Communists and Centrist Republicans.[36]

The spirit of resistance of the Spanish Republicans in Mauthausen and the work of resistance involved are fictionalised in the testimonial novel *K.L. Reich* (1946), written by camp survivor Joaquim Amat-Piniella. Its protagonist, Emili, is both a witness to this resistance and a participant in it. This character systematically witnesses the most abominable and inhuman acts committed within the camp: routine and arbitrary beatings meted out by the monstrously sadistic SS agents in the camp's public spaces; the torture of political prisoners in the camp prison; ritual massacres in the form of hangings to deter all thoughts of escape; the women forced to work as sex slaves for the camp's officers; the discovery that his best friend has been murdered in the clinic by a gasoline injection; the wearing down of comrades enslaved in the camp's notorious quarry until they died; his first-hand experience of these quarry jobs carrying extremely heavy rocks up the camp's hellish stairway; the allusions to the gas chamber; and the constant smell of human flesh from the crematorium's chimneys. After this much horror and suffering, Emili's need to survive becomes couched in both existential and political terms. His fight for survival becomes a fight against the 'spirit of the camp', which according to Emili, is intended to reduce human beings to a state of impassivity and indifference towards human monstrosity and to convert them into pure objects to be used, enjoyed and consumed by the Nazis. This apparent fate of humans being reduced by the

35 Wingeate Pike, *Spaniards in the Holocaust*, 383.
36 Constante and Razola, *Triángulo azul*, 126.

camp to a state of pure merchandise explains the title of the novel. 'K. L. Reich' is the 'brand' stamped on all the camp's materials, its clothes, tools, etc.

The temptation to succumb to the overwhelming triumphalism of the bestial 'spirit of the camp' in opposition to the universality of the human spirit, leads to an existential crisis throughout his existence in the camp in which he questions the sense of his nine long years fighting fascism, starting in the Spanish Civil War:

> He thought about the years of civil war when ordinary political rivals became mortal enemies, when he, a pacifist by nature, also took up arms to add to the carnage, although without much enthusiasm. And afterwards, in France, where the hunger and the lice in the refugee camp had propelled him into the 'Work Company' only to be captured a few months later with the collapse of the French army. Still later, in the prisoner-of-war camp, he hadn't had the courage to escape like some of his companions had done. And now, finally, in this Nazi concentration camp, where thousands of unfortunates were dying in the most horrifying ways. He couldn't come up with any justification for his life. 'Why?, Who am I?' he asked himself. 'Why am I alive?' Once free, he would find himself in the same world from which the civil war had torn him nine years before, and he would be just as vulnerable and naked. All the horrors he had witnessed, the suffering that had toughened his skin and aged his spirit, were they all for nothing? Was it all meaningless?[37]

Hence, throughout the whole novel, the character experiences a struggle between the negative and dehumanising force embodied by the camp and the positive force epitomised by his will not to succumb. One of the most effective means he finds to confront this struggle between the life instinct and the death instinct is to continue fighting the same political battle joining the Spanish Civil War with World War II by allying himself to the Spanish Republican resistance group in the Mauthausen camp.

Throughout the novel he is openly critical and sceptical of the Spanish resistance group's charitable and political actions. On the one hand, he suggests there are possible partisan motivations behind the actions of the majority Communist group, personified by the character Rubio, and on the other hand, he suspects that the altruistic acts performed by the main anarchist character, August, are motivated by personal interests and vanity. However, despite his

37 Joaquim Amat-Piniella, *K.L. Reich* (Waterloo: Wilfrid Laurier University Press, 2014), 202.

critical and sceptical position, Emili recognises that clandestine resistance is the most effective means of taking revenge on the dehumanising world of the camp and he decides to risk his life through active participation. An example of his activism is his infiltration of the photographic laboratory (alluding to the historical figures of Boix and García) to collect photographs and negatives documenting the barbarity of the camp to be used as evidence against Nazism in the future. The protagonist is aware of the risk: 'The task was certainly dangerous; the slightest slip could mean death'.[38] However, he is motivated by the desire instilled in him by his long fight:

> ... it would be an extraordinary graphic condemnation of the Nazi regime ... a collection of graphic evidence would be of greater value in the final accounting against Nazism than all the chatter of the camp conspirators.[39]

Hence, if for this group of witnesses their fight in World War II on the side of the allies was the logical continuation of the Spanish Civil War, then it follows for them that liberation from European fascism would logically lead to liberation from Spanish fascism. After his liberation from the Buchenwald camp, Semprún's narrator claims that: 'The end of the camps is the end of Nazism and therefore the end of Francoism, come on, there can't be the least shadow of doubt'.[40] However, Franco's Spain was not liberated after the end of World War II, perhaps as a logical part of the same premise that led to the Non-Intervention Agreement being signed by the democratic nations at the beginning of the Spanish Civil War: it was preferable to sacrifice Spain to Franco's fascist holocaust than to open up the possibility of another 'red' republic in Europe. After the reality dawned on Spanish Republicans in exile that the Allied forces did not plan to liberate fascist Spain, many Nazi camp survivors, including Vicente Moriones, Manuel Azaustre and Jorge Semprún, decided that the war had not finished for them and clandestinely crossed the Pyrenees to join the Spanish resistance against Franco.[41]

Therefore, the references to political identity in the republican testimonies of Nazi camps are so systematic that it is possible to postulate that a position which only takes into account the violation of human rights 'in general' in

38 Ibid., 200.

39 Ibid., 200–201.

40 Semprún, *El largo viaje*, 79.

41 Pons Prades, *Morir por la libertad*, 15.

the Nazi camps fails to do justice to the clamour of the demand for a specific historical memory. Žižek's reflections in this respect are important:

> I am deprived of human rights at the very moment at which I am reduced to a human being "in general", and thus become the ideal bearer of those universal human rights which belong to me independently of my profession, sex, citizenship, religion, identity, etc.[42]

The republican testimonies register the demand to recover the historical recognition of the Spanish republican cause, originally eradicated by the European fascist coalition and currently denied and forgotten by both the democratic heirs of the Non-Intervention Committee and the present Spanish democratic system in the wake of the Spanish democratic transition. The case of the deportation of Spanish Republicans to Nazi camps is in this sense relevant. At the time, Franco's authorities stripped the nationality of those Spanish Republicans captured by the Nazis and gave the green light to their deportation and disappearance. The socio-political identity of these persons was no longer recognised, converting them into beings whose sole identity consisted of belonging to the human species, that is to say, possessing the status of *homo sacer*. The deportation and internment of stateless persons branded with a blue triangle was thus the logical consequence of the existence of the Nazi concentration camp, the ontological destination, according to Agamben, of every totalitarian regime, and in the case of the Nazi state concerning us here, its bio-political strategy of making stateless persons' bodies disappear having stripped them of their specific socio-political identities as citizens.

5 Conclusion

The fight of these witnesses to survive in the Nazi camps was also a fight to ensure that the political identity giving their lives meaning within the Spanish and European historical process did not disappear either in the death camps or in official history. And that political identity was a Spanish Republican political identity. The fight for this identity, defined by republicans themselves, was a fight for a memory which has neither been recognised by any of the Western democratic nations' international authorities nor specifically by democratic memory in Spain.

42 Žižek, 'Against Human Rights', 127.

These democratic nations remain silent perhaps because in the end they must conceal the fact that the foundations of their democracy are partly based on the collaboration with Franco's anti-communist fascism during the three wars affecting Spain in the 20th century. During the Spanish Civil War the Non-Intervention Agreement declared by the democratic nations was not, according to many renowned historians, an act of neutrality, but rather a 'political and diplomatic farce' which ended up supporting Franco's victory and the defeat of the feared 'red' Spain.[43] Throughout World War II, the Allies preferred to ignore Franco's active collaboration with the Axis and for the second time preferred to abandon Spain to fascism for 'fear of communist destabilisation of the country'.[44] Finally, during the Cold War the allies ended up supporting Franco as the 'sentinel of the West' in his fight against communism.[45]

After the Cold War, the republican survivors of deportation to Nazi camps finally received honours and medals from France, the first country after World War II to offer them citizenship and therefore political rights. More recently, on the 16 of March 2015, the French government even awarded surviving republican deportees the Legion of Honour, the French state's highest medal. The current Spanish state is some way behind, although steps towards redress are now being tentatively initiated due to the 70th anniversary of the liberation of the Nazi camps. For example, on the day after the French medal ceremony, the Spanish Parliament approved a non-binding motion urging the government to

> organise as a form of moral redress a solemn ceremony individually and collectively recognising and honouring Spanish survivors of extermination camps for their dignity, bravery and the undeniable role they played as heroes in the fight for freedom and for the victims of totalitarianism.[46]

---

43 Enrique Moradielos, 'La No Intervención. Una farsa política y diplomatica', *En el combate por la historia. La República, la Guerra civil, el franquismo*, edited by Ángel Viñas (Barcelona: Pasado y presente, 2012), 221.

44 Carlos Collado Seidel, 'España en la Segunda Guerra Mundial. La "hábil prudencia" de un "neutral," ' *En el combate por la historia. La República, la Guerra civil, el franquismo*, edited by Ángel Viñas (Barcelona: Pasado y presente, 2012), 610.

45 Guixé Coromines, *La república perseguida*, 23.

46 Equipo Nizkor, 'Texto de la Proposición No de Ley a propuesta del PSOE para que el reconocimiento de los españoles prisioneros en los campos de exterminio del III Reich sea sólo moral', *Derechos*, viewed on 29 May 2015, http://www.derechos.org/nizkor/espana/doc/impuesp15.html.

Furthermore, on 29 of April of 2015, the Minister of Education and Culture, José Ignacio Wert, announced that the Government was ready to consider legal and material recognition of Spaniards deported to Nazi camps.

Given the tentativeness of the Spanish government's steps and in the absence of state initiatives, Spain still relies on key organisations funded by the survivors of Nazi deportation to create social projects. One such organisation is the 'Amical de Mauthausen and other camps and all victims of Nazism in Spain', which in 2015 launched the 'Fight against fascism memory network: Never Again', the objective of which is to 'preserve the historical memory of Republican deportation and resistance and to raise awareness about fascism' through actions such as 'providing support and advice to ex-deportees and their relatives', 'investigating and preserving repositories of documents', and 'dissemination and communication' in the form of 'talks in schools and colleges, film series about deportation, exhibitions, commemoration of International Holocaust Day and trips to camps'.[47]

These types of initiatives derive from the same demand for the historical rights of Republican memory made in the testimonies analysed here and they will continue to be urgent and necessary while the Spanish state still perpetuates an official version of history which favours its Francoist past and its collaboration with the Nazism at the same time that it marginalises those who fought in defence of the Second Spanish Republic and with the Allies in the two consecutive wars. The road towards this type of historical reconciliation in Spain has already begun, while France's reconciliatory efforts providing redress to Spanish Republicans must be construed as the first political act leading to the reconstruction of the historic bridge uniting the Spanish Civil War and World War II.

Bibliography

Agamben, Giorgio. *Homo Sacer: Sovereign Power and Bare Life.* Stanford: Stanford University Press, 1998.

'Amical de Mauthausen y otros campos y de todas las víctimas del nazismo', *Amical-Mauthausen*, viewed on 29 May 2015. http://www.amical-mauthausen.org

Archivo, Guerra y Exilio. 'Actos del memorial de Mauthausen-2013: El vergonzoso caso de la delegación española'. *Sociología crítica*, May 20 2013. Viewed 29 May 2015.

47 'Amical de Mauthausen y otros campos y de todas las víctimas del nazismo', *Amical-Mauthausen*, viewed on 29 May 2015, http://www.amical-mauthausen.org.

https://dedona.wordpress.com/2013/05/20/actos-del-memorial-de-mauthausen-austria-2013-el-vergonzoso-caso-de-la-delegacion-oficial-espanola-age-y-rps-cantabria/.

Arendt, Hannah. *The Origins of Totalitarianism*. New York: Harcourt Brace Jovanocich, 1979.

Català, Neus. *De la resistencia y la deportación: 50 testimonios de mujeres españolas*. Barcelona: Península, 2000.

Collado Seidel, Carlos. 'España en la Segunda Guerra Mundial. La "hábil Prudencia" de un "neutral" '. *En el combate por la historia. La República, la Guerra civil, el franquismo*, edited by Ángel Viñas, 593–612. Barcelona: Pasado y presente, 2012.

Constante, Mariano and Manuel Razola. *Triángulo azul*. Zaragoza: Gobierno de Aragón: Departamento de Educación, cultura y deporte, 2008.

Dimas, Florén. 'La division azul en el desfile del 12 de octubre en Madrid. Una Equidistancia histórica, anacrónica e inmoral'. *Foro por la Memoria*, 11 October 2015. Viewed on 29 May 2015. http://foroporlamemoria.info/documentos/2004/fdimas_11122004.htm.

Dreyfus-Armand, Geneviève. 'L'exili republicà i la seva significació dins del segle de les catàstrofes'. *Reflexionant l'exili. Aproximació a l'exili republicà: entre la història, l'art i el testimoniatge*, edited by Jordi Font Agulló, 27–45. Barcelona: Catarroja, 2010.

Equipo Nizkor. 'Texto de la Proposición No de Ley a propuesta del PSOE para que el reconocimiento de los españoles prisioneros en los campos de exterminio del III Reich sea sólo moral'. *Derechos*, March 30, 2015. Viewed on 29 May 2015. http://www.derechos.org/nizkor/espana/doc/impuesp15.html.

García Bilbao, Pedro A. 'Mauthausen, 12 de mayo de 2013: España ya no puede caer más bajo'. *Sociología crítica*, 20 May 2013. Viewed on 29 May 2015. https://dedona.wordpress.com/2013/05/20/mauthausen-12-de-mayo-de-2013-espana-ya-no-puede-caer-mas-bajo-pedro-a-garcia-bilbao/.

Graham, Hellen. *The Spanish Civil War: A Very Short Introduction*. New York: Oxford University Press, 2005.

Guixé Coromines, Jordi. *La república perseguida: Exilio y represión de la Francia de Franco, 1937–1951*. València: Universitat de València, 2012.

Moradielos, Enrique. 'La No Intervención. Una farsa política y diplomática'. *En el combate por la historia. La República, la Guerra civil, el franquismo*, edited by Ángel Viñas, 221–234. Barcelona: Pasado y presente, 2012.

Niewyk, Donald and Francis Nicosia. *The Columbia Guide to the Holocaust*. New York: Columbia University Press, 2000.

Pons Prades, Eduardo. *Morir por la libertad: Españoles en los campos de exterminio nazis*. Madrid: VOSA SL, 1995.

Preston, Paul, *The Spanish Holocaust: Inquisition and Extermination in the Twentieth-Century Spain*. New York: N.W. Norton & Co., 2012.

Semprún, Jorge. *El largo viaje.* Barcelona: Tusquets, 2011.

Todorov, Tzvetan. *Facing the Extreme. Moral Life in the Concentration Camps.* New York: Henry Hold and Company, 1996.

Wingeate Pike, David. *Spaniards in the Holocaust: Mauthausen, the Horror on the Danube.* London: Routledge, 2014.

Žižek, Slavoj. 'Against Human Rights'. *New Left Review* 34 (2005). Viewed on 29 May 2015. http://newleftreview.org/II/34/slavoj-zizek-against-human-rights.

CHAPTER 3

Writing Spain's Fraught History: Testimony or Fiction?

Olga Bezhanova

Abstract

In 2006, Benjamín Prado, one of Spain's leading novelists, published a novel titled *Mala gente que camina* (*Bad People Walking*) where he addressed in a fictionalized form one of the crimes of Franco's dictatorship in Spain that had been concealed from public knowledge for decades. During the Spanish Civil War (1936–1939) and in the post-war years, as many as 30,000 children of Republicans were abducted by the dictatorship with the goal of eradicating any possibility that the children would adopt the anti-fascist ideas of their Republican parents. Prado became familiar with the tragedy of the stolen children through the 2002 documentary titled *Franco's Forgotten Children* (*Els nens perduts del franquisme*) created by Montserrat Armengou and Ricard Belis. The documentary and, later, the collection of testimonial accounts published on its basis in collaboration with historian Ricard Vinyes presented the heart-rending testimony of the survivors who had been taken from their families and were still denied the truth about their origins decades after the dictator's death. In conjunction, the documentary and the novel managed to awaken interest in the issue that many people in Spain had considered a past long gone. This chapter discusses how different forms of creative production engage with historical memory and work together to preserve the testimonies of the survivors of traumatic events in history.

Keywords

Franco's dictatorship – Spain – literature – testimonial documentary – stolen – children

 | DOI:10.1163/9789004391130_005

1 The Genre of the Spanish Civil War Novel and the Recovery of Spain's Historical Memory

There is an enormous interest in Spain in the fraught era of the Spanish Civil War (1936–1939) and the subsequent dictatorship of Francisco Franco (1939–1975). Between 1989 and 2011, 181 novels on the subject of the war were published in Spain.[1] A significant number of these works of literature went through several editions and some were adapted to film with varying degrees of success.[2] Discussions of whether it is necessary to recover the historical memory of the war transcend the space of artistic creation and make a significant impact on Spain's political environment. To provide a single example, in the electoral campaign of 2015, the need to recover the historical memory of the war and the Franco era was used by political forces that wanted to emerge from relative obscurity and speak to the issues that were likely to attract voters. For instance, Albert Rivera, the leader of Ciudadanos, a party that has been trying to make itself relevant on the national level, has indicated that his party supported the exhumation of the victims of the Franco dictatorship whose bodies were still lying in unmarked graves in many different regions of Spain. 'A country's worth is measured by the dignity it accords to its dead', said Rivera in one of his campaign appearances, knowing very well that this statement was likely to attract the attention of his listeners and journalists.[3] This is precisely the attitude that has inspired many of Spain's leading writers and film-makers since the beginning of the 21st century to create works of art that addressed the crimes of the Franco regime.

By the end of the millennium, 'the Spanish crisis of memory became evident',[4] and addressing it could no longer be avoided. The creation of the

1 David Becerra Mayor, *La guerra civil como moda literaria* (Madrid: Clave Intelectual, 2015), 19.

2 Among the more successful film versions of Civil War novels, one could name *Soldados de Salamina* by the film-maker David Trueba based on a best-selling novel by Javier Cercas and *La voz dormida* by Benito Zambrano based on an extraordinarily successful novel by Dulce Chacón (2002). *Soldados de Salamina*, dir. David Trueba. España: Lolafilms/Fernando Trueba P.C., 2003, DVD.; *La voz dormida*, dir. Benito Zambrano. España: Audiovisual Aval SGR/Maestranza Films and Warner Bros., 2011, DVD.

3 Juan José Mateo, 'Rivera se compromete a apoyar las exhumaciones de la Guerra Civil', *El País*, November 18, 2015, Viewed on 20 November 2015, http://politica.elpais.com/politica/2015/11/17/actualidad/1447796568_381704.html

4 Michael Richards, 'Grand Narratives, Collective Memory, and Social History: Public Uses of the Past in Postwar Spain', *Unearthing Franco's Legacy: Mass Graves and the Recovery of Historical Memory in Spain*, edited by Carlos Jerez-Ferrán and Samuel Amago (Notre Dame: University of Notre Dame Press, 2010), 122–123.

Association for the Recovery of Historical Memory[5] *in December of 2000 opened an era when the need to recover lost memories of the past became a matter of passionate debates in Spanish media.*[6] *In the realm of literary production, the extraordinarily successful Soldados de Salamina (2001)/Soldiers of Salamis (2003) by Javier Cercas was followed by an explosion of novels about the Spanish Civil War. These novels adopted the model introduced by Cercas, depicting a 21st century protagonist who embarked on a search of truth about the past. Some of the novels that belong to this genre are Benjamín Prado's Mala gente que camina* (2006), Fernando Sánchez Dragó's *Muertes paralelas* (2006), Almudena Grandes's *Corazón helado* (2007), Julia Navarro's *Dime quién soy* (2010), and *Andrés* Trapiello's *Ayer no más* (2012). *Even writers who heretofore had no interest in history began exploring the genre of history writing during this time. The voracious appetite of the readers who did not seem to tire of the Civil War and were eager to buy a seemingly unlimited number of such novels made working in this genre profitable for artists:*

> In the decade 2000-09 remembering became not simply a trend but *the* trend … . One writes a novel of the Spanish civil war, therefore one is a Spanish novelist – or at least a remunerated one.[7]

The Civil War novels that rely on the model introduced by Cercas fictionalize historical events in a way that leaves it unclear as to how much of the story is true[8] and use history to question Spain's present and, possibly, influence its future.

The novel of the Spanish Civil War is not a new genre, of course.[9] Works of literature that draw on the experience of the civil conflict and the post-war era have been appearing in print in a steady stream for decades. The Civil War

---

5 In Spanish, the Association is known as *'Asociación para la Recuperación de la Memoria Histórica'*.

6 *Pedro Ruiz Torres, 'Los discursos de la memoria histórica en España', Generaciones y memoria de la represión franquista: Un balance de los movimientos por la memoria,* edited by Julio Aróstegui and Sergio Gálvez (Valencia: Universitat de València, 2010), 45.

7 Nathan Richardson, '*No pensar*, or Does the Contemporary Spanish Novel of Memory Really Want to Know? *Tiempo de silencio, Corazón tan blanco, Soldados de Salamina* and Beyond', *Letras Hispanas* 7.1 (2010): 6.

8 Carmen de Urioste, 'Memoria de la Guerra Civil y modernidad: el caso de *El corazón helado* de Almudena Grandes', *Bulletin of Hispanic Studies*, 87.8 (2010): 939.

9 For a discussion of why the novel on the Spanish Civil War merits being considered a genre see Isaac Rosa's prologue to *La guerra civil como moda literaria,* by David Becerra Mayor (Madrid: Clave Intelectual, 2015), 9–14.

novels published in the 1980s and 1990s, however, did not tend to approach the war as an issue that could still provoke debate. Instead, they aimed to explore it as a distant time in history that had acquired mythical dimensions but lost any ideological significance.[10] Bertrand de Muñoz attributes this lack of interest in the ideological facets of the civil conflict to the lengthy period of time that had passed since the war.[11] Still, although an even greater distance separates the first decades of the new millennium from the events of 1936–39, the ideological contradictions that inspired the war become central to the novelistic production of the 2000s. The Civil War is no longer a past long gone but, rather, a time when issues were debated that are still relevant today. In 1996, Joan Oleza Simó, a scholar and a novelist, predicted the emergence of a genre that would turn to history in order to address the present:

> The end of the millennium comes at a time when all of us feel the desire for a special kind of fiction … the kind that lets us be somebody else without renouncing the need to be ourselves, the kind that allows us to project ourselves onto the figures and situations of the past, sifting through history for something that we lack in the here and now. In other words, we long to alter history in order to possess it more fully. The popularity of historical fiction reveals our lack of conformity with the present.[12]

The enduring interest of the Spanish audience in the Civil War and Franco's dictatorship demonstrates that there are many people in Spain who are unhappy with the way in which the country's painful past was laid to rest during Spain's Transition to democracy after the death of the dictator in 1975. Contesting the interpretation of the country's 20th century history that was adopted during the Transition is a way to question the political, ideological and economic status quo in Spain. One of the writers who expresses his dissatisfaction

10 Maryse Bertrand de Muñoz, 'Novela histórica, autobiografía y mito (La novela y la guerra civil española desde la Transición)', *La novela histórica a finales del siglo XX: Actas del V Seminario Internacional del Instituto de Semiótica Literaria y Teatral de la UNED, Cuenca*, edited by José Nicolás Romera Castillo and Mario García-Page Sánchez (Cuenca: Visor, 1996), 28.

11 Ibid., 33.

12 Joan Oleza Simó, 'Una nueva alianza entre historia y novela: Historia y ficción en el pensamiento literario del fin de siglo', *La novela histórica a finales del siglo XX: Actas del V Seminario Internacional del Instituto de Semiótica Literaria y Teatral de la UNED, Cuenca*, edited by José Nicolás Romera Castillo and Mario García-Page Sánchez (Cuenca: Visor, 1996), 94.

with the state of Spain's political establishment through a re-evaluation of the official narratives of the Spanish Civil War is Benjamín Prado.

2 Benjamín Prado's Journey towards Engagement with Spain's History

Before 1999, Benjamín Prado's novelistic production was characterized by 'an escapist attitude on the part of almost all of his characters'.[13] Together with Ray Loriga, Prado is considered one of the most important representatives of the Peninsular Generation X movement characterized by the apolitical nature of its literary production. The novels produced by the writers of this artistic generation were, for the most part, divorced from Spanish realities.[14] In his 1996 discussion of Prado's writing, Manuel Vázquez Montalbán, a noted novelist of an older generation, pointed out that the writer's characters 'seem to be from a cultural galaxy where neither Spanish literature nor culture exist'.[15] The main criticism levelled against the writers of this artistic generation was precisely their incapacity to connect with the historic legacy of Spain that led to attempts to fill the resulting vacuum with pop culture references suggested by the global music and film industry. Generation X writers responded to the readers' desire to overcome the Franco-era isolation and position themselves as full-fledged citizens of the global cultural community. As a result, these writers' works were imbued with a 'self-conscious insistence on their association with a global (i.e. primarily Anglophone) culture [that] often carried with it an adamant rejection of an autochthonous tradition'.[16]

Benjamín Prado with the publication of *No sólo el fuego* (1999) effectuated a turn away from writing imbued by feelings of alienation and indifference towards Spain's historic memory. The novel brings together the experiences of

13 Eva Navarro Martínez, 'La novela de Benjamín Prado: Cómo construirse un mundo y una realidad propios', *Letras peninsulares* 14.3 (2001–2002): 405.

14 Paul D. Begin, 'The Pistols Strike Again! On the Function of Punk in the Peninsular '"Generation X" Fiction of Ray Loriga and Benjamín Prado', *Generation X Rocks: Contemporary Peninsular Fiction, Film, and Rock Culture*, edited Christine Henseler and Randolph D. Pope (Nashville: Vanderbilt University Press, 2007), 16.

15 Manuel Vázquez Montalbán, *Un polaco en la corte del Rey Juan Carlos* (Madrid: Alfaguara, 1996), 382.

16 Santana, Cintia. 'What We Talk about When We Talk about Dirty Realism in Spain', *Generation X Rocks: Contemporary Peninsular Fiction, Film, and Rock Culture*, edited by Christine Henseler and Randolph D. Pope (Nashville: Vanderbilt University Press, 2007), 34.

the Republicans who were forced to exile themselves from Spain in the aftermath of the war, the representatives of the post-war generation who participated in the anti-Franco resistance movements of the dictatorship's closing years, and the members of the younger generation who are finding it hard to relate to the issues that are of importance to their parents and grandparents. In his 2006 novel *Mala gente que camina*, Prado continued to explore the legacy of the Civil War. This novel addresses the post-war practice of removing the children of the Republican prisoners from their families with the goal of re-educating them in a way consistent with the ideology of the Nationalist Movement of Francisco Franco. *Mala gente que camina* is based on Prado's meticulous reading of testimonial accounts gathered by Tomasa Cuevas, a political prisoner during Franco's regime, and published by her under the title *Testimonios de mujeres en las cárceles franquistas* (*Testimonies of Women in Francoist Prisons*) and Juana Doña, who survived torture in Franco's jails and wrote *Desde la noche y la niebla: las mujeres en las cárceles franquistas* (*From Night and Fog: Women in Francoist Prisons*) *on the basis of the testimonies of female prisoners she met during her 18 years of incarceration.*[17] The information gleaned by Prado from these collections of testimonial accounts is seamlessly integrated into the narrative. The fictional universe of his novel gains substance, in the eyes of the readers, as a result of the integration of these non-fictional sources. At the same time, Prado manages to bring the testimonial accounts published by Cuevas and Doña to the attention of readers who would not know of their existence otherwise. The writer's fans who know him from his Generation X stage are likely to read a new novel by Prado and mimic the author's transition from politically disengaged literature to the kind of writing that is more deeply involved with Spain's history and politics. Prado is convinced that nine out of ten readers of *Mala gente que camina* will agree that it is crucial to bring to light the crimes committed by the Franco regime against the children of Republicans.[18]

Prado's curiosity towards the kidnapped Republican children was awakened by a documentary film that attracted great interest on the part of Spain's viewing audience. On January 20, 2002, the TV3 channel in Spain aired the first part of the documentary by film-makers Montse Armengou and Ricard

17 Tomasa Cuevas, *Testimonios de mujeres en las cárceles franquistas* (Huesca: Instituto de Estudios Altoaragoneses, 2004) and *Juana Doña, Desde la noche y la niebla: las mujeres en las cárceles franquistas* (Madrid: Ediciones de la Torre, *1977*).

18 Stacey Dolgin Casado, 'Benjamín Prado: La literatura es lo contrario del olvido', *Ojáncano* 33 (Apr 2008): 105.

Belis titled 'Els nens perduts del franquisme' ('Franco's Forgotten Children').[19] The film offered evidence that the dictatorship of Franco (1939–75) had consciously adopted policies aimed at separating the children of the defeated Republicans from their families with the goal of ensuring that they were not exposed to their parents' anti-fascist ideology. The documentary was aired at one o'clock in the morning in Catalonia, the Basque Country and Andalusia. Still, in spite of the late hour, only in Catalonia 900,000 viewers tuned in to watch the film, one of whom was Benjamín Prado. The writer was so astounded by what he saw that he immediately decided to write a novel about it.[20] For the next four years, Prado researched the subject and in 2006 published his novel *Mala gente que camina*. He was aided in his work by the book *Franco's Forgotten Children* that had been published by the creators of the documentary[21] and he included the testimonies of the survivors of this Francoist crime and the documents that had not been used in the film. The narrative structure of the novel prompts readers to engage in their own research of these events, filling in some of their lacunae in knowledge about the dictatorship. Both the novel by Prado and the collection of the survivor accounts published by the creators of the documentary combine testimonial evidence with fictional elements in order to enhance the readers' emotional engagement with history and prompt them to begin to investigate the events of the Civil War and the dictatorship on their own account.

3 Prado's *Mala gente que camina*: Unearthing Franco's Crimes

Prado's *Mala gente que camina* addresses one of the crimes of the dictatorship that remained hidden not only throughout Franco's rule but also during the thirty years of Spain's existence as a democratic state. The first-person narrator of Prado's *Mala gente que camina* is Juan Urbano, a middle-aged professor of literature whose research interests lie in the area of post-Civil War literary production. Urbano accidentally discovers a forgotten novel titled *Óxido* that contains references to the efforts by the Franco regime to separate children

19 The second part of the documentary was aired a week later, on January 27. The documentary can be accessed at the web site of TV3. 'Els nens perduts del franquisme', *Televisió Catalunya*, viewed on 3 May 2015, http://www.tv3.cat/30minuts/reportatges/333/ELS-NENS-PERDUTS-DEL-FRANQUISME-I

20 Dolgín Casado, 'Benjamín Prado: La literatura es lo contrario del olvido', 110.

21 Armengou and Belis were assisted in the writing of the book by Catalan historian Ricard Vinyes.

from their Republican families. As he begins to learn more about the novel's author, Dolores Serma, the scholar realizes that *Óxido* is based on the events that she experienced first-hand. Her sister Julia was jailed by the dictatorship for being married to a volunteer of the International Brigades that attracted anti-fascist volunteers from all over the world to come to Spain to fight against the spread of European fascism. Julia's son Carlos Lisvano was handed over by the authorities to a family that was faithful to the regime and promised to re-educate the boy according to the principles of Franco's Nationalist Movement. In order to find the boy and bring him back to his real family, Dolores Serma becomes part of Auxilio Social (Social Assistance), a beneficent organization loyal to Franco, and dedicates her life to concealing her true convictions that would have placed her in great danger in case of being discovered by the Franco authorities. The only way for Serma to let the truth be known is to relate it, in a veiled form, in her only published novel with the hope that someday the novel might find a reader who will want to decipher its true meaning. Nobody in Serma's family knows the secrets that her novel conceals, and Urbano needs to decode Serma's writing in order to recover her story from oblivion. As they follow Urbano's investigation of Serma's life, the novel's readers will likely wonder how many similar mysteries inherited from the Franco era are still hidden from view.

When Urbano reveals to Serma's nephew Carlos Lisvano the true story of his family, it becomes clear that Lisvano has no interest in learning the truth about his origins. Lisvano is now a rich and successful man who believes that there is no need 'to resuscitate these old stories'.[22] Lisvano's use of the word 'resuscitate' is not accidental. In her analysis of Spain's transition to democracy, Paloma Aguilar Fernández points out that words like 'forget' and 'bury' were used with great frequency by the representatives of all political forces at the time when Spain's democracy was being fashioned in 1977–9.[23] The 1977 Amnesty Law adopted as part of the country's transition to democracy was expected to bring about a definitive rupture with Francoist past:

> During parliamentary debates, almost all groups praised the law precisely because it was an instrument of "national reconciliation", intended to "close the past", "forget", and start a new phase. Even the communists

22 Benjamín Prado, *Mala gente que camina* (Madrid: Santillana, 2006), 314.

23 Paloma Aguilar Fernández, 'Justice, Politics, and Memory in the Spanish Transition', *The Politics of Memory: Transitional Justice in Democratizing Societies*, edited by Alexandra Barahona de Brito, Carmen González-Enríquez and Paloma Aguilar Fernández (Oxford: Oxford University Press, 2001), 103.

> boasted of wanting to forget the past and "bury the dead" and called for an amnesty that excluded no one.[24]

In the early 2000s, the time when Prado's novel is set, Carlos Lisvano is still reluctant to abandon the rhetoric that had currency during the Transition and start learning the truth about the past. Lisvano belongs to the political class that has enriched itself in the aftermath of the Transition and is not prepared to let go of the foundational myths of this era. Accepting that there is still a great amount of crucial information about his family's past that he does not know would lead him to question whether the Transition's philosophy of putting the past to rest was reasonable.

Urbano's research into the crimes of the dictatorship puts at risk Carlos Lisvano's narrative of his personal and familial identity. If Lisvano accepts that his parents were Republicans, he will have to get used to seeing himself as belonging to the category of the war's losers. A possibility of no longer being on the side of the powerful proves very disconcerting to Lisvano.[25] At the same time, his professional success hinges on the preservation of the philosophy of letting the past remain buried. From the beginning of Spain's transition to democracy, the decision was made to preserve 'the main civilian and military institutions inherited from the Franco dictatorship [that] were not purged after his death'.[26] The grievances of the victims of the dictatorship against these institutions might endanger their capacity to remain unchanged, and this is something that Lisvano does not want to happen. As an active member of a right-wing party, Lisvano is not prepared to put at risk his capacity to occupy positions of power within a political force that, at least to an extent, has inherited the ideology of Francoism.[27]

Unlike Carlos Lisvano, Urbano believes that the project of resisting the ideology of the dictatorship should be revived, taking the form of bringing to light the numerous ways in which the structures of oppression inherited from the Franco era remain present in Spain. At the time when Urbano reads Serma's novel and discovers the story of her struggle to save her sister and nephew, Dolores suffers from Alzheimer's and has lost her memory of the war and the dictatorship. She symbolizes, in Urbano's eyes, the generation of those who experienced the Civil War and whose capacity to transmit what they witnessed to the younger generations is fading. Urbano hopes to publish his book about

24 Ibid.

25 Prado, *Mala gente que camina*, 303.

26 Aguilar Fernández, 'Justice, Politics, and Memory in the Spanish Transition', 92.

27 Prado, *Mala gente que camina*, 217–218.

Serma in time to put it in her hands before she dies.[28] This is a tribute that, Urbano believes, is owed by those born after the war to the survivors. Accessing the Republican memory of the Civil War is the only way to ensure that the structures of oppression inherited from the dictatorship of Franco are revealed for what they are and, eventually, removed. The discussion of the seemingly distant past is crucial for understanding the present and transforming the future.[29]

Urbano feels happy and at peace as a result of learning about the past,[30] even though publishing his research will expose him to grave legal and economic repercussions. Carlos Lisvano promises to initiate legal proceedings against Urbano if the truth about his family's experiences during the dictatorship appears in print.[31] Lisvano is not willing to allow Dolores to play any other role than that of his caretaker and refuses to accept his connection to those who lost the war. Lisvano's narrative of self cannot accommodate the revelation about the true identity of his parents because his professional and economic success in neoliberal Spain is based on a triumphalist account of his own, as well as the country's, history that has no space for political stories of trauma and loss. Urbano realizes that unearthing the past always comes at a price because this is an act that disturbs the certainties of the present and challenges the status quo.

What Urbano has learned from Dolores is that political engagement might bring painful consequences. Carlos Lisvano sues him for revealing the truth about his family[32], and Urbano finds himself in a paradoxical situation of having to imitate Dolores Serma and, instead of a scholarly essay that he initially hoped to publish, having to write a work of fiction about the events of 1939. Urbano remarks sardonically that 'fiction is one of the only two territories where one can hide from lawyers. The other one is a cemetery'.[33] Like Dolores, he cannot afford to publish the story of the Serma family openly and has to live with the uncertainty of whether the novel he is writing will be confiscated at the behest of Lisvano before anybody gets a chance to read it.[34] The difficulties

28 Ibid., 460.

29 Ibid., 282–283.

30 Ibid., 254.

31 Ibid., 448–449.

32 In order to access Dolores Serma's personal archives, Urbano signs a contract promising not to publish any of the information he found there without Lisvano's permission. Breaking the terms of the contract exposes Urbano to a lawsuit filed against him by Lisvano. Ibid., 420–421.

33 Ibid., 421.

34 Ibid., 444.

Urbano faces as a result of his engagement with history serve as a reminder that even today recovering the truth about the Civil War and the dictatorship might be fraught with danger. Still, this is a risk that has to be assumed if there is any hope of bringing meaningful change to the country and ensuring that all vestiges of the dictatorship are eradicated in full. The fear of another civil conflict was ever-present during the years of Spain's Transition to democracy and often led to compromises that endangered the very nature of the newly democratic society:

> Fear of a right wing coup, even a return to civil war, that might be provoked by democratization strategies that were too quick or too conflictual was … an ever-present feature of the transition and one that led Spaniards to prioritize peace, order and stability over other values such as justice, freedom, and democracy.[35]

Today, it has become clear that the edifice of Spanish democracy cannot be erected on a foundation of forgetfulness and denial of the Republican accounts of the past. In order for Spain's democracy to be meaningful, memories of those who lost the war have to be disinterred and incorporated into the narrative of the country's past.

Dolores Serma, the writer who sacrificed her literary career to Lisvano's well-being, is a product of Prado's imagination. The author, however, goes to great lengths to make Serma appear real to his readers. He even inserts references to Serma into quotes from several well-known books on the subject of post-war Spain,[36] prompting the more curious among his readers to access these sources on their own to verify whether Dolores Serma is, indeed, mentioned there. In his 2007 interview with Blas Vives, Prado confessed that he considered it 'a triumph' that 90% of journalists who interviewed him about the novel had searched for Dolores Serma in Google.[37] Serma's story is neither more nor less poignant than the testimonies of the survivors collected by Armengou, Vinyes and Belis in *Franco's Forgotten Children*, yet Prado chooses to construct a fictional character instead of placing one of these testimonial

35 Madeleine Davis, 'Is Spain Recovering Its Memory? Breaking the Pacto del Olvido', *Human Rights Quarterly* 27.3 (August 2005): 864.

36 Pablo Gil Casado, 'Benjamín Prado: de "la nueva novela" al realismo documental', *Ojáncano* 35 (April 2009): 78–79.

37 Damián Blas Vives, 'Entrevista a Benjamín Prado: Literatura y derechos humanos', *Evaristo Cultural: Revista Virtual de Arte y Literatura* 7 (2007): np., viewed on 29 September, 2016, http://www.evaristocultural.com.ar/-%20EVARISTO%20Nro.%2007%20-/prado.htm.

accounts at the centre of his novel. Instead of engaging with history in the role of passive consumers of information, the readers of the novel are prompted to start questioning the veracity of their knowledge about the war and the post-war era. The confusion between fiction and reality in Prado's novel aims to motivate the readers to embark on their own research of what happened to the lost children of Francoism and become engaged in a search for historical truth. Trivial as it might seem, a Google search for Dolores Serma's name might lead to other searches and produce a more active involvement with the country's history. In the era of cyberactivism and the proliferation of participatory web experiences, political engagement increasingly begins online[38], and *Mala gente que camina* offers readers a reason to make research into Franco-era repression part of their online experiences.

Instead of offering definitive answers, Prado's novel poses questions and entices the readers to respond to them on their own. The realization that their own family history might have been falsified in the same way as Carlos Lisvano's has the potential of unsettling the readers and awakening in them the need to learn more about their country's past. In Prado's own words,

> at this very moment, there are many people of seventy years of age or older who go about their lives and who might not be who they think they are, who might not be the children of the people they consider their parents, who might have been brought up by their parents' killers. I believe that this is what will have the greatest impact on the novel's readers.[39]

While Carlos Lisvano refuses to accept the revelations about the true history of his family, Prado hopes that most readers will feel reluctant to identify with this character and will feel curious about the past. The first-person narrator of the novel informs the readers that Lisvano has threatened to take him to court for publishing the truth about Dolores Serma.[40] The very act of reading the novel makes those who hold a copy of *Mala gente que camina* in their hands complicit in resisting the pact of silence[41] defended by those who, like Lisvano, believe that Spain's future should not involve looking back at the past.

---

38 Martha McCaughey, *Cyberactivism on the Participatory Web* (New York: Routledge, 2014), 2–3.

39 Dolgín Casado, 'Benjamín Prado: La literatura es lo contrario del olvido', 105.

40 Prado, *Mala gente que camina,* 446.

41 The term 'the pact of silence' refers to the tacit agreement among the representatives of all political forces in Spain after the death of Francisco Franco in 1975 to abstain from bringing to light the crimes of the dictatorship. According to Espinosa Maestre, the first

The genre of Civil War novel has enjoyed enormous popularity in Spain, reaching a peak after the passage of the Historical Memory Law[42] in 2007. More often than not, however, in these novels the experiences of those who lost the war were emptied of all political content and used to titillate the jaded sensibilities of consumers:

> Victimhood has ... been absorbed by an all-encompassing consumer society that is eager to experience safely controlled aseptic "emotions" but that does not have the taste to analyse the implications and contradictions behind them.[43]

Prado's novel attempts to push the readers out of this familiar mode of approaching the Spanish Civil War genre and encourage them to engage with the memory of the war in a more active manner. The writer works fairly extensive quotes from the testimonial sources he uses into the text of *Mala gente que camina* and refuses to end the novel in a way that would create feelings of catharsis for the readers and, in this manner, liberate them from any obligation towards the past. At the end of the novel, there is still no clarity as to whether Lisvano will be able to take Juan Urbano to court for disinterring the truth about his family, and the readers are left with the responsibility to disseminate the knowledge unearthed by Urbano about the way Republican children were treated during the dictatorship.

---

usage of the term in this context can be traced back to José Vidal-Beneyto's article in the leading Spanish newspaper *El País* published in November of 1980. Since then, the term has entered common usage and is still hotly debated in Spain. Francisco Espinosa Maestre, Francisco, 'De saturaciones y olvidos. Reflexiones en torno a un pasado que no puede pasar'. *Hispania Nova* 7 (2007): np, viewed on 29 September, 2016, http://hispanianova.rediris.es/7/HISPANIANOVA-2007.pdf

42 In Spanish it is known as 'Ley de Memoria Histórica'. The full name of this piece of legislation is 'Ley 52/2007, de 26 de diciembre, por la que se reconocen y amplían derechos y se establecen medidas en favor de quienes padecieron persecución o violencia durante la Guerra Civil y la Dictadura'.

43 Antonio Cazorla-Sánchez, 'From Anti-Fascism to Humanism: The Spanish Civil War as a Crisis of Memory', *Memory and Cultural History of the Spanish Civil War: Realms of Oblivion*, edited by Aurora G. Morcillo (Boston: Brill, 2001), 445.

4 *Franco's Forgotten Children*: a Collection of Testimonial Accounts

The authors of *Franco's Forgotten Children*, the collection of testimonial accounts that served as the basis for Prado's novel, brought together their expertise in different areas to create the documentary and, later, the book with the same title. Ricard Vinyes is a professor of modern and contemporary history at the University of Barcelona. He contributed to the project of creating *Franco's Forgotten Children* his expertise as a scholar specializing in the prison system of the Franco regime. Montse Armengou is an award-winning journalist and film-maker whose documentaries on the crimes of the dictatorship have attracted large audiences. Ricard Belis is a journalist who has participated in creating documentaries on the subject of the Franco-era repression of political dissent. Initially, the documentary that Armengou and Belis were planning to create was going to cover the experiences of the adult prisoners of Franco's repressive apparatus. In the course of their research, however, the film-makers realized that the dictatorship jailed not only adults but also children.[44] Armengou and Belis reached out to Ricard Vinyes who informed them of the research he was conducting into the subject of the measures relied upon by the Franco authorities in their efforts to ensure that the children of 'the Reds' did not adopt their parents' political convictions. The children who fell under the scope of these measures ranged from newborn infants who were often separated from their mothers to teenagers who had gone into exile but were repatriated, mostly against their will, by the dictatorship.

Vinyes, Armengou and Belis state in the preface to their book that only the victims themselves and some of the historians researching the war knew about the tragedy of the children separated from their parents by the dictatorship. What was lacking was a general awareness among Spaniards that this had taken place.[45] One of the viewers of the documentary *Franco's Forgotten Children* commented:

> Why is it that we know so much better what happened in Argentina or Germany during their dictatorship than what took place here during the forty years of dictatorship, and especially since it ended over twenty-five years ago?[46]

---

44 Ricard Vinyes, Montse Armengou and Ricard Belis, *Los niños perdidos del franquismo*, translated by Daniel Royo (Barcelona: Plaza & Janés, 2002), 15–16.

45 Vinyes, Armengou and Belis, *Los niños perdidos del franquismo*, 17.

46 Ibid., 18.

The protagonist of Prado's novel also draws parallels between the disappearances of children in Spain after the Civil War and in Argentina or Uruguay several decades later because testimonies that have emerged from Latin America have set the frame of reference currently used within testimonial literature in Spanish-speaking countries.[47]

Testimonial literature genre arose as a result of 'the civil conflicts in Latin America in the 1970s and 1980s and represented the political act of denouncing injustices against members of marginalized groups'.[48] The existing testimonial literature of Spain has not been studied in depth,[49] and consequently, public awareness of the ways in which Franco's dictatorship treated the children of the defeated Republicans has been minimal. The makers of the documentary believe that the reluctance to explore all of the crimes of the dictatorship during the transition to democracy contributed to creating an environment of civic disengagement and emptied the political process of any meaning.[50] Only through a sustained effort to recover the country's historical memory will it become possible for Spaniards to create a truly democratic society where there will be no place for the structures of oppression inherited from the dictatorship of Franco.

In Latin America, the genre of *testimonio* reached the peak of its popularity in the decade of the 1990s. In 1992, Rigoberta Menchú, a Guatemalan human rights activist, won the Nobel Peace Prize. Menchú's testimonial account was recorded by Elisabeth Burgos-Debray and published under the title *I, Rigoberta Menchú* and provoked an intense debate on the limitations of the genre of testimonial literature. In the aftermath of this controversy, the discussions of testimonial literature have often been limited to the attempts to determine the degree to which the authors might have injected their subjective view of the events they relate into the narrative. According to Kimberly Nance, the critical reaction to the genre of testimony 'has consisted in the main of thirty years of celebration and ten of suspicion, all focused more on the contexts, character and motives of *testimonio*'s speakers and collaborating writers than on the texts themselves'.[51] More often than not, the response to testimonial literature

47 Prado, *Mala gente que camina*, 127.

48 Erik Ching, Christina Buckley and Angélica Lozano-Alonso, *Reframing Latin America: A Cultural Theory Reading of the Nineteenth and Twentieth Centuries* (Austin: University of Texas Press, 2007), 318.

49 Cristina Dupláa, 'Mujeres, escritura de resistencia y testimonios antifranquistas', *Monographic Review/Revista monográfica* xi (1995): 139.

50 Vinyes, Armengou and Belis, *Los niños perdidos del franquismo*, 16.

51 Kimberly Nance, *Can Literature Promote Justice? Trauma Narrative and Social Action in Latin American Testimonio* (Nashville: Vanderbilt University Press, 2006), 5.

centres on the degree of the author's objectivity and the presence of fictional elements in the account. Of course, no evidence of authenticity will ever prove sufficient for those who are politically motivated to reject the testimonial account in question. As a result, it has become easy to dismiss testimony as 'false' whenever it becomes politically expedient to do so. For instance, doubts as to the veracity of some of Menchú's statements in her testimonial account have been used to discredit her testimony altogether:

> The tribunes of culture and opinion can breezily dismiss [*I, Rigoberta Menchú*] as a hoax, or as an example of 'social or political witness stories that turns out to be works of fiction', as the New Yorker recently did … . This is regrettable, for subsequent research – by individual scholars … as well as sprawling, multi-year investigations by two truth commissions, one run by the Catholic Church and the other by the United Nations – has largely vindicated Menchú's version of events.[52]

The excoriation to which Menchú was subjected was politically motivated, yet it succeeded in casting doubt over the value of her entire testimony.[53]

In Spain, the public's interest in the testimonial accounts of the survivors of the Civil War and the post-war repression is only now becoming strong. In order to pre-empt possible accusations of falsehood of the kind that have plagued Latin American *testimonio*, Spanish writers are openly blending fact and fiction in their novels on the subject of the Civil War and the post-war persecution of Republicans and their family members. The need to effectuate a 'movement away from fiction'[54] that characterized the discussions of Latin American testimony in the 1990s is being subverted in the peninsular approaches to the genre. Even in a collection of testimonial accounts, such as *Franco's Forgotten Children*, there is no effort, on the part of the authors, to draw a strict demarcation line between fact and fiction. No longer do the authors who collect and record testimonial accounts feel the need to defend their veracity in order for the testimony to be considered legitimate. These authors affirm the right of testimonial accounts to be steeped in subjectivity and demonstrate that the subjective nature of testimony in no way detracts from its value. Vinyes, Armengou and Belis, the authors of *Franco's Forgotten Children*, carry out a movement towards fiction as they abandon the detached tone

52 Greg Grandin, *Who Is Rigoberta Menchú?* (London: Verso, 2011), v.

53 Ibid., 8–9.

54 Georg Gugelberger and Michael Kearney, 'Voices for the Voiceless: Testimonial Literature in Latin America', *Latin American Perspectives* 18.3 (Summer 1991): 10.

of scholarly analysis used in the first part of the book and adopt a more conversational tone that is closer to novelistic environment in the second part. The opening chapters of *Franco's Forgotten Children* discuss the legislation adopted in Franco's Spain that made possible the forced separation of Republican children from their parents, and the tone of the narrative mimics the subject matter. This part of the book is narrated in the third person and offers an example of scholarly writing. The narrator's voice is detached, unemotional and presents objective facts about post-war repression without expressing a personal opinion on these events. The title of this part of the book is 'The Mechanisms of Loss', which underscores the authors' efforts to make this part of the book data-driven and scholarly in tone.

However, the tone of the narrative changes dramatically in the second part of the book titled 'The Voices'. Most of the fifteen chapters' titles in this part of the book include the name of the survivor whose testimony inspired the chapter: Tomasa Cuevas, Carme Riera, Teresa Martín, Uxenu Álvarez, the Aguirre sisters, Emilia Girón, and others. The stories that the survivors had to share about the forcible separation of Republican parents from their children remained hidden from the public view for over sixty years. Learning about the private dramas of the survivors can allow the readers to connect with their experience on a profoundly personal level. Vinyes, Armengou and Belis make every effort to ensure that the victims of the dictatorship never become an undifferentiated group of nameless and faceless sufferers. The Republicans who were separated from their families by the Franco authorities are described in a way that makes the readers empathize and even identify with them.

This part of *Franco's Forgotten Children* is narrated in the first person plural. Instead of relating the events of a distant past in a dispassionate tone, the authors talk of their own emotions during the meetings with the survivors of Franco's prisons and orphanages. At several points throughout the text, the authors of the book slip into the indirect free style in which the perspectives of the researchers and of the survivors mesh:

> Tomasa, the one who was insulted so many times, tortured. "Whore", "Red", "Communist" ... .She can still hear these words in her head. During those times, when many of the prisoners did not know where fear ended and bravery began, little could she imagine that today she would be sitting here as the absolute protagonist.[55]

55 Vinyes, Armengou and Belis, *Los niños perdidos del franquismo*, 85.

This narrative style allows the readers to experience the impact of the survivors' accounts in a much more powerful way. As journalists, Armengou and Belis realize that any attempt to position themselves as fully objective observers will ultimately be dishonest. In the words of Rosalind Coward,

> 'objectivity' assumes detachment from the world that is unattainable; no one is able to detach their emotions, their fundamental beliefs and their world view from every situation creating themselves as a sort of tabula rasa. Neither is 'neutrality' a genuine possibility.[56]

Like Benjamín Prado whose novel leaves no doubt as to his political sympathies, Vinyes, Armengou and Belis renounce, from the very beginning, any claim to dispassionate objectivity. They do not attempt to conceal the compassion they feel towards the survivors, and their identification with the people who offer their testimony for the book is profound.

The journalists strive to guide the readers towards an emotional identification with the survivors whose testimony they present in each chapter. For instance, for the chapter titled 'Concentration Camps and Death Trains', they interviewed Juana Doña, a political activist and victim advocate who spent over twenty years in Franco's jails for her affiliation with the Communist Party of Spain.[57] In order to make the readers' encounter with Doña resonate on an emotional level, Vinyes, Armengou and Belis carefully describe the setting where the interview took place. The readers are invited to imagine the little hot room whose walls are covered with newspaper cuttings, Republican propaganda art, and paintings.[58] This is where Juana Doña, an 83-year-old survivor, is writing her book on the persecution suffered by Republicans after the war. A glimpse into Doña's apartment and the possibility of witnessing, through the journalists' narrative, the environment in which she lives and works enhance the emotional impact of the woman's devastating story of the horrors visited upon Republican women and their children in the concentration camps of the dictatorship and on the trains that carried prisoners to their tragic destinations.

56 Rosalind Coward, *Speaking Personally. The Rise of Subjectivity and Confessional Journalism* (London: Palgrave Macmillan, 2013), 20.

57 Vinyes, Armengou and Belis, *Los niños perdidos del franquismo*, 93.

58 Ibid.

The narrative part of *Franco's Forgotten Children*[59] ends with the story of Mercedes Sanz Bachiller, the founder of Auxilio Social (Social Assistance), the beneficent organization that mitigated some of the harshest social problems that arose as a result of the war in the Nationalist zone and where Prado's Dolores Serma worked in order to find her stolen nephew. Auxilio Social was a vehicle for political propaganda and social control that often separated children of Republicans from their families and subjected them to harsh punishments and ideological brainwashing.[60] For Dolores, the decision to work for an organization that was so crucial for the success of the Franco regime's project of eradicating dissent[61] represents a betrayal of her political convictions. Prado's novel is heavily indebted to the research that Vinyes, Armengou and Belis conducted of Auxilio Social. The authors of *Franco's Forgotten Children* interviewed Sanz Bachiller at the age of 91, long after the regime to whose stability she dedicated so much of her energy had ended.[62] The chapter opens with an epigraph quoting Sanz Bachiller's words: 'This never existed',[63] and these words can resume her attitude towards the testimonies of those who underwent ideological conditioning in one of the orphanages of her beneficent organization. Sanz Bachiller flatly refuses to accept the validity or even the existence of the testimonial evidence that casts doubt on her claims that Auxilio Social never engaged in indoctrination or strove to punish Republican families for their political beliefs. The journalists make no attempt to conceal their feelings of shock and incredulity when they realize that Sanz Bachiller dismisses the testimonies of the survivors as if they never existed. Speaking in the first person plural, Armengou and Belis signal their desire to ally themselves with the survivors whose testimony is rejected by Sanz Bachiller:

> If it weren't for the lucidity, the coherence and the good memory that [Sanz Bachiller] has demonstrated throughout the interview, we could say that she is delirious. But no. This is simply one more example of a denialist discourse that conceals what really happened.[64]

59 The third part of the book is constituted by the archival documents that further clarify the extent of the crimes committed by the dictatorship against the children of the Republican prisoners.

60 Vinyes, Armengou and Belis, *Los niños perdidos del franquismo*, 190–191.

61 Ibid., 191.

62 Mercedes Sanz Bachiller died in 2007, five years after the book was published.

63 Vinyes, Armengou and Belis, *Los niños perdidos del franquismo*, 187.

64 Ibid.

There will be no possibility of a dialogue between the winners and the losers of the Civil War until the crimes of the dictatorship are recognized in full. The journalists who interview Sanz Bachiller insert themselves into the conflict between those who want the lost memory of the past to be recovered in full and those who refuse to admit the validity of this claim. As representatives of a younger generation of Spaniards with no personal memory of the war, Vinyes, Armengou and Belis signal, through their emotional involvement with the story, the continued relevance of the Civil War to their understanding of their country's history.

5 Testimony as a Path to Healing

In his novel, Benjamín Prado takes the movement towards fiction in an exploration of testimonial accounts even further than the creators *Franco's Forgotten Children*. The novel's first-person narrator makes it very clear that he identifies strongly with those who lost the war and makes no attempt to lay claim either to objectivity or neutrality. Since Spain's Transition to democracy, calls for giving equal treatment to both the war's winners and its losers have concealed the desire to silence the victims of the dictatorship. No truly equal treatment was possible in a society that, for decades, had exalted the memory of the Nationalists and erased the remembrances of the Republicans in a way that contributed to creating a mentality that could not be undone without great effort:

> The acknowledgment only of the sacrifice made for the Francoist side during the war made the post-war dismantling of wartime mentalities problematic. Memories of the republican war effort were denied expression, representation and public ritualisation. This was essentially a symbolic continuation of the war.[65]

It has become impossible to deny the crimes of the Franco dictatorship, and very few voices in Spain attempt to construct a narrative of the Nationalists' innocence. This does not mean, however, that there are no efforts to justify the Franco regime and, consequently, everything that it did in the name of

65 Michael Richards and Chris Ealham, 'History, Memory and the Spanish Civil War: Recent Perspectives', *The Splintering of Spain: Cultural History and the Spanish Civil War, 1936–1939*, edited by Chris Ealham and Michael Richards (Cambridge: Cambridge University Press, 2005), 6.

consolidating its power. Today, the crimes of the dictatorship are erased through assertions that both sides of the civil conflict were equally guilty of the war's atrocities.[66] The belief in 'a fundamental similarity between the winners and the losers of the Civil War' was introduced by the Franco propaganda machine in the 1950s as a way of downplaying the persecution that was still going on.[67] Prado's Juan Urbano realizes that this approach perpetuates the Franco-era mentality. In his opinion, there are enormous differences between the crimes committed by the Nationalists and the Republicans during the war:

> An isolated case of violence ... is one thing but institutionalized crime is something quite different. And there is no comparison: while in the Nationalist zone Queipo de Llano encouraged crime and torture in his radio broadcasts, in the Republican zone Indalecio Prieto asked members of the militias to show courage in battle and compassion in the rearguard.[68]

Urbano is convinced that time has finally come to bring to light the decades of persecution visited on the Republicans and their descendants by the dictatorship and dispel the myth that both sides of the conflict were equally guilty in the war's atrocities.[69]

Prado's novel and the collection of testimonies by Vinyes, Armengou and Belis break down barriers between fiction and documentary in their search for a way to transmit the memory of the crimes of the Franco dictatorship in a way that will invite the readers to engage with history on a profound and personal level. This is all the more urgent given that several decades distance Spaniards from the events of the Civil War. As George Yúdice points out,

> the modern institution of literature traditionally has functioned as a gatekeeper, permitting certain classes of individuals to establish standards of taste within the public sphere and excluding others. This

66 Txetxu Aguado, 'A vueltas con el pasado: disidencias de la memoria en la historia', *Estudios culturales y de los medios de comunicación*, ed. María Pilar Rodríguez Pérez (Bilbao: Universidad de Deusto, 2009), 113.

67 Ulrich Winter, 'Asymmetry and the Political: Paradigms for a Cultural History of the Iberian Twentieth Century', *Iberian Modalities: A Relational Approach to the Study of Culture in the Iberian Peninsula*, edited by Joan Ramón Resina (Liverpool: Liverpool University Press, 2013), 140.

68 Prado, *Mala gente que camina*, 159.

69 Ibid., 160.

> explains why … .the expression of those deemed non-literary … .has been assigned to the genres of other disciplines … .or to substandard discursive forms.[70]

There seems to be a consensus among the peninsular authors who are interested in the Spanish Civil War that testimonial literature will not benefit from continued efforts either to draw a strict demarcation line between the literary and the non-literary or to present testimony as fully objective. These authors refuse to reproduce, in their writing, the strict separation between the public and the private forms of memory which served as a basis for post-war repression:

> The defeated cast no reflection. No public space was theirs … . The silent knowledge of unquiet graves necessarily produced a devastating schism between public and private memory in Spain.[71]

It is only by bridging this divide that the scars left by the dictatorship might finally begin to heal. Accessing the testimonial evidence left by those who lost the war will be crucial to this task.

Even though the hostilities of the Spanish Civil War officially ended on 1st April 1939, the war on the Spaniards who were seen as potentially dangerous to the regime continued, not sparing even children and infants. The state of war that had been declared on 18 July 1936, continued until 1948 and allowed Franco's officials to jail, torture and kill Republicans and their family members at will. In the 1950s, the dictatorship turned its attention to economic growth and reduced the volume of the repression of Republicans and their families. Throughout the 1950s, 1960s and until the dictator's death in 1975, Franco's authorities engaged in political persecution that was qualitatively extreme yet quantitatively limited.[72] Still, the narrative of the supposedly anti-Spanish nature of Republicanism remained in place. Vincent points out that, on the level of rhetoric, the war did not end until well into the 1970s:

---

70 George Yúdice, 'Testimonio and Postmodernism', *The Real Thing: Testimonial Discourse and Latin America*, ed. Georg M. Gugelberger (Durham: Duke University Press, 1996), 47.

71 Helen Graham, 'Coming to Terms with the Past: Spain's Memory Wars', *History Today* 54.5 (May 2004): 30.

72 Helen Graham, *La guerra y su sombra: una visión de la tragedia española en el largo siglo XX europeo*, translated by Sandra Souto Kustrin (Barcelona: Crítica, 2013), 210.

> Rhetorically, the regime continued to fight the Civil War. The division of Spain and, in particular, the threat posed by 'anti-Spain' remained a trope of official discourse even down to the 1970s.[73]

Today, the symbolic continuation of the war is present in the attempts to prevent a discussion of the past. Spain's Historical Memory Law adopted by the Socialist government of Rodríguez Zapatero was, from the very beginning, rejected by the conservative Partido Popular. The opponents of the law insisted that it undermined the legitimacy of the Transition and, consequently, cast doubt on the entire constitutional system that arose from it.[74] During the municipal elections of 2007, José María Aznar, the former President of Spain's government, gave a talk in Calatayud, Zaragoza, suggesting that the recovery of historical memory of the war and the dictatorship would undermine the country's capacity to build a better future. The Transition-era belief that inquiries into the crimes of the Franco dictatorship would bring Spain to the brink of another civil conflict reappeared in Aznar's discussion of historical memory. Aznar positioned the need to forget the past as a necessary precondition to entering a better future and dismissed the Civil War of 1936–9 as one of many indistinguishable civil conflicts.[75]

Paradoxically, it is not the debate over the issues surrounding the war and its legacy which keeps alive the wartime hostilities but, rather, the insistence that such a discussion is needless or dangerous. Juan Urbano's combative stance and the journalism of Vinyes, Armengou and Belis are more likely to put an end to the antagonism of the war and the post-war era than attempts to silence the debates about the war. In order for the past to be laid to rest, the graves of the victims will have to be disinterred and the importance of their memories will have to be acknowledged. Testimony can lead to national reconciliation but only after the voices of the victims are heard.

---

73 Mary Vincent, 'Breaking the Silence? Memory and Oblivion since the Spanish Civil War', *Shadows of War: A Social History of Silence in the Twentieth Century*, edited by Efrat Ben-Ze'ev, Ruth Ginio, and Jay Winter (Cambridge: Cambridge University Press, 2010), 53.

74 Rafael Escudero, Patricia Campelo, Carmen Pérez González and Emilio Silva, *Qué hacemos por la memoria histórica* (Madrid: Ediciones Akal, 2013), 38.

75 Marina Llorente, 'Exile and Erasure: A Poetic Reconstruction of the Spanish Past in Antonio Crespo Massieu's *Elegía en Portbou*', *Sites of Memory in Spain and Latin America: Trauma, Politics, and Resistance*, edited by Aída Díaz de León, Marina Llorente, and Marcella Salvi (Lanham: Lexington Books, 2015), 73, n. 15.

Bibliography

Aguado, Txetxu. 'A vueltas con el pasado: disidencias de la memoria en la historia'. *Estudios culturales y de los medios de comunicación*, edited by María Pilar Rodríguez Pérez, 105–22. Bilbao: Universidad de Deusto, 2009.

Aguilar Fernández, Paloma. 'Justice, Politics, and Memory in the Spanish Transition'. *The Politics of Memory: Transitional Justice in Democratizing Societies*, edited by Alexandra Barahona de Brito, Carmen González-Enríquez and Paloma Aguilar. 92–118. Oxford: Oxford University Press, 2001.

Becerra Mayor, David. *La guerra civil como moda literaria*. Madrid: Clave Intelectual, 2015.

Begin, Paul D. 'The Pistols Strike Again! On the Function of Punk in the Peninsular "Generation X" Fiction of Ray Loriga and Benjamín Prado'. *Generation X Rocks: Contemporary Peninsular Fiction, Film, and Rock Culture*, edited by Christine Henseler and Randolph D. Pope. 15–32. Nashville: Vanderbilt University Press, 2007.

Bertrand de Muñoz, Maryse. 'Novela histórica, autobiografía y mito (La novela y la guerra civil española desde la Transición)'. *La novela histórica a finales del siglo XX: Actas del V Seminario Internacional del Instituto de Semiótica Literaria y Teatral de la UNED, Cuenca*, edited by José Nicolás Romera Castillo and Mario García-Page Sánchez. 19–38. Cuenca: Visor, 1996.

Blas Vives, Damián. 'Entrevista a Benjamín Prado: Literatura y derechos humanos'. *Evaristo Cultural: Revista Virtual de Arte y Literatura* 7 (2007): np. Viewed on 29 September 2016. http://www.evaristocultural.com.ar/-%20EVARISTO%20Nro.%2007%20-/prado.htm.

Cazorla-Sánchez, Antonio. 'From Anti-Fascism to Humanism: The Spanish Civil War as a Crisis of Memory'. *Memory and Cultural History of the Spanish Civil War: Realms of Oblivion*, edited by Aurora G. Morcillo. 21–50. Boston: Brill, 2014.

Cercas, Javier. *Soldados de Salamina*. Barcelona, Tusquets, 2001.

Chacón. Dulce. *La voz dormida*. Madrid: Alfaguara, 2002.

Ching, Erik, Christina Buckley and Angélica Lozano-Alonso. *Reframing Latin America: A Cultural Theory Reading of the Nineteenth and Twentieth Centuries*. Austin: University of Texas Press, 2007.

Coward, Rosalind. *Speaking Personally. The Rise of Subjectivity and Confessional Journalism*. London: Palgrave Macmillan, 2013.

Davis, Madeleine. 'Is Spain Recovering Its Memory? Breaking the Pacto del Olvido.' *Human Rights Quarterly* 27.3 (August 2005): 858–80.

Dolgin Casado, Stacey. 'Benjamín Prado: La literatura es lo contrario del olvido'. *Oján-cano* 33 (April 2008): 103–13.

Doña, Juana. *Desde la noche y la niebla: las mujeres en las cárceles franquistas*. Madrid: Ediciones de la Torre, 1977.

Dupláa, Cristina. 'Mujeres, escritura de resistencia y testimonios antifranquistas'. *Monographic Review/Revista monográfica* XI (1995): 137–45.

Els nens perduts del franquisme ('Franco's Forgotten Children). Directed by Montse Armengou and Ricard Belis. España: Muntsa Tarrés, 2002.

Escudero, Rafael, Patricia Campelo, Carmen Pérez González, and Emilio Silva. *Qué hacemos por la memoria histórica*. Madrid: Ediciones Akal, 2013.

Espinosa Maestre, Francisco. 'De saturaciones y olvidos. Reflexiones en torno a un pasado que no puede pasar'. *Hispania Nova* 7 (2007): np. Viewed on 29 September 2016. http://hispanianova.rediris.es/7/HISPANIANOVA-2007.pdf

Gil Casado, Pablo. 'Benjamín Prado: de "la nueva novela" al realismo documental'. *Ojáncano* 35 (April 2009): 67–88.

Graham, Helen. 'Coming to Terms with the Past: Spain's Memory Wars'. *History Today* 54.5 (May 2004): 29–31.

Graham, Helen. *La guerra y su sombra: una visión de la tragedia española en el largo siglo XX europeo*, translated by Sandra Souto Kustrin. Barcelona: Crítica, 2013.

Grandes, Almudena. *Corazón helado*. Barcelona: Tusquets Editores, 2007.

Grandin, Greg. *Who Is Rigoberta Menchú?* London: Verso, 2011.

Gugelberger, Georg and Michael Kearney. 'Voices for the Voiceless: Testimonial Literature in Latin America'. *Latin American Perspectives* 18.3 (Summer 1991): 3–14.

La voz dormida. Directed by Benito Zambrano. España: Audiovisual Aval SGR/Maestranza Films and Warner Bros., 2011. DVD.

Llorente, Marina. 'Exile and Erasure: A Poetic Reconstruction of the Spanish Past in Antonio Crespo Massieu's *Elegía en Portbou*'. *Sites of Memory in Spain and Latin America: Trauma, Politics, and Resistance*, edited by Aída Díaz de León, Marina Llorente, and Marcella Salvi, 63–76. Lanham: Lexington Books, 2015.

Mateo, Juan José. 'Rivera se compromete a apoyar las exhumaciones de la Guerra Civil'. *El País*, November 18, 2015. Viewed on 20 November 2015. http://politica.elpais.com/politica/2015/11/17/actualidad/1447796568_381704.html

McCaughcy, Martha. *Cyberactivism on the Participatory Web*. New York: Routledge, 2014.

Nance, Kimberly A. *Can Literature Promote Justice? Trauma Narrative and Social Action in Latin American Testimonio*. Nashville: Vanderbilt UP, 2006.

Navarro Martínez, Eva. 'La novela de Benjamín Prado: Cómo construirse un mundo y una realidad propios'. *Letras peninsulares* 14.3 (Winter 2001–2002): 405–426.

Oleza Simó, Joan. 'Una nueva alianza entre historia y novela: Historia y ficción en el pensamiento literario del fin de siglo'. *La novela histórica a finales del siglo XX: Actas del V Seminario Internacional del Instituto de Semiótica Literaria y Teatral de la UNED, Cuenca*, edited by José Nicolás Romera Castillo and Mario García-Page Sánchez, 81–95. Cuenca: Visor, 1996.

Prado, Benjamín. *No sólo el fuego*. Madrid: Alfaguara, 1999.

Prado, Benjamín. *Mala gente que camina*. Madrid: Santillana, 2006.

Richards, Michael. 'Grand Narratives, Collective Memory, and Social History: Public Uses of the Past in Postwar Spain'. *Unearthing Franco's Legacy: Mass Graves and the Recovery of Historical Memory in Spain*, edited by Carlos Jerez-Ferrán and Samuel Amago, 121–45. Notre Dame: University of Notre Dame Press, 2010.

Richards, Michael and Chris Ealham. 'History, Memory and the Spanish Civil War: Recent Perspectives'. *The Splintering of Spain: Cultural History and the Spanish Civil War, 1936–1939*, edited by Chris Ealham and Michael Richards, 1–20. Cambridge: Cambridge University Press, 2005.

Richardson, Nathan. '*No pensar*, or Does the Contemporary Spanish Novel of Memory Really Want to Know?: *Tiempo de silencio, Corazón tan blanco, Soldados de Salamina* and Beyond'. *Letras Hispanas* 7.1 (2010): 2–16.

Rosa, Isaac. Prologue to *La guerra civil como moda literaria,* by David Becerra Mayor, 9–14. Madrid: Clave Intelectual, 2015.

Ruiz Torres, Pedro. '*Los discursos de la memoria histórica en España*'. *Generaciones y memoria de la represión franquista: Un balance de los movimientos por la memoria*, edited by Julio Aróstegui and Sergio Gálvez, 39–74. Valencia: Universitat de València, 2010.

Sánchez Dragó, Fernando. *Muertes paralelas*. Barcelona: Planeta, 2006.

Santana, Cintia. 'What We Talk about When We Talk about Dirty Realism in Spain'. *Generation X Rocks: Contemporary Peninsular Fiction, Film, and Rock Culture*, edited by Christine Henseler and Randolph D. Pope, 33–56. Nashville: Vanderbilt University Press, 2007.

Soldados de Salamina. Directed by David Trueba. España, Lolafilms/Fernando Trueba P.C., 2003. DVD.

Trapiello, Andrés. *Ayer no más* Destino: Barcelona, 2012.

Urioste, Carmen de. 'Memoria de la Guerra Civil y modernidad: el caso de *El corazón helado* de Almudena Grandes'. *Bulletin of Hispanic Studies* 87.8 (2010): 939–959.

Vázquez Montalbán, Manuel. *Un polaco en la corte del Rey Juan Carlos*. Madrid: Alfaguara, 1996.

Vincent, Mary. 'Breaking the Silence? Memory and Oblivion since the Spanish Civil War'. *Shadows of War: A Social History of Silence in the Twentieth Century*, edited by Efrat Ben-Ze'ev, Ruth Ginio, and Jay Winter, 47–67. Cambridge: Cambridge University Press, 2010.

Vinyes, Ricard, Montse Armengou, and Ricard Belis. *Los niños perdidos del franquismo*. Translated by Daniel Royo. Barcelona: Plaza & Janés, 2002.

Winter, Ulrich. 'Asymmetry and the Political: Paradigms for a Cultural History of the Iberian Twentieth Century'. *Iberian Modalities: A Relational Approach to the Study of Culture in the Iberian Peninsula*, edited by Joan Ramon Resina, 129–142. Liverpool: Liverpool UP, 2013.

Yúdice, George. 'Testimonio and Postmodernism'. *The Real Thing: Testimonial Discourse and Latin America*, edited by Georg M. Gugelberger, 42–57. Durham: Duke University Press, 1996.

PART 2

Suffer the Children

CHAPTER 4

When the Personal Becomes Collective: a Mother's Re-Membering of a Disappeared Daughter in *Madre de Mendoza*

Cristina Santos

Abstract

Historically relegated to the private sphere of Latin American society, women's entrance into the public arena of politics took place primarily under the military-authoritarian governments during the second half of the twentieth century. In *Madre de Mendoza* the reader is presented with the life story of María Isabel Figueroa, an Argentine mother who began her activism after her daughter disappeared. We will see how María Isabel's social activism develops during the various stages of the Argentinean Dirty War and how in being an active militant or *guerrera* in search of her missing daughter the personal, enters the arena of the collective. This testimony works through not only personal and collective trauma but also acknowledges and vindicates the number of disappeared. Although she did not begin as a revolutionary, María Isabel, becomes a militant mother who not only searched for her disappeared daughter, but in the end, mothered many other revolutionary children.

Keywords

Argentina Dirty War – social activism – militant – mothers – testimony – *desaparecidos*/disappeared – trauma – mourning

Historically relegated to the private sphere of Latin American society, women's militancy reappeared with a stronger impetus into the public arena of politics primarily under the military-authoritarian governments during the second half of the twentieth century. In *Madre de Mendoza* (2013) the reader is presented with the life story of María Isabel Figueroa (1918–2012), an Argentine mother who began her activism after her daughter, Lila, was taken as a political prisoner and disappeared during the last dictatorship in Argentina (1976–1983).

 | DOI:10.1163/9789004391130_006

At first María Isabel did not necessarily take her daughter's militancy seriously but became involved in social activism because of Lila's disappearance and her children's own political convictions, she did not necessarily accept their socio-political philosophy in its entirety. Even though María Isabel's social activism develops during the various stages of the Argentinean Dirty War, María Isabel's active militancy focused always on her disappeared daughter and thus did not seek to become a political figure; but in her social activism she becomes a 'emblematic mother' to many.[1] Antonius Robben has remarked that in the context of the political violence suffered in Argentina 'the political becomes personal' and 'the personal becomes political'.[2] For the purposes of this study I would propose that *the personal becomes the collective* and *the collective is personal.* This testimony works through not only personal and collective trauma but also acknowledges and vindicates the number of disappeared by putting into question official histories. Although she did not begin as a revolutionary, María Isabel, in the end, becomes a militant mother who not only searched for her disappeared daughter, but unselfishly mothered many other revolutionary children.

Historically those women who became involved in the public arena were primarily '[e]ducated, middle-class feminists, female guerrilla fighters, activist Mothers, and militant urban homemakers from class-oriented, grassroots organizations'.[3] The majority of critical studies on Latin American female militancy have tended to focus on the activism and mobilization of mothers in human rights groups, such as the Mothers of the Plaza de Mayo.[4] This is largely due to their reception and promotion from international solidarity organizations and the fact that these groups were based primarily in Buenos Aires, the capital city of Argentina. However, María Isabel belonged to a different group from the province of Mendoza located in the interior of Argentina. Regardless of geographical location, these women came to exemplify how, at any given moment,

1 "Dirty war" is the term used predominantly by the military forces to refer to this time period but not by the opposing organization. The term implies armed 'dirty' warfare on both sides which was not the truth of the matter.

2 Antonius C. G. M. Robben, *Political Violence and Trauma in Argentina* (Philadelphia: University of Pennsylvania Press, 2005), 297.

3 Elizabeth Maier, 'Accommodating the Private into the Public Domain. Experiences and Legacies of the Past Four Decades', in *Women's Activism in Latin America and the Caribbean: Engendering Social Justice, Democratizing Citizenship*, edited by Elizabeth Maier and Nathalie Lebon (New Brunswick, NJ: Rutgers University Press, 2010), 27.

4 Other organizations include the Grandmothers of the Plaza de Mayo (founded 1977) and Hijos por la identidad y la justicia contra el olvido y el silencio (HIJOS, Sons and Daughters for Identity and Justice against Oblivion and Silence) founded in 1995.

women are able to mobilize, personally and collectively, to begin to take command away from men to pursue an agenda of re-membering the disappeared.[5]

María Isabel's story incorporates a discussion of testimonial literature as not only bearing witness but engaging with the implicit question of ethical testimony. It draws on the concept Tsvetan Todorov called the 'duty of remembering and bearing testimony' and Rodolfo Walsh's idea of 'contar para sobrevivir' [to tell to survive] and 'sobrevivir para contar' [to survive to tell].[6] That is, how do we continue to remember as witnesses of a time when 'the unbelievable and the quotidian became blurred' are either dead or disappeared?[7] Especially since, as Robben points out: the 'practice of disappearance was systematic, premeditated strategy based on a firm ideological foundation' resulting in the 'traumatization of Argentine society last[ing] longer than the culture of fear'.[8] It becomes an inter-generational cycle of trauma relived through the gap in the social and familial fabric left by the disappeared and cemented in a generation of 'living victims' who, despite not having a direct memory of the time of dictatorship suffer the inter-generational trauma of those who did.[9]

Essential to María Isabel's quest to find her daughter Lila—and subsequent fight for human rights—is the quintessential question of 'How do we make the disappeared speak?' In a personal conversation with one of the authors of *Madre de Mendoza*, Adriana Spahr, clarified that, for her, it was a question more so of 'allowing for the disappeared to *speak through her* and not her *speaking for* them'.[10] In the end, the authors seek to reconstruct María Isabel's life through her own testimony and other's stories about her while 'forging her identity and building her belonging to the community'.[11] Herein are the narratological innovations that De Marinis and Spahr bring to the genre of testimony—it constructs the life of the disappeared daughter through the testimonies of her activist mother and

5 See Nora Stejilevich, *Una sola muerte numerosa* (Córdoba, Argentina: Alción Editora, 2006), 34.

6 Quoted in María del Carmen Sillato, *Huellas: Memorias de Resistencia (Argentina 1974–1983)* (San Luis: Nueva Editorial Universitaria, 2008), 7. Translation mine.

7 'una épica donde lo asombroso y lo cotidiano se mezclan'. Hugo De Marinis and Adriana Spahr, *Madre de Mendoza: Vida de María Isabel Figueroa* (Buenos Aires: Corregidor, 2013), 11. This and all subsequent English translations from this text are mine.

8 Robben, *Political Violence and Trauma in Argentina*, 265.

9 Term coined by Antonius Robben in 'How Traumatized Societies Remember', in *Cultural Critique* 59 (2005): 121.

10 Personal conversation 8 May 2014.

11 'contar lo suyo, que no significa sino forjar identidad y construir la pertenencia a la comunidad'. De Marinis and Spahr, *Madre de Mendoza*, 11.

community members that knew both women. As testimonial literature, *Madre de Mendoza* fulfils what Nora Strejilevich has indicated as a primary role of testimony: that is, 'as a means for working through traumatic memories and for social and cultural resistance'.[12] Strejilevich, a survivor herself of the Argentinean state of terror, further indicates that: 'A truthful way of giving testimony should allow for disruptive memories, discontinuities, blanks, silences and ambiguities; it should become literary'.[13] De Marinis and Spahr use the testimonies from multiple testimonialists around María Isabel and Lila to overlap and complement each other—providing a literary testimony where the disruptive memories of the collective (family and friends) inform the blanks, silences and ambiguities.

Madre de Mendoza engages the voices and memories of many to shape a symphony of voices and memories that succeed in (re)constructing María Isabel as militant mother and Lila as disappeared daughter. It is a communal exercise of re-membering the lost Lila while piecing together a mother's 'accidental' activism in her struggle to give meaning, shape and dignity to her missing daughter's life. It is a communal exercise in memory so that the past may be examined that it not be repeated and underlined by a social responsibility of sharing these testimonial voices while also confronting the cultural trauma that has marked generations of Argentines.[14] De Marinis and Spahr allow 'for the past to become part of the pastinstead of remaining a haunting present' and reincorporate the name of the disappeared Lila with her mother's commitment to defeat 'annihilation by working through loss'.[15] It is interesting to point out that Adriana Spahr's chapter contribution to this volume picks up on testimonies of the children of militants during this time in Argentinean history in which the children work through their own process of recovery from losing a relative due to exile (internal and external) as well as discrimination and suspicion.

These testimonies are not only trauma-stories of personal embodiment—but incorporate the ideal of in-corporating the body into the experience, despite attempts to maintain and/or impose silence. The post-traumatic re-opening of the wound must consider if the testimonialist is prepared to deal with possibility of post-trauma. That is, will the testimonialist be ready to disinfect the re-opening of the wound of this past trauma so that it does not fester and become newly infected?[16] Avoiding the risk of that 'haunting'–when the

12 Nora Strejilevich, 'Testimony: Beyond the Language of Truth', *Human Rights Quarterly* 28.3 (2006): 701.

13 Ibid., 704.

14 Sillato, *Huellas*, 26.

15 Strejilevich, 'Testimony', 706.

16 Berta Horen, personal interview 14 May 2015.

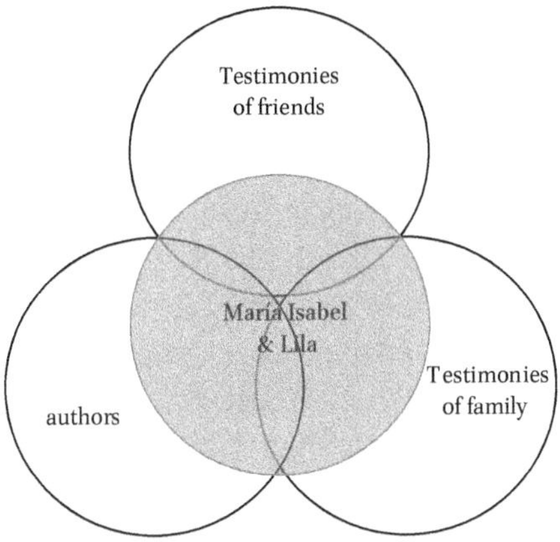

FIGURE 4.1 Testimonial (re)construction in *Madre de Mendoza*

wound has not been opened to allow it to be healed–or at least be properly 'disinfected'. De Marinis and Spahr recognize the relationship between trauma experience through language and thought processing so that the story is no longer denied nor forgotten—that it becomes a part of history. *Madre de Mendoza* is an affirmation of the personal experience as part of a collective history through personal and social memory–to tell the story, to contextualize, to understand and most importantly, to not forget.

A tripartite mimetic process that links telling one's story to the metaphor of a wound–parallels the same metaphoric representations used at the *Parque de la memoria* in the construction of a scar-like three walled edifice populated by the 30,000 names of the disappeared. Both look at 'the wound' as a prompt towards 'belonging' via symbolic reparation in which the[17] wound cannot fully heal. Working from Paul Ricoeur's mimesis, I propose:

Mimesis1 →	prefigurative → the wounding 'the infecting'
Mimesis2 →	configurative → sharing/telling the story 'the disinfecting'
Mimesis3 →	refigurative → catharsis via acknowledgment 'the healing over the scar'

17 See Ricoeur, Paul. *Time and Narrative*. Vol. I. Trans. Kathleen McLaughlin and David Pellauer. Chicago: Chicago UP, 1984.

It is crucial that the healing occurs *over the scar*, not the wound, since the scar forever remains as a reminder written on the body, on the psyche, on the self and on the other. This is especially important since the unscarred wound re-opens the body to infection and to a 'haunting' when the wound which is re-opened has not been opened to allow it to heal. Healing from a trauma, physical or psychological, must recognize that, as Cathy Caruth points out, 'trauma is not simply an effect of destruction but also, fundamentally, an enigma of survival'.[18] It is in testimonial writing that the wound of past pain, suffering and victimization is re-opened with the hope of working through the traumatic experience but giving voice and historical presence to both the personal and collective experience. Similar to scriptotherapy, by giving testimony the testimonialist works through the *wounding* and moves into *healing* by 'embarking on a calculated exercise in scriptotherapy [or literary testimony in this case]—a graphic and detailed reiteration of earlier traumatic experiences that threatened to kill her but strengthened her instead'.[19] Although Henke is describing Audre Lorde's own scriptotherapy as an 'impassioned *testimonio*' it is interesting that this African American woman's text incorporates the same aims as *Madre de Mendoza* in that it 'will offer a healing narrative for those who come after her and for all women engaged in political, economic, psychological, or physiological struggles'.[20]

Elaine Scarry in *The Body in Pain* adds that regaining one's voice can be the prelude to the task of diminishing one's pain and that art (in our case the oral and written testimony) provides an alternative forum to afford visibility (outside) the courtroom, to the sensation of pain.[21] It resonates with Freud's 'talking cure'/catharsis when experience skips the rational directly to the psyche. Similar to the wounding metaphor—it is in recalling the trauma, the re-construction, the re-identification of the disappeared–that one does not allow it to destroy the self, the memory—the disappeared. Because, although 'the *body* [is] the locus of *pain* ...the *voice* [is] the locus of *power*'.[22] It is the rebirth of language when pain [both personal and collective] re-discovers speech/enunciation.[23]

18 Cathy Caruth, *Unclaimed Experience: Trauma, Narrative and History* (Baltimore: John Hopkins University Press, 1996), 58.

19 Suzette A. Henke, *Shattered Subjects: Trauma and Testimony in Women's Life Writing* (New York: St. Martin's Press, 2000), 115.

20 Ibid., 119, 118.

21 Elaine Scarry, *The Body in Pain: The Making and Unmaking of the World* (New York: Oxford University Press, 1985), 9–11.

22 Ibid., 51. Emphasis mine.

23 Ibid., 172.

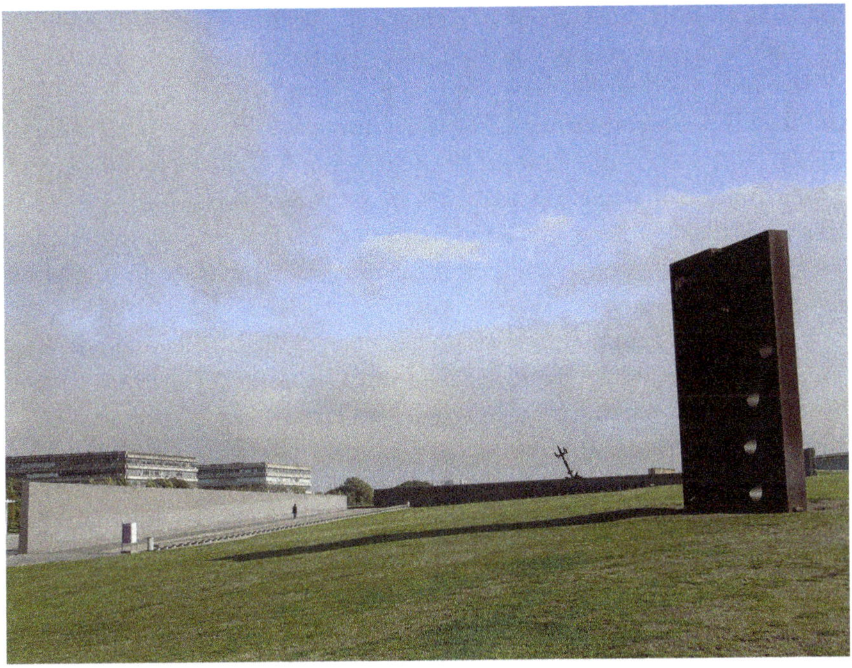

FIGURE 4.2 Parque de la memoria, two of the four walls forming the scar formation
© 2015 PHOTOGRAPHER CRISTINA SANTOS. USED WITH PERMISSION.

In capturing María Isabel's struggle, De Marinis and Spahr construct the testimonial subject by way of a collectivized testimony of those in her family and community and not just by a first person narrative. It is a methodology that embodies María Isabel's own militant motivation: that the focus be placed on her disappeared daughter and constructed as part of a national social memory.

Yet, returning to the past is not always a freeing experience and consists of a refiguration of the present that Beatriz Sarlo describes as 'the immediacy of the body's voice favour[ing] testimony' in 'that which is lived is told, what is told is what is lived'.[24] *Madre de Mendoza* in its compilation of testimonies around Lila and María Isabel's search for answers brings about the retelling of a story of loss that in the search for meaning becomes incomprehensible, yet to a certain degree, restores the social and collective that once was lost in the cult(ure) of terror.[25] The process of rememorialization

24 'la inmediatez de la voz del cuerpo favorece el testimonio' Beatriz Sarlo, *Tiempo pasado: Cultura de la memoria y giro subjetivo. Una discusión* (Buenos Aires: Siglo veintiuno, 2006), 23. All translations mine. 'la que se vive relata, lo que se relata es lo que se vive'. Ibid., 33.

25 Ibid., 59.

connotes a use of this exercise in memory and testimony in an affective dimension with a sense of collective moral responsibility.[26] However, *Madre de Mendoza* does not become part of a post-memory because the authors are careful not to construct it as history turned story, turned movement. Similar to the focus of *El parque de la memoria*, it is the re-membering of disappeared so that their identity can be restored—even if it is just symbolically.[27] Furthermore, it is an exercise in inter-generational trauma and memorialization where a conflict of memory sometimes emerges around an unresolved trauma.

It becomes evident that motherhood in much of the critical literature written on testimony has been one of the most complex and controversial negotiations for women in socio-political and cultural environments of most Latin American countries. Meg Samuelson notes that:

> [t]wo strands of feminist thought diverge ... one finds in war a potential realm of gendered equality and female liberation; another associates women with nurturing and life-giving qualities, linking them to an ethos of peace and pitting them and their interests against war.[28]

When placed alongside Western traditions of motherhood and war, the acceptance of the female militant becomes inherently unsettling since:

> '[m]othering' and 'war' have often been twinned in a sort of lethal symbiosis: whether collusive or oppositional, conceptual or practical, life giving and death dealing are seen to be connected.[29]

In Latin America, there is a similar tradition of female militancy that has provided both controversy as well as sources of inspiration for revolutionaries in the latter half of the twentieth century since: 'Militancy was a type of uterus that enveloped you from all sides: political, cultural and

26 Ibid., 74, 84.

27 Ibid., 126–129.

28 Meg Samuelson, 'The Disfigured Body of the Female Guerrilla: (De)Militarization, Sexual Violence, and Redomestication in Zoë Wicomb's *David's Story*', in *War and Terror. Feminist Perspectives*, edited by Karen Alexander and Mary Hawkesworth (Chicago: U of Chicago P, 2008), 89.

29 Irene Matthews. 'Daughtering in War: Two "Case Studies" from Mexico and Guatemala', in *Gendering War Talk*, edited by Miriam Cooke and Angela Woollacott (Princeton, N.J.: Princeton UP, 1993), 148.

affective'.[30] A militancy that co-existed in what Pilar de Calveiro classifies as a 'binary universe' where the militant other is made out to be dangerous, threatening and potentially destructive.[31] In becoming a 'total' threat to 'I'/military powers the 'I'/subversives must be 'totally' persecuted.[32] Notwithstanding, the heightened culture of terror also gave way to a more pronounced resistance not only with within the militant organizations but, as in the case of María Isabel, for the family members of the disappeared who had no prior interest in the socio-political movements of their loved ones.

It is important to note that María Isabel comes from this tradition of militant women that recognized the gendered power relation and combated it by embracing it as an intrinsic part of their militant mothering: 'the strength I had in that moment ... kept me strong in many other situations, was born out of my feminine condition'.[33] It is a sense of power based on their political and cultural role that Robben sees as 'cultural transgressors' because they are able to overstep their socially gendered roles to assume both public political roles as well as politicizing their domestic roles.[34] María Isabel, via her own admission and the testimonies of those who knew her, embodied a maternal thinking of socio-politicizing of her private pain in order to bring attention to the case of her disappeared daughter. This was accomplished with a certain ideological neutrality because, as women, they were not perceived as political actors but as 'just mothers' seeking disappeared children.[35] This embodies not only a removal of the woman from the private sphere of the home but also her repositioning as the active mother figure as an intrinsic part of a 'new' home—the revolutionary movement:

> But we are here alive. We form part of a chain, vital and feminine, that began with the indigenous peoples (who hardly exist anymore), primitive

30 '[l]a militancia era una especie de útero que te contenía en todos los terrenos: político, cultural, afectivo'. Marta Diana, *Mujeres guerrilleras: sus testimonios en la militancia de los setenta.* 3rd ed. (Buenos Aires: Booket, 2011), 273.

31 Calveiro situates the 'binary universe' within the concentration camp, however one can also apply it to the exterior world outside the walls of the detention centers (88–89). Pilar de Calveiro, *Poder y desaparición: Los campos de concentración en Argentina* (Buenos Aires: Ediciones Colihue, 2001).

32 Ibid., 89.

33 'la fuerza que tuve en ese momento [...] y mantenerme firme en muchos otros, nacieron de mi condición femenina'. Ibid., 37.

34 Robben, *Political Violence and Trauma in Argentina,* 304–305.

35 Ibid., 305–306.

> residents of these lands, whose next link in the chain includes those women who boarded those ships in Europe for unknown lands to embark on an even more uncertain destiny. The Argentine guerrillas (who hardly exist anymore) also belonged to this chain. This is not a question of politics. It is a historic, social, and human question. What is political is the treatment that has been given to this topic: heroine or delinquent.[36]

There is, as Scarry notes a conflation of inside/outside; the private/public, a combination of both isolation and exposure.[37] It is this well-established prefigurative that allows for the evolution of this new sense of *guerrera* mothering that integrates an awareness of solidarity where 'they are all that immense family that one never had'.[38] For many of the women there was also a sense of sisterhood together with the notion of communal mothering.[39] María Isabel relates that at the demonstrations many of the mothers of the disappeared would get together and 'we would chat, console one another, each one would tell how their children had been taken away from them and we would cry'.[40] This, we shall see, has been the legacy created by María Isabel as well as many of *las madres guerreras* as described by her granddaughter, Paula: 'the image of my grandmother as the nucleus. She is a mother, but in the most profound sense of the word mother'.[41]

In *Madre de Mendoza* the reader is presented with the life story of María Isabel Figueroa, an Argentine mother who 'was born' and 'transformed' by her activism after her daughter disappeared, bearing in mind that her own past had much bearing on how she dealt with Lila's kidnapping. Giving testimony to Lila's disappearance not to create heroes or heroic stories but to break the silence and enforce memory as collective memory–to give name and history to those

36 'Pero nosotras estamos sí estamos vivas. Formamos parte de una cadena, vital y femenina, que se inició con las indígenas (que casi ya no existen), primitivas habitantes de estas tierras, cuyo próximo eslabón integran esas otras mujeres que un día en Europa abordaron inciertas naves para desembarcar en un destino más incierto todavía. De esa cadena, las que fueron guerrilleras argentinas (que casi ya no existen) también forman parte. Esta no es una cuestión política. Es una cuestión histórica, social, y humana. Lo que es político es el tratamiento que se ha dado al tema: heroínas o delincuentes'. Ibid., 444.

37 Scarry, *The Body in Pain*, 53.

38 'son esa familia inmensa que no tuvo'. De Marinis and Spahr, *Madre de Mendoza*, 179.

39 Diana, *Mujeres guerrilleras*, 280.

40 'Conversábamos, nos consolábamos, cada una contaba la historia de cómo les habían llevado a los hijos, llorábamos'. De Marinis and Spahr, *Madre de Mendoza*, 114.

41 'la imagen de la abuela como un núcleo. Es una madre, pero en el sentido más profundo de la palabra madre'. Ibid., 157.

who have been denied both—to breakdown the *collective amnesia*.[42] In this case family members admit that María Isabel at first did not necessarily take Lila's militancy seriously but becomes involved because of Lila's and her other children's own personal commitment, even though she did not necessarily accept what they did in its entirety.[43] Figueroa admits:

> I didn't really belong to any particular party. My father was a radical, I was a radical, and my mother belonged to one party one day and to another party the following day. We didn't trust any of them.[44]

It is important to point out that although María Isabel did not share in the political outlook of her children she came from a family history in which its women were not afraid to break from tradition in order to stand up for themselves and for their loved ones. María Isabel's mother, for instance, fought to educate all of her children during a time when it was difficult to do so all the while being vocal of her own radical socio-political beliefs.[45] Notwithstanding, it is the early death of María Isabel's brother, Hector, from tuberculosis when she sees her mother fight to care for her brother despite the medical prognosis given to him. It is most telling that María Isabel refers to the moment of his death, when she was only 18 years old, as 'the moment that marked her path of how the rest of her life would be'.[46]

Mothers were critical in shaping how their militant children were able to contribute to the revolutionary movements. Finding inspiration and/or support from their own mothers was a common feature for many families across the spectrum of revolutionary movements in Latin America. Collective memory in this context can serve as a safeguard that serves as both a tool of empowerment and a self- protection. Keeping in mind, as Beatriz Sarlo underlines, memory questions a reconstruction that focuses only on the rights of memory.[47] In her militancy María Isabel, like many other mothers, brings the focus back onto the identity and name of the disappeared—maintaining the human link on a process that has sought the dehumanization and desocialization of the militant. That is, the

42 Ibid., *Poder y desaparición*, 11.

43 Ibid., 76–77, 80.

44 'Yo no era de ningún partido realmente. Mi papá era radical, yo era radical, y mi mamá era de un partido un día y después del otro. A todos les desconfiaba'. Ibid., 92.

45 Ibid., 31–33.

46 'Eso fue un episodio de mi vida muy fulero, que me marcó la cancha acerca de cómo iba a ser el resto'. Ibid., 35.

47 Sarlo, *Tiempo pasado*, 9.

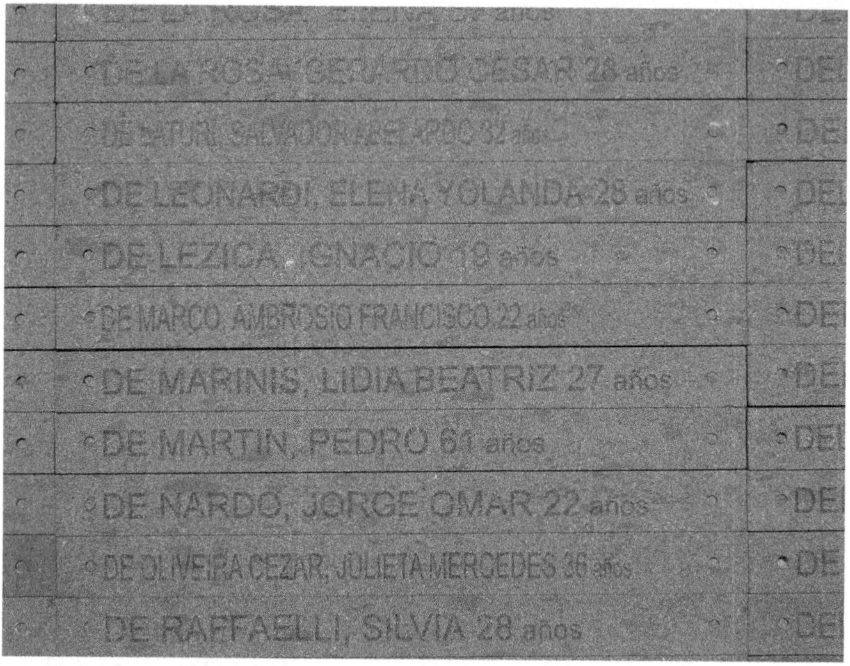

FIGURE 4.3 Wall of memorialization at Parque de la memoria

mother's *visible* body in the politicized space brings the attention back onto the *invisibility* of the disappeared child's body. It also places the name as the center of importance—it signals an existence; by naming the disappeared they *exist* since the name is the symbol of belonging to a society or community, of citizenship and of the rights to which one is entitled as a citizen. María Isabel fought against the erasure of Lila's name so that Lila's person would not be forgotten; in recovering the name of the disappeared daughter she recovers her identity and, ultimately, her place in history.

María Isabel is an exemplary case of 'la madre emblemática' (emblematic mother) within various human rights organizations such as the Mothers of the Plaza de Mayo and Relatives of Disappeared and Imprisoned for Political Reasons (Familiares de Desaparecidos y Detenidos por Razones Políticas). Moving her role as mother from the private sphere of the home to the public sphere of political mobilization provided many women like María Isabel with the opportunity

> [to come] together to mourn, to bear witness to loss and atrocity, and to demand redress, accomplish[ing] still another important goal. It

> allowed us [mothers] to keep connection with the child we [had] lost.[48]

It created 'communities of resistance, based on the primary demand of mothering' in which the mothers 'could be seen as the mothers of a new form of nationhood, based on principles of justice, community, and the preservation of life'.[49] This role as 'emblematic mother' was assigned to María Isabel, as she admits: 'Because I am old, I must be the oldest one and because ever since they took my daughter I haven't stopped looking for her, never slowing down'.[50] It is important to point out that even though María Isabel had a common goal with the organization of the Mothers of Plaza de Mayo she chose to not wear the white head scarf associated with the movement—preferring the focus to be on the image of her disappeared daughter.[51] Furthermore, the key to María Isabel's 'emblematic mother' role was the fact that her own personal fight for justice for her disappeared daughter Lila rose, of its own volition, to a level of militancy for the larger collective seeking a universal social justice in which she chose individuality over the option of being part of Mother of Plaza de Mayo movement. That is, to avoid getting lost in the 'political machine' she focuses on the personal stories and memories of the disappeared, educating others on the real history so that the fight can be taken up by others; in this way, it becomes a transgenerational commitment to social justice and the upholding of human rights. This is best summarized by Lila's son Lisandro:

> …we cannot allow the criminal events of the dictatorship to be repeated. We must practice an active and collective memory and for that one must be militant and work. … The new generations need to know what happened. For that … each social group needs to commit themselves to memory.[52]

---

48 Regina Edmonds, 'Transforming Loss into Action: Mothers from the Plaza de Mayo to Juarez, Mexico', *Journal of the Motherhood Initiative for Research and Community Involvement.* Special Issue: *Mothering, Violence, Militarism, War and Social Justice* 1.1 (2010): 59.

49 Ibid., 60.

50 'Porque tengo mucha edad, debo ser la más vieja y porque desde que se llevaron mi hija, he caminado sin flojar'. Ibid., 174.

51 In *Una sola muerte numerosa* Nora Strejilevich opines that the Mother of Plaza de Mayo 'becomes famous on the backs of the subverssives – reflective of a society that is also to blame' (16–17).

52 '…no dejar que se repitan acontecimientos criminals como los que ocurrieron durante la dictadura. Debemos practicar siempre una memoria active, colectiva y para eso hay que

It should also be noted that María Isabel formed part of the organization "Familiares de desaparecidos y detenidos por razones políticas" [Relatives of Disappeared and Political Prisoners] which gave guidance and support to all mothers and relatives of the disappeared prior to the creation of the Mothers of Plaza de Mayo. Even though many left the group "Relatives of the Disappeared" regarding its affiliation with the Communist party and fear of being accused of being communist, María Isabel decided to remain with the group that helped her from the beginning. María Isabel never accepted a position in any organization and she remained with the "Relatives of the Disappeared" until the day she died.

Most importantly, María Isabel's militancy and perseverance come specifically out of her role as mother looking for her disappeared daughter and giving voice to her child so that she (and her sacrifice) would not be forgotten. Her militancy is two-fold: social justice for the collective and personal justice for Lila. It is what Nora Strejilevich has termed as 'Uno sola muerte numerosa' ('a single numerous death') referring to the individual being able to represent and speak for the collective—where one stands for many who cannot speak because they are not present or unable.[53] For that reason, to write is equated to surviving since it is in writing and telling that one is able to acknowledge the many that died, were imprisoned, missing and tortured and where the individual can speak for the collective and the collective for the individual.[54] It can be seen as a 'mothering' role, but one that is done not only for the individual, but for the larger community in the attempt to heal the community through the individual. María Isabel, therefore, took on the mothering role for her larger 'human family' out of 'a profound sense of social responsibility toward born or yet unborn children, whether biologically their own or those of the community at large'.[55] It is a militant mothering that seeks to recover not only the physical bodies of the disappeared but also the social bonds destroyed by the political violence of the time. Diana remarks on the irony of the situation for many militant mothers: 'We either lost as militants or we lost as mothers'.[56] Some

military y trabajar. ... Las nuevas generaciones tienen que saber lo que pasó. Para eso ... cada grupo social tiene que comprometerse con la memoria'. De Marinis and Spahr, *La Madre de Mendoza* 183.

53 Strejilevich, *Una sola muerte numerosa*, 13.

54 Ibid., 150.

55 Gisela Norat, 'Up in Arms! A Brief Women's History of Militancy in Latin America', *Journal of the Motherhood Initiative for Research and Community Involvement*. Special Issue: *Mothering, Violence, Militarism, War and Social Justice* 1.1 (2010): 44.

56 'O perdíamos como militantes o perdíamos como madres'. Diana, *Mujeres guerrilleras*, 19.

believed that in this new socio-political mechanism there is an inherent risk of the disappeared becoming a path to political power rather than the focus—ultimately resulting in a re-victimization because of their loss of identity and name once more.[57] As a mother, María Isabel chose to bring her private pain as a mother in to the socialized public arena in order to raise awareness around the disappeared and she did so with what was perceived as an 'ideological neutrality', since she, like many other mothers, were not seen as political actors by the security forces because they were 'just mothers' seeking their children.[58]

Yet, there subsists a 'cult/ure of the absent mother'—a term that a patriarchal and middle class perspective supersedes and equates as the 'bad mother': 'The official culture can ultimately label her as a bad mother'.[59] María Isabel faced a difficult choice as described to her by her husband: 'look, you're not going to be a good teacher nor a good mother nor a good daughter, so you're better off to quit teaching'.[60] Furthermore, when María Isabel goes looking for Lila at various police stations and other clandestine centres she finds herself emphasizing that the disappeared women were not 'bad mothers.' A member of the military makes the following comment:

> This lady has come looking for her daughter, like we are here to know where these daughters go when they leave their houses. 'She definitely went out dancing'. Me, with Lila's baby in my arms, could not keep my mouth shut: 'You are making fun of me and my daughter may have been killed; they could have killed her and you don't find anything better than to make fun of a mother's anguish.[61]

In an article with Tracy Crowe Morey we explore the very similar ethos: that the militant mothers that were absent from their biological child's life were actually 'mothering', in a communal sense, a new generation of children.[62]

---

57 Spahr, personal interview.

58 Robben, *Political Violence and Trauma in Argentina*, 306.

59 'La cultural oficial puede llegar a decir que era una mala madre'. Ibid., 187.

60 'mirá, no vas a ser ni buena maestra ni buena madre ni buena hija, mejor renunciá'. De Marinis and Spahr, *Madre de Mendoza*, 46.

61 'Esta señora viene a buscar a su hija, como si nosotros estuviéramos acá para saber adónde se van las hijas que se ausentan de sus casas. Seguro que se habrá ido a bailar'. Yo con el nene de la Lila en brazos no me pude quedar callada: 'Usted se está burlando de mí y a mi hija la pueden haber matado; la pueden haber matado y usted no encuentra nada mejor que burlarse de la angustia de una madre'. Ibid., 102.

62 Tracy Crowe Morey and Cristina Santos, '*Las madres guerreras* [The Warrior Mothers]: Testimonial Writing on Political Motherhood in Latin America', in *Motherhood*

In *Madre de Mendoza,* María Isabel is the inversion of this paradigm: she is the mother whose child has disappeared and, as a result, takes on a different militancy—that of the emblematic mother figure. For those mothers who lost a child during this dictatorship their trauma symbolized 'a new birth, but inverted: the children in their martyrdom, allowed for the birth of their mothers to another life on this earth'.[63] That is, María Isabel took on the broader task of mothering, as educating the masses, and extended her mothering to the wider community in the form of solidarity marking her sacrifices not only for her biological child but for all future generations—including Lila's son, her grandson. In the end, as stated by María Isabel's other daughter, Dora: 'How are you going to repair the lives of the children of the disappeared? They have the entire weight of history on their shoulders'.[64] Yet it is through 'cultural potential of these stories of memory' that Sarlo believes that one is able to include the disappeared in the process of reconstruction—of restoring the disappeared to their political sphere for the generations that follow.

The most telling section in *Madre de Mendoza* in constructing María Isabel as the social activist emblematic mother figure is entitled 'The gaze of the others' ['La mirada de los otros']. This chapter consists of a collection of testimonies gathered to comment on María Isabel's remark: 'I don't know why everyone makes such a fuss, I'm nobody'.[65] Throughout her struggle to find Lila the focus of her efforts always remained on locating Lila and wanting to combat the culture of forgetting and further silencing of the disappeared. In so doing a process of memorialization emerged that focused on the healing process and re-incorporation of the disappeared as part of the collective conscience and national memory. Fulata L. Moyo speaks to such healing and hope:

> ...whatever manifestation hope bears, it has to lead to healing and wholeness. It cannot be negatively about revenge and therefore a threat to life and wholeness. ... One clear connecting thread is how loss has to either coexist with, or be preceded by, genuine—and not cheap—hope for life to be livable in a meaningful way in the face of pain and violence.[66]

---

and War: International Perspectives, edited by Dana Cooper and Claire Phelan (New York: Palgrave MacMillan, 2014), 61–83.

63 De Marinis and Spahr, *Madre de Mendoza,* 10–11.

64 '¿Cómo vas a reparar la vida de los hijos de los desaparecidos? Tienen todo el peso de la historia encima'. Ibid., 206.

65 '[Y]o no sé por qué me premian tanto si yo no soy nadie'. Ibid., 215.

66 Fulata L. Moyo, 'Afterword: What Shape Does Hope Take When Loss is Embodied in Death?', in *Loss and Hope: Global, Interreligious and Interdisciplinary Program,* edited by Peter Admirand (New York: Bloomsbury, 2014), 196.

María Isabel did not set out to become a political figure although many of her activities were intrinsically linked to the political mechanisms of the Truth and Reconciliation process. She was first, and foremost, Lila's mother who, in giving voice to her daughter's disappearance became an emblematic mother figure and a symbol of hope, resistance and revindication fuelled by 'the spiritual force that mothers have'.[67] Alicia Partnoy, a political prisoner survivor herself, adds that 'building a discourse of solidarity with the victims is what ultimately will empower those who chose to tell and will encourage others to share their experiences'.[68] This fighting spirit proved doubly useful in the face of the dictatorship but also in the face of isolation, abandonment and vigilance felt by many of the families of disappeared. This is, intrinsically, a part of the broader process of the ethics of testimony–to tell the story so that the fight can be taken up by others based on a real history of the events.

De Marinis and Spahr pull together in *Madre de Mendoza* a collection of personal first and third person testimonies that adeptly construct how María Isabel Figueroa worked through not only her personal sense of loss and mourning but also a collective trauma that sought to vindicate the injustices suffered by many during the Argentine dictatorship of 1976–1983. Both María Isabel and the other testimonialists that participate in telling her story repeatedly insist that this was *her* particular response to *her* situation and not a universal response or type of mothering for *all* women in a similar situation. *Madre de Mendoza* encompasses the principle that the political is personal and the personal is political as insinuated in the title of this chapter. María Isabel like other activist mothers seeking their disappeared loved ones moved her 'social trauma through symbolic and spiritual expansion into the political arena'.[69] Not only was it a response to the military invading their private domain but an active coping mechanism of the official denials of the disappeared loved ones. As a result, the experience of personal sorrow becomes a small group protest of mothers which ultimately mobilize into larger oppositional crowds. Her emblematic mother role was not undertaken intentionally but rather developed from her commitment to fighting social injustice and defending human rights without any sense of self-aggrandisement or financial gain.[70] María

67 'Pienso que tiene una fuerza espiritual impresionante como todas las madres que sufrieron algo parecido'. Ibid., 216.

68 Alicia Partnoy, 'A Collective Testimony by Argentine Genocide Survivors: "The Prison Walls Cry and We Laugh"', in *Loss and Hope: Global, Interreligious and Interdisciplinary Program*, edited by Peter Admirand (New York: Bloomsbury, 2014), 11.

69 Robben, *Political Violence and Trauma in Argentina*, 317.

70 Ibid., 215–216.

Isabel spoke up for a daughter who had been silenced in the hopes of educating, inspiring and motivating others so that her own personal dark period of family history would not be blurred nor erased from the 'official' record books of Argentine history.

Bibliography

Calveiro, Pilar de. *Poder y desaparición: Los campos de concentración en Argentina.* Buenos Aires: Ediciones Colihue, 2001.

Caruth, Cathy. *Unclaimed Experience: Trauma, Narrative and History.* Baltimore: John Hopkins University Press, 1996.

Crowe Morey, Tracy and Cristina Santos. '*Las madres guerreras* [The Warrior Mothers]: Testimonial Writing on Political Motherhood in Latin America'. *Motherhood and War: International Perspectives*, edited by Dana Cooper and Claire Phelan, 61–83. New York: Palgrave MacMillan, 2014.

De Marinis, Hugo and Adriana Spahr. *Madre de Mendoza: Vida de María Isabel Figueroa.* Buenos Aires: Corregidor, 2013.

Diana, Marta. *Mujeres guerrilleras: sus testimonios en la militancia de los setenta.* 3rd ed. Buenos Aires: Booket, 2011.

Edmonds, Regina. 'Transforming Loss into Action: Mothers from the Plaza de Mayo to Juarez, Mexico'. *Journal of the Motherhood Initiative for Research and Community Involvement.* Special Issue: *Mothering, Violence, Militarism, War and Social Justice* 1.1 (2010): 52–63.

Henke, Suzette. *Shattered Subjects: Trauma and Testimony in Women's Life Writing.* New York: St. Martin's Press, 2000.

Maier, Elizabeth. 'Accommodating the Private into the Public Domain. Experiences and Legacies of the Past Four Decades'. *Women's Activism in Latin America and the Caribbean: Engendering Social Justice, Democratizing Citizenship*, edited by Elizabeth Maier and Nathalie Lebon, 26–43. New Brunswick, NJ: Rutgers University Press, 2010.

Matthews, Irene. 'Daughtering in War: Two 'Case Studies' from Mexico and Guatemala'. *Gendering War Talk*, edited by Miriam Cooke and Angela Woollacott, 148–176. Princeton, N.J.: Princeton University Press, 1993.

Moyo, Fulata L. 'Afterword: What Shape Does Hope Take When Loss Is Embodied in Death?' *Loss and Hope: Global, Interreligious and Interdisciplinary Program*, edited by Peter Admirand, 191–196. New York: Bloomsbury, 2014.

Norat, Gisela. 'Up in Arms! A Brief Women's History of Militancy in Latin America'. *Journal of the Motherhood Initiative for Research and Community Involvement.* Special Issue: *Mothering, Violence, Militarism, War and Social Justice* 1.1 (2010): 31–50.

Partnoy, Alicia. 'A Collective Testimony by Argentine Genocide Survivors: "The Prison Walls Cry and We Laugh" '. *Loss and Hope: Global, Interreligious and Interdisciplinary Program*, edited by Peter Admirand, 9–17. New York: Bloomsbury, 2014.

Ricoeur, Paul. *Time and Narrative*. Vol. I. Trans. Kathleen McLaughlin and David Pellauer. Chicago: Chicago UP, 1984. Print.

Robben, Antonius C. G. M. 'How Traumatized Societies Remember: The Aftermath of Argentina's Dirty War'. *Cultural Critique* 59 (2005): 120–164.

Robben, Antonius C. G. M. *Political Violence and Trauma in Argentina*. Philadelphia: University of Pennsylvania Press, 2005.

Samuelson, Meg. 'The Disfigured Body of the Female Guerrilla: (De)Militarization, Sexual Violence, and Redomestication in Zoë Wicomb's *David's Story*'. *War and Terror. Feminist Perspectives*, edited by Karen Alexander and Mary Hawkesworth, 89–112. Chicago: University of Chicago Press, 2008.

Sarlo, Beatriz. *Tiempo pasado: Cultura de la memoria y giro subjetivo. Una discusión*. Buenos Aires: Siglo veintiuno, 2006.

Scarry, Elaine. *The Body in Pain: The Making and Unmaking of the World*. New York: Oxford University Press, 1985.

Sillato, María del Carmen. *Huellas: Memorias de Resistencia (Argentina 1974–1983)*. San Luis: Nueva Editorial Universitaria, 2008.

Strejilevich, Nora. 'Testimony: Beyond the Language of Truth'. *Human Rights Quarterly* 28.3 (2006): 701–13.

Strejilevich, Nora. *Una sola muerte numerosa*. Córdoba, Argentina: Alción Editora, 2006.

CHAPTER 5

Growing Up in Pain: Children of the Victims of the Argentinean Dictatorship

Adriana Spahr

Abstract

Between 1976 and 1983, state terrorism ruled Argentina. After the coup d'état the regime crushed political, social and student organizations – many of which were associated with the guerrillas. As a result, these people were persecuted, incarcerated and exterminated in brutal ways by the military and other members of the Argentine security forces. Many children, whose parents were persecuted and killed, were made prisoners or went into exile. They suffered a similar fate as their parents. Human rights violations during this period had repercussions worldwide. As a result, a great deal of literature was produced at home and internationally. However, little attention has been given to the children who were born in jail, in exile, or went as children into exile with their parents. Yet, despite of their parents' political involvement they did not become politically active. The aim of this work is to examine how the political persecution of the children's family members affected their growth and their attitudes toward life in Argentina and in Canada as a place of exile.

Keywords

children – trauma – testimony – Argentina – exile – Canada – dictatorship 1976–1983 – disappeared

Dictatorships were not unusual in the life of Argentina before 1976. However, what distinguished the last coup d'état from others in the past, was the brutality to which people in general and rebellious groups in particular were subjected. As a result, many people had to go into exile. While some opponents of the regime were arrested, ten thousand to thirty thousand were killed by paramilitary groups and security forces led by the Armed Forces of

 | DOI:10.1163/9789004391130_007

the country.[1] Some of the women who were imprisoned, kidnapped or disappeared were pregnant or had young children. In some cases the children born in captivity or who were detained with their parents, were then delivered to their immediate families. In other instances, they were adopted illegally by the armed forces or their friends to be raised as their own.

The focus of this chapter is to present some of my findings based on the interviews I conducted with some of these children during the summer of 2013 and 2014 in Argentina and Canada (the place of exile of their parents and the present residence of those children). The political impact on the interviewees, despite their parents' political involvement as young adults, was not of significant relevance in their lives. It is the purpose of this chapter to shed light on the effect of this traumatic period on the children's lives (as a child, as youth and as adults). I will also discuss their positive perception, despite an important quota of criticism, in some of them, about their parents' political participation during their militant years. It is important to note that none of the interviewees is a restored child. This name is given to the children who were kidnapped and adopted illegally, and later restored to the biological family. Their exclusion from this project is justified by the fact that when it started, a good number of publications focused on them. This study included children born in the years of internal conflict in Argentina, or up to five years after the military dictatorship ended (since the psychological effect of the repression persisted for many more years). They grew up and/or spent most of their lives in Argentina or chose to remain in Canada. In order to better understand the context in which these children grew up, I will briefly contextualize the political situation in which the parents of these children lived.

The military *coup*, understood as the overturning of the popular will as expressed at the ballot box, began as early as 1930, when the Radical party was

---

1 The first number is based on cases of persons who were reported as missing by their relatives or acquaintances before official organizations, such as the National Commission on the Disappearance of Persons (CONADEP). The second number represents the number given to human rights organizations in the country. These numbers take into account that at ESMA, La Perla, and Campo de Mayo (the three more emblematic detention centres) where about 5000 people were detained in each of them. Duhalde expresses that we should add to the number of detainees those of 336 clandestine centres and also include the number from those centres whose existence is still unknown. Eduardo Luis Duhalde, 'Carta de Eduardo Luis Duhalde a Graciela Fernández Meijide', *Perfil*, August 4, 2009, viewed on 8 February 2016, http://www.perfil.com/politica/Carta-de-Eduardo-Luis-Duhalde-a-Fernandez-Meijide-20090804-0037.html. Given that those involved in the genocide continue to maintain silence, the number of victims remains a mystery.

overthrown. The Radical party, a centrist formation founded at the beginning of the last century, won the second national election in 1928. In the intervening 53 years, until the end of the last coup in 1983, there were a total of 19 presidents, of whom 17 were installed as a result of coups.[2]

The political dynamics of Argentina centred on a main contradiction which developed since the beginning of the country as a nation. In the 20th century this contradiction took form in two irreconcilable economic models which were in power after each other after 1930. One was the model of the aristocracy supported by the authoritarianism of the military, and the other was the power of the people represented by the majority of the population as expressed in popular elections.

The dynamics of *coups d'état* since the foundation of the country, with some degree of variation depending on the international political situation in which Argentina was situated, was as follows: the military forces tended to assume the role of *protective patriarchs* of the country and the defenders of *Western and Christian values*, whenever the elite believed that its economic interests were in jeopardy. The aim of these military coups, was in fact, to dismantle any kind of opposition that resisted the development, expansion or maintenance of the privileges of the traditional agricultural exporting oligarchy with the ideological support of the Roman Catholic Church. Since these elements are not enough to guarantee the success of any *coup d'etat*, they gathered support as well from different sectors of the population.[3]

The 1976 coup developed within these parameters. Most of the radicalized youth were influenced by the excitement that existed in the international arena, and by independence and anti-systemic movements. Within these influences were the French May movement of 1968, the anti-war and anarchist hippie movement of the late 1960s in the United States, the end of colonialism in countries such as Algeria, Angola, the Cuban Revolution of 1959, and the Pacem in Terris encyclical of John XXIII in 1963. All of these movements proposed an alternative to the prevailing capitalist model in the hegemonic core countries at that time (USA and Europe).

2 Sixteen were military men. In this period, the following completed their mandate: Agustín Justo (1932–38) of the Partido Demócrata Nacional [National Democratic Party] and General Juan Domingo Perón (1946–1951). He was deposed in 1955.

3 The 1976 coup had the support of sectors of the middle class, traditional union leaders and centre and right political organizations. For more information see Adriana Spahr, 'Unveiling the Truth through Testimony: The Argentinean Dirty War', *Disgust and Desire: Humanity's Paradoxical Relationship with Monsters*, edited by Kristen Wright (Amsterdam: Brill Rodopi, 2018), 21–41.

Within that international commotion many young Argentines became involved in politics, and in social movements along with leftist guerrillas groups in the belief that social changes in favour of the dispossessed were possible. In 1974, with the return of Juan Perón (undisputed leader of the majority of the population) who spent 18 years in exile, optimism for change increased, not only within the Peronist guerrilla groups, but in the entire population. When the death of the leader occurred there was an intensification of the political repression. With the help of the media, groups opposed to the new reactionary forces in power were demonized. Before long, they were completely destroyed, by the use of mechanisms of repression and violence hitherto unknown in the country.

The armed forces, as in previous dictatorships, suspended constitutional guarantees which put all power in their hands. Not satisfied, as their predecessors were with the *legality* granted within institutional frameworks, they chose unlawfulness for their actions. Security forces, without identification, entered the homes of suspected guerrillas; they also broke into their places of work and other public dwellings. The military perpetrators took prisoners and beat them on the way to clandestine detention centres. In these centres, scattered throughout the country, detainees were subjected to terrible physical and psychological torture (electric prods, mutilation, waterboarding, impaling, hitting, attacks with dogs, rape, and torture of children) for an unlimited time. Some there were killed and their remains burnt, others were thrown alive into rivers and into the Atlantic Ocean. It is estimated that less than 10% of them came out alive from these places. The remaining 90%, whose final destination is not known, were given the name of *disappeared*. Other people were imprisoned and between 20,000 and 40,000 went into exile due to persecution. Many of them did not return to the country after the dictatorship ended (1983).[4]

People who were interviewed for this study are surviving victims of the previously described state of terror. The ages of the participants (7 men and 5 women), range from 32 to 42. Four were born before the dictatorship, five during the dictatorship, and three after it. Three spent time in jail with their mothers, two of whom were born when their mothers where in captivity (one of them was born in a clandestine detention centre). Three of the participants went into exile as children and came back to Argentina immediately after 1983,

---

4 Marcos Novaro and Vicente Palermo, *La dictadura militar 1976/1983. Del golpe de Estado a la restauración democrática* (Buenos Aires: Paidós), 76, cited by María Soledad Catoggio, 'Case Study: La última dictadura militar argentina (1976–1983): la ingeniería del terrorismo de Estado', *Mass Violence.org*, September 30, 2014, 6,7,11, viewed on 4 June 2015, http://www.mass-violence.org/la-ultima-dictadura-militar-argentina-1976-1983-la.

at the end of the dictatorship. Three did not return to Argentina (one was born during the exile of his parents).

None of the interviewees fully participate in politics, unlike many Argentineans of the same age and situation living in Argentina, whose political participation is noticeable.

A high level of education distinguishes the participants. Eighty-three per cent have completed post-secondary education,[5] which corresponds to their parents' level of education as well as to the education of the majority of the members of the targeted opposition political groups in Argentina of the 70s.[6]

The first memories of these children born before and during the dictatorship are related to sensory impressions, always enclosed by a climate of fear, confusion and uncertainty due to political issues. This situation occurred as a consequence of visiting their parents in prison, having as a parent a missing or disappeared person, and because of displacements and/or a continued change of residence.

5 The parents of the generation of the 1970s were, in general, hard-working people who passed on to their children the importance of post-secondary education as the only way of succeeding in life.

6 The social structure of the guerrilla fighters was mostly small factions of the wealthy petite bourgeoisie and urban workers with higher levels of education. The average age of the guerrilla movement at the time of their disappearance was under 30 years of age, and 33% of them were women. But it is difficult to determine the number of people who made up the social and guerrilla movements in the country. One of its most significant characteristics was its clandestine mode of operating. The majority of the studies done on this topic are based on the number of disappeared people denounced by relatives or acquaintances. The following study shows two numbers for each category. The first number corresponds to the period of the 1970s in which the repression was more indiscriminate. The second figure corresponds to the last period of the dictatorship when the repression was focused on the guerrilla organizations as well as on the dictatorship's allies: for example, the murders of dictatorship diplomats (Elena Angélica Holmberg Lanusse, ex-dictator's niece and the ambassador Héctor Hidalgo Solá). The following is from the study done by Inés Izaguirre: Fractions of the wealthy bourgeoisie: 4.7% and 9.6%; middle and petite bourgeoisie (professionals, university students) 8.8% and 4.1%; self-employed 13.2% and 21.8%; qualified urban employees with some conditions as the petite bourgeoisie 21%-22%; qualified urban and rural workers 50.8% and 45.9%. Ines Izaguirre, 'Los desaparecidos. Recuperación de una identidad expropiada', *Programa de Investigaciones sobre Conflicto Social. Instituto de Investigaciones Gino Germani, Facultad de Ciencias Sociales*, UBA, viewed on 6 May 2015, http://webiigg.sociales.uba.ar/conflictosocial/libros/izaguirre/losdesaparecidos/index.htm and Débora D'Antonio, 'Represión y resistencia en las cárceles de la última dictadura militar argentina', *La revista del CCC*. 2, Jan/April 2008, 3, viewed on 8 June 2014, http://www.centrocultural.coop/revista/articulo/29/represion_y_resistencia_en_las_carceles_de_la_ultima_dictadura_militar_argentina.html.

The following is a memory of Eduardo Veiga, who lives in Canada. Eduardo, as a baby shared prison with his mother. His memory seems to suggest that he was in a game, but obviously it was not that playful:

> I have a vague memory of running through a corridor surrounded by bars. I slipped between the bars and crossed into the other side and felt the cold. But I have no memory of my parents … Years later, when both of my parents were released from prison, we left [Argentina]. Canada was terrible [because of] the separation from my grandparents with whom I lived. … Only, after a long time is that I began to feel that my parents were my new family.[7]

Lucía Bertone was 10 months old when her parents were detained. She never lived outside the country. She recalls her visit to her parents in prison:

> [The prison] Caseros was the worst prison. It smelled of disinfectant. … I remember one Christmas the guards would not let us in because I could not take off an earring: in the end they cut it. It seemed that my father was going to kill someone with it … Devoto was terrible, I remember the screeching of the bars and giant latches, the sound of shoes echoing in the gigantic empty halls. There was a metal pipe to talk to my mom. The tube smelled of something between arse and metal. … My grandmother would put a handkerchief over the pipe to [in order not to smell] [the foul] vapours accumulated during years … The frisking was horrible because they would run their hands up and down everywhere; they would touch you all over, pull down your panties. It was worse for the older ladies to go through all this … I remember the bar, before entering. The bar was nice and fun. We were all there with all the mothers and the kids' grandmothers. The one I liked the most was La Plata. I remember all the games I played with my dad, raising me in the air, swinging me up (very much like a dance). Creating a performance with it has always kept crossing my mind … something exciting … It was two hours in a yard with the

7 All testimonies recorded in Spanish were translated into English by the author unless otherwise indicated. 'Tengo vaga memoria de haber estado corriendo en un pasillo rodeado de rejas. Me voy por un lado, me deslizo por las barras y me voy del otro lado de la reja y siento algo frío. Pero no tengo recuerdos de mis padres. Años después, cuando mis padres salieron de la cárcel, salimos del país. Canadá fue terrible [debido a] la separación de mis abuelos con quienes viví … Con el tiempo, después de mucho empecé a tener el sentido de que mis padres eran mi familia nueva'. Eduardo Veiga, Interview with the author, 16 December 2014.

> kids jumping up and down with the parents, all of us totally out of control. It was two hours when we seemed to say, *I got to touch him as much as I can.*[8]

Pablo Martínez recounts:

> We moved from my mother's grandparents' home that had been destroyed by the Argentinean Anti-Communist Alliance (right-wing paramilitary group), then my grandparents ... had to leave their neighbourhood and move to a different province. I was a year old when a navy officer spotted my mom, and then, again we had to move Talking openly about myself or my family was out of the question. We lived in an internal exile.[9]

Alejandra Fernández was born in a clandestine detention centre. Her parents immigrated to Canada after their release from jail:

> I remember one particular incident; this one always stuck in my head. I remember a huge courtyard and my grandmother and I were walking through and all of a sudden there was a gunfight and my grandmother and I had to hide behind a pillar. I just remember her hiding me and

8 '[La cárcel de] Caseros fue la peor cárcel a la que fui. Tenía olor a desinfectante ... Había un tubo de metal para hablar con mi mamá. El tubo tenía olor a culo y metal mezclado. ... Mi abuela le ponía un pañuelo para [no oler el] vapor [nauseabundo] de años acumulados. ... La requisa era horrible porque te ponían las manos por todos lados, te tocaban todo, te hacían bajar al bombacha. Para las señoras era peor pasar todo esto ... Me acuerdo del bar, antes de entrar. El bar era bueno y divertido. Estábamos ahí con todas las madres y las abuelas de los pibes. La que más me gustaba era La Plata. Todos los juegos que hacíamos con mi papá, me levantaba, me revoleaba, (muy así como la danza). Siempre que quedó dando vuelta en la cabeza como hacer algo performativo con eso ... algo animado ... Eran dos horas en un patio, los chicos saltando arriba de los padres, todo un descontrol. Eran dos horas donde parecíamos decir 'tengo que tocarlo todo lo que pueda'. Lucía Bertone, Interview with the author, 13 June 2013.

9 'Nos mudamos de la casa materna que fue destrozada por la Alianza Anticomunista Argentina (un grupo paramilitar de ultraderecha) y mis abuelos ... tuvieron que [mudarse] de barrio y de provincia. Nos mudamos. Tenía un año cuando un miembro de la fuerzas de seguridad reconoce a mi mamá y nos tenemos que mudar nuevamente. Lo que se hablaba dentro de mi casa, quedaba dentro de la casa, no hablaba ni de mi familia ni de mí fuera de ella. Vivíamos en exilio dentro del país.' Interview with the author, 15 July, 2014.

> I guess that would be a memory that you would remember only of all memories. I remember visiting my mother and, one time she made me this beautiful house out of cardboard and I just loved it. I just remember her giving it to me and I took it. It was hard for me to leave it in my uncle's place … . There were more visits but I do not remember details. When I was almost four we went to Canada. It was hard for me. I missed my family in Argentina. As I grew older I understood my parents' position of leaving Argentina. I loved living in Canada. Parts of me would still like to live in Argentina, just to get more of a grounding of where I came from. Also to know my family a bit better. It is strange how life works. The language barriers I felt when arrived to Canada, exist today but on the other direction.[10]

In the case of Paula Isla, her parents were detained when her mother was pregnant. She was born in jail. She was 4 years old when her mother was released from jail under the condition of leaving the country. Finally the entire family reunited in Italy, when her father was released after eight years in prison. After 1983 the family returned to Argentina. Her own memory was the day in which her mother left the country:

> I was not very aware of what was happening. Back then, I had the feeling I had good times. One bad memory I have is when my mom was given the option to leave the country. After she left jail she was welcomed as a political exile in Italy. On the way to the airport she was taken in handcuffs. In my mind I thought, *There she is, finally she is free, finally she left jail.* Then, I remember that we got to the Ezeiza airport [in Buenos Aires] where we waited for her. She was taken there by a soldier. As we acknowledged her, I thought to myself, 'my mom is out again'. They took her away. And I repeated 'they took her away again'. I imagine they tried to explain to me the next steps but I couldn't understand (I was too young). I noticed a disconnection between the message and the image. As I got back to my home I placed a sofa chair close by the door. There I sat for long times in anguish, crying and very sad. I had the illusion my mom was going to return.[11]

---

10 This interview was conducted in English.

11 'No tenía mucha conciencia de todo lo que pasaba. Yo tengo la sensación de pasarlo bien. Un recuerdo que la pasé muy mal es cuando mi vieja le dan la opción para salir del país.

The situations told by the interviewees occurred more than thirty years ago. However, they remain clear in their memories. Through their memories a situation of terror and instability lived by society is perceived. But the eyes of these children offer a distressing and perplexing vision—disconcerting is the situation being experienced by Paula when she saw her mother out of prison yet again disappearing. They took her mother to board a plane and then she was abandoned once again. The hide and seek game, which should have been supplemented with complicit chuckles between Alexandra and her grandmother transformed into a state of terror, where a young Alejandra could not have known what was happening around her. Yet, she most certainly sensed the terror her grandmother felt and subsequent desire to protect her from any stray bullet.

A never fulfilled state of confusion or happiness took hold of Alejandra and Eduardo when their parents left prison. They suffered another tear in their lives when they left their grandparents who had given them protection and stability in their first years of life.

This is also perceived in Pablo's case who, although never separated from his parents, lived continuously changing locations after a bomb destroyed the house of his maternal grandparents. In the meantime he learned to be wary of strangers as one of them could have snatched his mother. Meanwhile Lucía was steeped in prison odors, loud noises, unknown adults groping her which her grandmother could not stop. Their world as children challenges the limits of what is socially *normal*. Yet, behind this crazy world, and in constant change, there were also moments of fleeting joy in the personal contact with their parents. Behind all this, there was a children's world where monsters hiding under the bed coexisted with a world of insecurity and terror. It is not surprising that all participants in this study, suffered anxiety and anguish derived from the instability produced by the repression not through their parents' experiences and conditions but from their own experience. This situation is worsened by the separation from the loved ones who formed their first childhood world. Only in the case of Paula was this separation avoided because the children

---

Italia la recibe como exiliada política y sale de la cárcel. Y la sacan de ahí esposada. En mi cabeza la soltaban *ya está, la soltaron, mi mamá salió*. Llegamos a Ezeiza y ahí la esperábamos. La trae un militar, la saludamos y en mi cabeza *volvió a salir mamá*. Pero ahí se la llevaron. Y yo dije *se la llevaron*. Con tres autos, cuando la sacaron del auto fue para subirla al avión. Imagino que me explicaron que la iba a ver luego, pero no entendí. Hubo una desconexión entre el mensaje y la imagen. Llegué a la casa de mi abuela y me puse el sillón en la puerta. Ahí estuve mucho tiempo angustiada, llorando muy triste. Tenía la ilusión de que llegaba mi vieja'. Paula Isla, interview with the author, 15 June 2013.

went into exile accompanied by their grandparents who had raised them until and after their parents were freed.

Children who had a parent or parents who were *disappeared* deserve special attention because of the cruel definition of the disappeared or missing people. Jorge Videla, who took power in 1976, defined the disappeared as follows:

> [The disappeared are an unknown entity]. If they reappeared they would receive treatment x, and if their disappearance becomes definitive in the certainty of their death, they would receive treatment z. But while they are disappeared, they can't have any special treatment, they are an unknown entity, neither dead nor alive, they are disappeared.[12]

A new *legal* category was thus created, the disappeared. In her contribution in this volume Cristina Santos examines the inhuman effects of the category of the "disappeared" in the life of Mrs. Figueroa and her family. Santos investigates how Mrs. Figueroa exemplifies the dedication of thousands of families in the country who dedicated her lives relentlessly, to no avail, to the search of their disappeared loved ones. Mrs. Figueroa search for her disappeared daughter continued for decades after the end of the dictatorship. How would you explain this frightening situation to a child, like Martina, when it is so difficult for even an adult to understand?

Martina Martínez was born ten days after her father was kidnapped by the security forces. Even today, his whereabouts are unknown:

> I was always a very introverted, very quiet and weird girl. I felt that way. My mom always told me about my father. We had his picture on the bedside table. We sang for his birthday, and for Father's Day. My mother wrote a diary of everything I did for him for when he would return …
>
> I think at first my dad had gone on a trip, or to work. That he had had an accident after work and therefore we did not know where he was.

12 '[Es una incógnita el desaparecido]. Si reapareciera tendría un tratamiento X, y si la desaparición se convirtiera en certeza de su fallecimiento tendría un tratamiento Z. Pero mientras sea desaparecido no puede tener ningún tratamiento especial, es una incógnita, es un desaparecido, no tiene entidad, no está ni muerto ni vivo, está desaparecido'. *Clarín*, 14 December 1979, cited by Archivo Histórico, 'Declaraciones del presidente de facto general Jorge Rafael Videla sobre los detenidos desaparecidos en 1979', *Testimonio y Documentos*, Buenos Aires, Oficina de Publicaciones del CBC – UBA, 1996, viewed on 1 June 2015, http://archivohistorico.educ.ar/content/j-r-videla-sobre-detenidos-desaparecidos-en-1979?frame=1&lista=indice#sthash.jKnlob3R.dpuf.

> I did not quite understand. I asked myself, *If we did not have the body it was because in the accident he did not have his identification papers* ... In the school where one would normally ask for a record of the father and mother, they did not have a record of his name. Neither was it on my birth certificate ... I saw the situation as an injustice but could not tell others. It was confusing to me; it should have been either *alive or not alive*, period. ... No one talked about him ... I grew up with the unknown, with that uncertainty ... I kept waiting, but always silence, feeling strange in society, and ... I still feel that way. For the first time, while in fourth grade, I said something. Pope (John Paul II) was coming and the school teacher proposed that we should give him a message of peace and a message with our wishes. I said I wanted my dad, who was missing, and that I wanted him to be back. Everyone in the class looked at me weird. All was always the same, everything was weird. Nobody talked about anything. So I went back to saying nothing. ... At 25 I got my surname back (before I used my mother's maiden name). After that, I started to reconstruct my dad ... My mother helped me remember. ... Friends and comrades of my father gave me details about his life ... By reconstructing him, I reconstruct myself.[13]

Martina as a child was given the ambiguity in which the family was living: a father whose whereabouts nobody knew nor whether he ever would be back.

---

13 'Yo siempre fui una chica muy introvertida, muy callada y rara. Me sentía así. Mi mamá siempre me hablaba de mi papá. Teníamos su foto en la mesita de luz. Le cantábamos para el día de su cumpleaños, y para el día del padre. Mi mamá escribió un diario de todo lo que yo hacía para él, cuando volviera. ... Creo que al principio me había que mi papá se había ido de viaje, o a trabajar. Había tenido un accidente a la salida del trabajo y, por eso no sabíamos dónde estaba. Yo no terminaba de entender. Le preguntaba no teníamos el cuerpo porque cuando tiene el accidente no tenido documentos. ... En las planillas de la escuela donde se preguntaba el nombre del padre y de la madre, no estaba su nombre. Tampoco en mi partida de nacimiento ... Yo veía la situación como una injusticia pero no podía decirlo. Era confuso para mí, debería ser *vive o no vive y punto*. ... Nadie hablaba de él ... Crecí con esa incógnita, con esa incertidumbre ... Seguía esperando, pero siempre en silencio, sintiéndome rara en la sociedad, y ... me sigo sintiendo así. En cuarto grado fue la primera vez que yo dije algo. Venía el papa (Juan Pablo II) y la maestra propone en clase que debíamos dar un mensaje de paz, un mensaje de deseos. Yo digo que quería que mi papá, que era un desaparecido, volviera. Todos en la clase me miraron raro Todo era así, todo quedaba en la rareza. Nadie hablaba de nada. Así que no lo volví a hablar. ... A los 25 años recuperé mi apellido. Después de esto, empecé a reconstruir a mi padre ... mi madre empieza a recordar. ... los compañeros me dan datos.. sobre su vida. Al reconstruirlo a él, me reconstruyo yo'. Martina Martínez interview with the author, 11 June 2014.

Martina's mother, in order to protect her daughter, pretended not to know the father's identity. She therefore identified herself as a single mother. The confusion and the anguish of Martina stemmed from a dual situation: on the one hand, according to the mother, she had a father who loved her. On the other hand, her father was not present anywhere or under any circumstances, not even on her birth certificate. In this case, Martina as a child felt that hers was an incomplete identity that she only began to recover in adulthood when she re-acquired her father's family name. In order to do that, mother and daughter reconnected with the father's past. This reconnection with Martina's father's past was facilitated by the political opening that happened in Argentina after 2003, twenty years after the ending of the dictatorship.

One factor that accelerated the end of military impunity was the international outcry led by human rights organizations, which demanded the Armed Forces and the government to account for the fate of the missing people. Due to the strong pressure of these organizations, the democratic government that emerged after the dictatorship created the National Commission on the Disappearance of Persons (CONADEP). The statements given by the victims led to the prosecution and conviction of the military leadership. However, the subsequent arrival of conservative governments not only prevented the deepening and repairing of the damage caused to the population by the excesses, but those convicted were pardoned. Silence and frustration again saddened the victims of state terror. On March 24, 2004, the new president Néstor Kirchner (2003–2007) apologized on behalf of the state for the atrocities committed during the dictatorship. This statement marked the commitment of the new government on human rights. With government support, the discussion about what happened resumed. In other words, the victim can now express his plight and be heard. His word goes to court, to schools, to the media. In this context Martina investigated and reconstructed the figure of her father, the *black Martínez* (nickname) and began to feel her full identity.

Argentinean society mostly recognized the violations of human rights and the atrocities committed by security forces during the military dictatorship. Martina, Laura, Paula and the rest of the participants in Argentina, felt the discriminatory gaze of *the other* (society) toward them start to dissipate, even though their feeling of being *strange/different* never went away. They certainly felt that they were different from the rest. Their childhoods were not similar to those of their classmates or friends. Some differences came from conversations at home around the family table, from political discussions, from the types of music played and heard, from the large number of *uncles*, *aunt*s and *cousins* (who in reality were political activists like their parents), etc.

The parents created a closed world in order to protect their children from the effects of a society in which parents and children represented the different OTHER. This *demonization* justified to society the atrocities committed by the dictatorship.

Juan Bampín, born in 1986, remembers as a child when a friend of his threw a cruel insult at him, *your mother was raped by the military*! Obviously, the friend did not understand what he was saying. He had simply reproduced an insult he had heard, to make his friend feel bad. Here, one can visualize how the victim is blamed: the mother of Juan deserved and even sought to be raped. The *alleged impurity of the mother went further and marked her son too.*

The children's world did not differ tremendously whether they lived in Argentina or abroad. But, the type of aggressiveness pointed out by Juan is not expressed by any of the respondents in Canada, or the feeling of being different and weird. One of the answers given on this is that in the Canadian environment those differences are contained within the multiculturalist perspective. Families keep their languages, different cultural traditions, and the longing for the home country. In this context the differences between home and the outside world are expected. As one of the interviewees, Natalia Veiga,[14] born in Canada, said: '*in Canada everyone comes from somewhere else, we are all different*'. However, neither in Argentina nor in Canada, could the children share their experiences with their friends. As a result, not only did the military dictatorship have a strong impact on the parents but also on the children who could never ignore what had happened to their parents.

Perhaps because of the traumatic situation experienced, none of the participants would take the militant way of their parents. They also believe that a violent course was not an acceptable path to follow, neither in the past nor in the present. Other criticism focuses on the parents' lack of care and protection of the children:

> My parents left the prison, closed their eyes and entered life as they could. They had two other children, after feeling their failure, with my sister and me … In my parents' house, the words trade union, comrade, were said all the time, 12 hours later they would still be talking about the same. They never ask how you were, or how is your daughter. (Lucia)
>
> [My mother] went to work after she was released from prison. She continued her studies. She felt much anguish and sadness because she also lost many comrades. Both were strong sympathizers for the cause … For

14 Natalia Veiga, interview with the Author, 19 December, 2014.

> me, it was also ideal when *mom came back* but she quickly began a very busy life doing a thousand things. They could not assume the family responsibilities. (Paula)[15]

As in Paula's and Lucia's cases, some of the interviewees felt abandoned when their parents prioritized political activism over them, both during the 1970s and after obtaining freedom [a common criticism amongst the children who lost both parents to the disappearances].

Here, two irreconcilable needs overlap.

On the one hand, there are the parents who lived before and during their detention in a world where political commitment was at the centre of life. The children in this context were part of a project in which the welfare of children depended on the triumph of these ideals. And, if parents learn to be parents through contact with their children, then it follows that [under prohibitive circumstances] these parents lacked the parenting ability and therefore were unable to assume parenting properly. Thus, they could not meet the expectations and needs of their children, who in turn, idealized meeting with their parents for the first time, in order to have a normal daily and school life.

On the other hand, these deficiencies are compensated by the children born after the dictatorship. Parents, as in the case of Lucia's parents, assumed the [political] role society expected of them, while the children with parents involved in politics, also expected to be part of that activity.

Laura Burgos, was born after her parents were released from prison. She is one of two interviewees in this account who identifies herself as a *political activist*.[16] She states:

15 'Mis viejos salieron de la cárcel, cerraron los ojos y entraron a la vida como pudieron. Tuvieron otros dos hijos. Al sentirse tan fracasados (con mi hermana y conmigo). En la casa de mis viejos, la palabra compañeros, sindicato, se decía a cada momento, hasta que ibas 12 horas después. Nunca te preguntaban *cómo estás, cómo está tu hija*' (Lucía). '[Mi mamá] salió de la cárcel se puso a trabajar. Siguió estudiando. Con mucha angustia y tristeza porque también perdió a muchos compañeros. Eran supermilitantes los dos. … Para mí también fue ideal cuando *llegó mamá* pero salió y se puso a ser mil cosas. No podían asumir la cuestión familiar' (Paula).

16 In the Argentinean context a political activist is any individual who carries out an ideological project. Laura has always participated in student centres, demonstrations, open and general assemblies, and of social groups. Participation in all activities is voluntary; therefore there is no money received. She has an administrative job and is a mechanical engineering student.

> My parents always actively belonged politically, and took me everywhere with them. I was five years old when they would take me with them to political rallies to the congress building, and everywhere ... I'd get bored ... I saw my parents' old friends who left their children at home and I thought, that's wrong.[17]

In the case of children living abroad, this difference was not evident. The political affiliation of the parents did not interfere with the attention given to the children.

Moreover, it is interesting to note that all participants seemed to feel responsible for the sufferings of the parents and assumed the role of protectors, especially of their mothers. They also considered that their parents and their generation took the right path in their youth by offering their lives to ensure equality and justice for all citizens. In Argentina, especially, where politics is part of the everyday life for everyone, the participants felt so proud of their parents and their parents' generation to the point of seeing them as heroes, not people of flesh and blood who made mistakes, but as heroes.

How do we understand this phenomenon of heroes versus the criticism toward their parents? Two events that occurred in the country allowed us to get closer to an answer: 1) the tireless work of human rights organizations that since the dictatorship have continued to investigate the fate of the disappeared, and that of the babies illegally appropriated by the forces of repression; 2) the official emphasis given to human rights since 2003. This not only condemned those responsible for committing atrocities belonging to the armed forces but also some civilians (judges, entrepreneurs) and institutions such as the hierarchy of the Argentinean Catholic Church, as accomplices of the dictatorship; 3) artefacts which represent visible presences of the state terrorism to the general public disseminated in the whole country such as a) tiles and drawings on the street indicating the place from where a disappeared person was taken by military or paramilitary forces (see image 1), b) clandestine detention centres (there were at least 340 in the country) that are now memory sites that students from elementary, secondary, and university and people visit every day (see image 2), and c) rooms at schools and universities named after a disappeared person; 4) Parque de la memoria (The Memorial Park) where three memorial walls containing 30,000 plates for the 30,000 disappeared. Only 9000

17 'Mis padres siempre militaron y me llevaban a todas partes. A los cinco años me llevaban al congreso, a las marchas, a todos lados. Yo me aburría. ... Vi a compañeros de mis viejos que dejaban a sus hijos y pensaba *está mal*' (Laura).

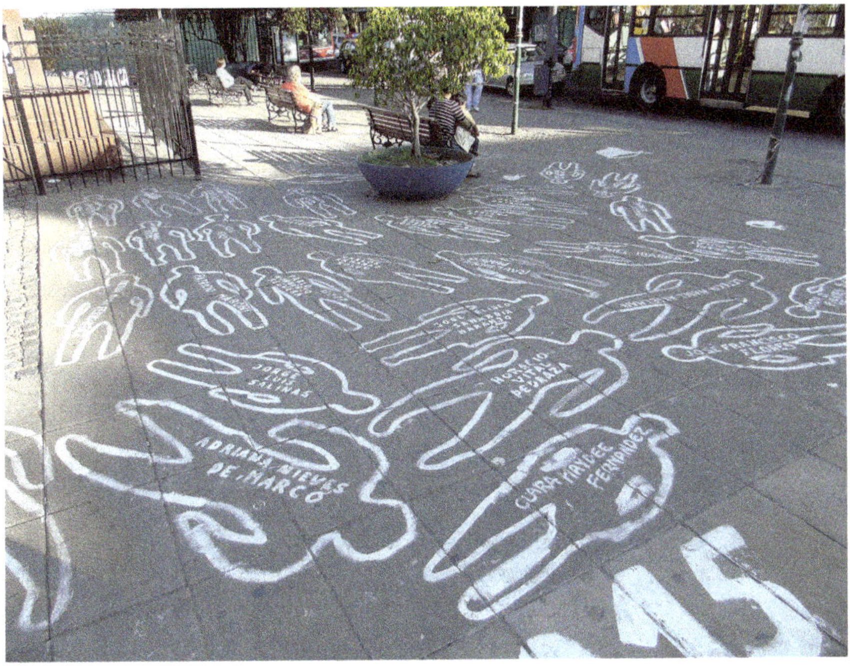

FIGURE 5.1 Artefacts in Buenos Aires
© 2015. PHOTOGRAPHER CRISTINA SANTOS. USED WITH PERMISSION.

are engraved with the names of the missing (dead women, men and children, all victims of the state violence during the dictatorship (see image 3).

All of this generated an almost full understanding of society in regards to the atrocities committed. This large part of the society also assumed the redemption of the guerrilla figure as an opponent of the dictatorship, and as a champion of justice, not as the destroyer of Western and Christian society. This acknowledgement by society gave the children, especially in Argentina, a sense of pride, distinguishing them from the rest of society. Although these children have a positive view towards their parents' struggle, they continued to carry the political activities of their parents as an extra burden with a great psychological impact on them.

In conclusion, as many critics agree, the recognition of a given society of past atrocities is the first step to rebuild the society after a mass atrocity.[18] It is undisputed that the Argentinean society accomplished this recognition. This acknowledgement helped the children whose parents suffered political

18 Carlos Martín Beristain, *Justicia y reconciliación: El papel de la verdad y la justicia en la reconstrucción de sociedades fracturadas por la violencia* (Bilbao: Henoa, 2000), 7–9.

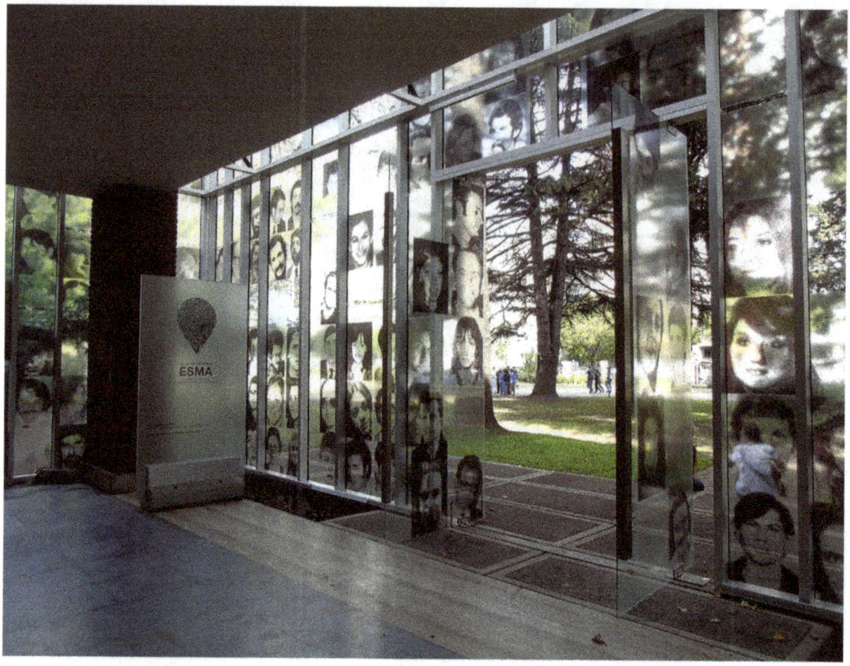

FIGURE 5.2 ESMA
© 2015. PHOTOGRAPHER CRISTINA SANTOS. USED WITH PERMISSION.

persecution to increase their self-esteem since their parents were not the criminals that military had claimed them to be. However, a deeper analysis is required to determine—especially in the case of the children who were born before and during the dictatorship–to what extent this positive gaze towards the militants of the 1970s prevents these children from detaching themselves from the political trajectory of their parents and from recognizing their own traumatic situation. These children have to reconcile the social admiration for their parents with the drama through which they lived; they must reconcile the collective and the personal. Until the children are able to speak more deeply about their anguish and losses, they will not be able to find the path to a full identity. In other words, Argentinean society has to help these children to resolve their internal/external reality: an external reality which results in a kind of fairy tale where the parents are flawless and epic characters and an internal reality in which the surviving children frequently end in tragic situations such as suicide, addiction or psychological trauma. One of the aims of my work and interviews is to understand the complex situation in the present lives of these children/adults as a means of collaborating in healing their traumas. Can we talk about community resilience or individual resilience? This term is defined

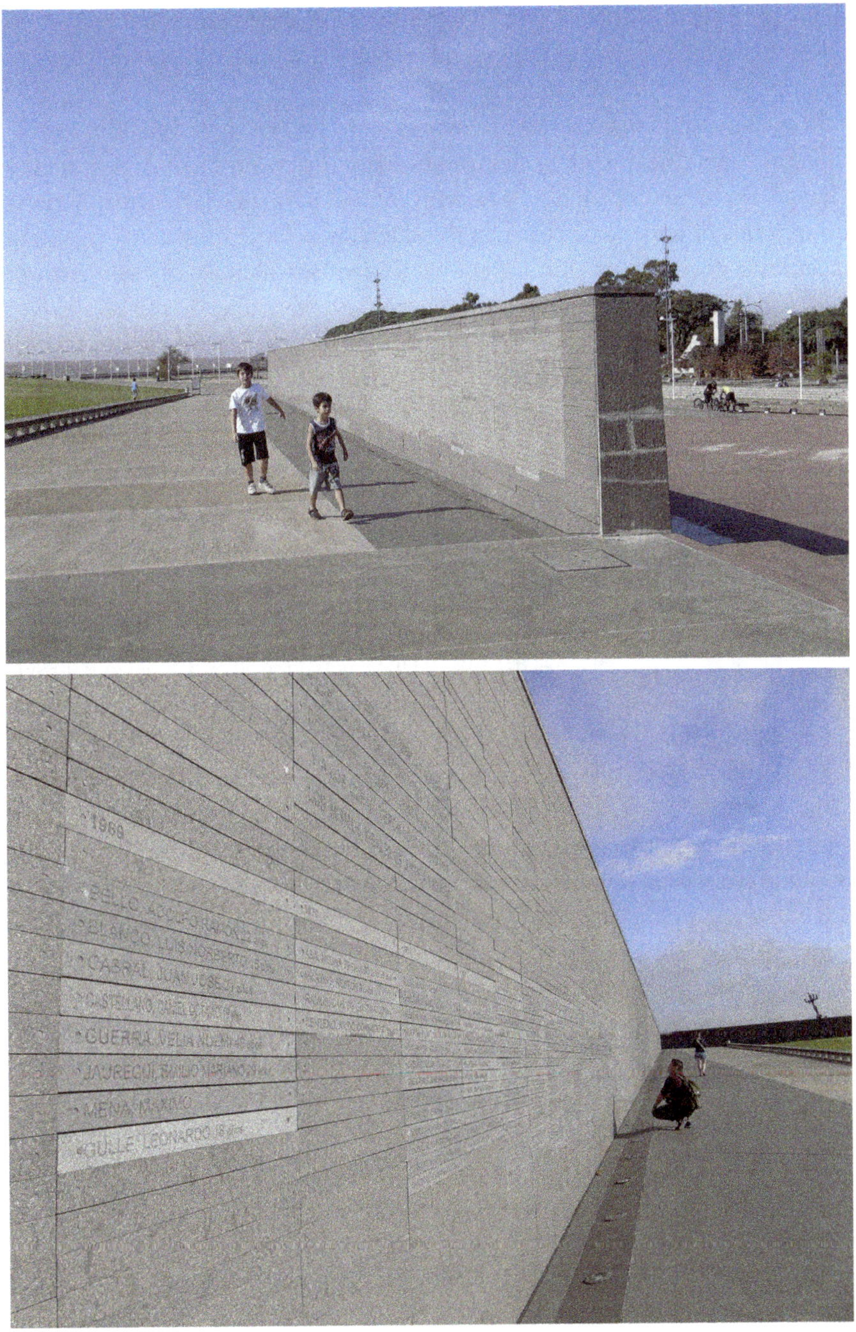

FIGURE 5.3 Parque de la memoria I and II, Buenos Aires.

often as 'a positive trajectory of adaptation after disturbance, distress or an adversity as the capacity of the individual's ability to maintain a stable level of functioning following traumatic events'.[19]

It is impossible to separate the two, as they are closely linked. The assessment of Argentinean society changed because the government supported the change. Up to now, much has been achieved, yet more needs to be done. However, clouds of uncertainty loom in the skies. Since December 2015, Argentina is led by a government with a right-wing agenda, which clearly sympathises with former human rights' abusers, dictators and their allies. In this context we ask ourselves: Will society keep making further progress on human rights? Will the children move forward in their healing process? Or, on the contrary, will they again get society's old accusatory gaze?

Bibliography

Archivo Histórico. 'Declaraciones del presidente de facto general Jorge Rafael Videla sobre los detenidos desaparecidos en 1979'. *Testimonio y Documentos*. Buenos Aires, Oficina de Publicaciones del CBC – UBA, 1996. Viewed on 1 June 2015. http://archivohistorico.educ.ar/content/j-r-videla-sobre-detenidos-desaparecidos-en-1979?frame=1&lista=indice#sthash.jKnlob3R.dpuf Telam.

Beristain, Carlos Martín. *Justicia y reconciliación: El papel de la verdad y la justicia en la reconstrucción de sociedades fracturadas por la violencia*. Bilbao: Henoa, 2000.

Catoggio, María Soledad. 'Case Study: La última dictadura militar argentina (1976-[1983): la ingeniería del terrorismo de Estado'. *Mass Violence.org*, September 30, 2014, 1–20. Viewed on 4 June 2015. http://www.massviolence.org/la-ultima-dictadura-militar-argentina-1976-1983-la.

D'Antonio, Débora. 'Represión y resistencia en las cárceles de la última dictadura militar argentina'. *La revista del CCC* 2.1 (Jan/April 2008). Viewed on 8 June 2015. http://www.centrocultural.coop/revista/articulo/29/represion_y_resistencia_en_las_carceles_de_la_ultima_dictadura_militar_argentina.html.

Duhalde, Eduardo Luis. 'Carta de Eduardo Luis Duhalde a Graciela Fernández Meijide'. *Perfil.* August 4 2009. Viewed 8 February 2016. http://www.perfil.com/politica/Carta-de-Eduardo-Luis-Duhalde-a-Fernandez-Meijide-20090804-0037.html.

Izaguirre, Ines. 'Los desaparecidos. Recuperación de una identidad expropiada'. *Programa de Investigaciones sobre Conflicto Social. Instituto de Investigaciones Gino*

19 Shaul Kimhi, 'Levels of Resilience: Associations among Individual, Community and National Resilience', *Journal of Health Psychology* (*JHP*) 21.2 (2016): 164–165.

Germani, 1–9. Universidad de Buenos Aires: Facultad de Ciencias Sociales. Viewed on 6 May 2015. http://webiigg.sociales.uba.ar/conflictosocial/libros/izaguirre/los-desaparecidos/index.htm.

Kimhi, Shaul. 'Levels of Resilience: Associations among Individual, Community and National Resilience'. *Journal of Health Psychology (JHP)*. 21.2 (2016): 164–170.

Novaro, Marcos and Vicente Palermo. *La dictadura militar 1976/1983. Del golpe de Estado a la restauración democrática*. Buenos Aires: Paidós, 2003.

Spahr, Adriana. 'Unveiling the Truth through Testimony: The Argentinean Dirty War'. *Disgust and Desire: Humanity's Paradoxical Relationship with Monsters*, edited by Kristen Wright, 21–41. Amsterdam: Brill Rodopi, 2018.

CHAPTER 6

Non-Standard Witness: Lessons from Working with/for Traumatized Children

Melissa Burchard

Abstract

Testimony is standardly defined as a relatively straightforward autobiographical narrative or account of personal experience. Working with traumatized children shows how testimony cannot always be straightforward. My claim is that exploring testimony of traumatized children leads us to conclude that both our understanding of what testimony is and our responsibilities to those who give testimony need to be reconsidered. I first argue several points regarding children's speaking capabilities, including that children's testimony is often not autobiographical, because children may not have the vocabulary to narrate their history. When children are traumatized pre-verbally, words are not even associated with the experience, so that testimony may take the form of a 'performance' rather than a telling. Further, children often cannot tell the story by themselves. Certain epistemological concepts will not function 'normally' in such children's testimony, e.g., truth, certainty, knowing. Children's testimony also challenges standard moral concepts, such as duty and honesty. I then claim that we should recognize a distinction in testimonial purposes: 'straightforward' testimony may be directed at justice, but the kind of narrative speaking that is necessary for healing is very different and more complex, requiring different modes of speaking and different responses from hearers. Having recognized this distinction, we can then make more sense out of the trend in testimony theory that conceptualizes it as an effort to express that which is inexpressible, or characterizes atrocities as paradoxical and impossible to know. I argue that because standard testimony is aimed at restoring justice, it places burdens on testifiers of all ages, appearing to encourage an unhealthy dissociation. Although the work of testifying for justice is necessary, it should give ample consideration to these extra burdens and provide accommodations to aid children who testify, but also adults, whenever this is appropriate.

 | DOI:10.1163/9789004391130_008

Keywords

legal testimony – trauma – children – epistemological – moral – second-order witnessing – justice – dissociation

1 Testimonial Discourses

A standard definition of testimony is 'an autobiographical narrative that presents evidence of first-person accounts of human rights abuses, violence and war, and life under conditions of social oppression'.[1] However, working with traumatized children shows that testimony cannot always be a straightforward 'autobiographical narrative'. Instead, epistemological and moral concepts associated with testimony must be reconsidered in terms of the context under which and the purpose for which the testimony is given, whether by children or adults. The definition above indicates a form of testimony that is directed at justice, but that form should not be conflated with testimonial speaking that is really the expression of experience for the purposes of *understanding and recovery*. I argue that looking at the testimony of young children helps show the importance of this distinction and how it should be made, because young children are generally not able to construct a coherent narrative account but are attempting, through their testimonial speaking, to create meaning.

The definition given above refers, broadly, to the kind of testimonial speaking used in reports of rights violations and other abuses to legal and political organizations such as rights commissions and treaty monitoring bodies, as well as courts. In seeking redress for wrongs committed against them, survivors are required, in such settings, to present an account of their experiences that obeys the conventions that have been established for their telling. These conventions are responsive to certain directives: namely, that the testimony be verifiable, and that it be presented objectively.

Verifiability refers to the idea that the events being testified to may be confirmed or corroborated by others. It is not the case that testimony always is corroborated, merely that what is being testified to is the kind of thing that could

1 Cristina Santos, Adriana Spahr and Tracy Crowe Morey, '1st Global Conference – Testimony, Truth, Trauma, Memory, Engagement, Conference Announcement' *Inter-Disciplinary.Net*, viewed 2 May 2016. https://www.facebook.com/events/475985079187816/.

be independently verified. So, for example, testimony is of actions or events rather than only of the testifier's experience of or beliefs about those events, except insofar as he or she is making allegations regarding the wrongness of them. What must be verifiable is that the events occurred, and that the facts of those events could be discoverable if an investigation were made.

The requirement that testimony be presented objectively is somewhat more complex. In one sense it means that the testifier should provide his or her story in a controlled way. Given that such stories are sometimes presentations of abuses that are horrific, this may in fact represent something of a difficulty, as the testifier may have to struggle to keep her emotions or pain from disrupting the story and making it confusing. This is the sense mentioned above of the coherent narrative, the balanced presentation that provides necessary detail, but avoids being side-tracked away from the facts of the events, and maintains the correct chronological sequence.

In another sense, objectivity is a matter of what the audience is willing and capable of hearing. Although a sympathetic commission or jury will of course recognize that a certain level of emotion or passion frequently accompanies testimony of abuses and injuries, there are also expectations of formality of procedure that may lead listeners to unconsciously reject a telling that is too emotionally fraught. The association of emotionally laden speech with hysteria encourages an expectation that even in telling their stories of terrible experiences, speakers must maintain a calm and stable demeanour if they are to appear credible. A further complication along these lines is that if testimony places too heavy an emotional burden on the listeners, their own need to protect themselves from the reality of the horrors being described may lead them to respond, however unintentionally, with scepticism.[2]

Testimony given in a court of law has further requirements. Consistency is key among them, and is determined in large part by the testifier's ability to maintain the accuracy of their story under sometimes harsh and deliberately confusing cross-examination. Further, because the definition of testimony in the courts is somewhat different, emphasizing the need for the testifier to recognize and accept the seriousness of their speech and the consequences it may have for themselves and others, there is a kind of 'informed consent' testifiers are required to give in witnessing. It has been put in the following way:

2 Roberta Culbertson, 'Embodied Memory, Transcendence and Telling: Recounting Trauma, Re-Establishing the Self', *New Literary History* 26.1 (1995): 180–182.

> [A] person must be able to recognize and understand the truth of the propositions in the following causal chain:
>
> As a result of my statement, my listeners may believe that what I say happened did in fact happen; as a result of that belief they may take action; and as an ultimate result of that action, the person whose conduct I am describing may suffer serious adverse consequences. Accordingly, my listeners, or others, regard it as important that I speak truthfully.[3]

In sum, what we see from examining the standard, official definitions of testimony is that it is a particular type of narrative, subject to certain conventions, with specific purposes. This standard picture of testimony indicates quite clearly that it is conceptually and pragmatically ordered by the requirements of justice.

2 (Young) Children's Speaking

A *Technicalities*

Many aspects of young children's speaking show that they are generally not fully capable of constructing the kind of narrative that is needed for the pursuit of justice in human rights abuses. This is acknowledged in fields that work with children's development and psychology, obviously, but also in legal thought and practice, where we see a tremendous literature devoted to the question of whether children, especially abused children, are capable of telling the truth in court or being reliable witnesses. The question may be focused in one of two ways: in terms of strict courtroom practice and procedure, it can be examined in terms of the Confrontation Clause of the Constitution, which requires that the accused have access to their accusers to confront them. Children's ability to testify can then be questioned on the grounds that they are not equal to such a confrontation; again, this will be especially difficult in cases of abuse, and when the alleged abuser is a family member or other person the child is or was attached to. But further, the child's ability may be challenged in terms of the cognitive and moral requirements of testifying: so, for example, Richard Friedman and Stephen Ceci explain:

3 Richard D. Friedman and Stephen J. Ceci, 'The Child Quasi Witness', *The University of Chicago Law Review* 82.1 (Winter 2015): 91.

> most children under the age of four are unaware that other people might have false beliefs. Indeed, below this age, most children do not recognize that the information that is available to them from their observations is not known by other people; therefore, the basic concept of *informing* another person, and adding to that other person's state of knowledge, is foreign to them.[4]

Carole Peterson and Brenda Parsons raise a further issue regarding cognitive abilities, pointing out that

> in many jurisdictions, for a case to be successfully prosecuted it is crucial for children to be able to differentiate various experiences. In fact, in most jurisdictions children must be able to specify the details of where, who, when, and what happened for each event, regardless of how often they are repeated.[5]

This difficulty for children arises from their observed tendency to blur events that are similar when they occur regularly over a period of time. Thus a child abused regularly over a year may not distinguish easily, for example, between an abuse event that happened on Tuesday of one week and a similar event that occurred on Thursday of the following week.[6]

Related to this last point is another way in which children's ability to testify is non-standard, giving rise to controversy. It refers to the accuracy and authenticity of children's memories. Very young children, like pre-schoolers, may indeed have some memory difficulties. However, much research, such as that by John Myers et al., shows even these youngsters as having 'quite accurate' recall, roughly as good as older children of 10 and 11.[7] The concern about accuracy is less controversial than authenticity, the worry here being that children's memories may somehow have been tampered with or imposed on them. The accusation is less about deliberate lying on the part of child witnesses than

---

4 Ibid., 98, italics in original.

5 Carole Peterson and Brenda Parsons, 'Interviewing Former 1- and 2-Year Olds about Medical Emergencies 5 Years Later', *Law and Human Behavior* 29.6 (Dec. 2005): 752.

6 Pedro Paz-Alonso, Christine M. Ogle, and Gail S. Goodman, 'Children's Memory in "Scientific Case Studies" of Child Sexual Abuse: A Review', *Applied Issues in Investigative Interviewing, Eyewitness Memory, and Credibility Assessment*, eds. Barry S. Cooper, Dorothee Griesel and Marguerite Ternes. (New York: Springer, 2013), 163.

7 John E. B. Myers, 'Adjudication of Child Sexual Abuse Cases', *The Future of Children* 4(2) (Summer-Autumn 1994): 86.

about claiming that overzealous therapists or prosecutors may have worked on a child's relatively high level of suggestibility to 'make' her[8] 'remember' events that never actually took place. Again, although research cannot dispel the possibility of this, it does show that such instances are rare, and are usually a matter of what Myers refers to as 'poor interviewing skills' on the part of therapist or attorney. Because young children often need support to 'bring [a] memory to the surface', a very careful level of suggestive or probing questioning may be required to help her articulate her experience of abuse. 'Thus, during interviews of young children, it is often necessary – for developmental reasons – to ask specific questions, some of which are suggestive'.[9]

B *Narrative Matters*

Beyond these technical issues, there are simply difficulties for children in constructing coherent narratives. For one thing, young children have not yet developed a strong sense of self to place in such a narrative. Although adults typically have a 'continuing, integrated story of the self', this is not something children have developed.[10] The child's 'sense of self and its embededness [*sic*] in an awareness of cultural realities is new, relatively primitive perhaps'.[11] They often do not have the vocabulary or the standard time sense to narrate a history of events. Aida Alayarian explains that adults typically have 'the ability to place it in a time perspective and also situate it in relation to different social and psychological contexts', but this is exactly what young children may be unable to manage.[12] Further, when children are traumatized pre-verbally, words are not even associated with the experience. In cases like this testimony may take the form of a 'performance' rather than a telling, an acting out that may come spontaneously rather than in response to a setting in which they are being formally questioned. Other factors as disparate as whether a child has healthy attachment with caregivers and time delay from the event to disclosure affect their ability to produce a narrative account of traumatic experiences.[13]

---

8 I choose to use the feminine pronouns to counter the more usual practice of assuming that masculine pronouns function as 'generic' for all humans. This usage is becoming more frequent in feminist philosophy.

9 Myers, 'Adjudication of Child Sexual Abuse Cases', 87.

10 Culbertson, 'Embodied Memory', 174.

11 Ibid., 180.

12 Aida Alayarian, *Trauma, Torture and Dissociation: A Psychoanalytic View* (London: Karnac Books, 2011), 54.

13 Paz-Alonso, Ogle and Goodman, 'Children's Memory', 164.

My own work with and research on sexually abused children has shown me that understanding children's testimony requires a non-standard epistemology because the experience of sexual abuse is essentially unintelligible. The truth of many traumatic experiences is neither straightforwardly nor easily told because they are not easily comprehended. Cathy Caruth goes to the heart of this in saying 'the most direct seeing of a violent event may occur as an absolute inability to know it'.[14] This inability to know may be a matter of adaptive mechanisms brought into play by the traumatic events, as a child's mind shields her from a knowing which would make it impossible for her to continue functioning. As expressed by Roland Summit, the typical, healthy response of children to severe abuse is to dissociate – to 'set it aside and keep it out of consciousness and to learn one way or another to get distance from that experience, even as it's happening'.[15] Especially when the child is in the position of having to maintain an at least minimally successful relationship with her abuser, as when that person is a parent the child must live with and depend on for whatever safety, attachment and good she receives, an epistemology of ignorance and forgetting is a survival mechanism.[16]

The logic of sexually abused children is also non-standard, becoming what I call 'circuitous' as they attempt to reconcile their lived experiences with what they are told to believe about the world. Children who have been subjected to brutal and prolonged abuse have an epistemological framework that is different from the 'ordinary', and from what philosophy tends to say about knowing. Children who have suffered abuse need to tell someone about it, but most often are not able to do this directly. A number of reasons may prompt this: aside from the one already noted, that they may be too young to even articulate it, they may have been too effectively threatened. Or they may re-experience too much of the events when they even think about them to be able to verbalize them.

The experience of abuse and the imperative of secrecy that comes with it means that their world jumps from one reality to another. One is what we

14 Anne Cubilié, *Women Witnessing Terror: Testimony and the Cultural Politics of Human Rights* (New York: Fordham University Press, 2005), 15.

15 David L. Corwin, 'An Interview with Roland Summit', *Critical Issues in Child Sexual Abuse: Historical, Legal and Psychological Perspectives,* edited by Jon R. Conte (Thousand Oaks, California: Sage Publications, 2002), 14.

16 Jennifer J. Freyd, 'Memory and Dimensions of Trauma: Terror May Be "All-Too-Well Remembered" and Betrayal Buried', *Critical Issues in Child Sexual Abuse: Historical, Legal and Psychological Perspectives,* edited by Jon R. Conte (Thousand Oaks, California: Sage Publications, 2002), 145–149.

would call the ordinary world, which they must learn to negotiate at least to some extent, but which is not the primary focus of their concern. The other is the world of double-speak, false appearances, constant threat, unpredictable violence and a love that both sustains and destroys at the same time. In that world, which is more real to them than the other, the real is unspeakable.

Further, the rules for survival are different in each world, and children have to learn to watch carefully for any potential indicators that they are about to be flung into a hell (or more hellish) dimension. Sensing that they are under constant threat, they cannot be sure that anything or anyone is truly 'safe'. Within this framework it makes sense to say that whatever one experiences is real, that what one feels is in fact what is true, and there is no other basis for truth. I believe Candace Couse puts this well when she says, in her chapter in this volume, that the body becomes a site of knowledge, and that 'the felt comes first, leading one into thought'.[17] Under this embodied epistemology of abuse, nothing but what you feel/experience yourself can be true, real, or trusted. But even this cannot be ultimately relied on, because of abusers' tendencies to undermine the abused by insisting that they are wrong, crazy, spiteful or otherwise not to be believed. So what can become of the experience of knowing when the only foundation for knowledge is riddled with uncertainty to start with, and then is deliberately submarined?

Obviously, then, certain epistemological concepts do not function 'normally' in such children's testimony, e.g., truth, knowing, 'the real'. Further, we need to reconsider standard claims about what counts as evidence in these cases. For example, child therapists such as Lenore Terr argue that expressions other than speech may be what we need to look to as evidence.[18] Terr talks about ways that traumatized children express their experiences as play and/or reenactment. These behaviours are highly repetitive and extremely literal and can consequently be interpreted easily and directly in terms of the facts of the child's trauma. She cites examples of children who experienced kidnapping on a school bus repeatedly playing games of driving dolls to mysterious locations.[19] She gives other examples of child sexual abuse victims 'playing' in ways that explicitly recreate the sex acts they were subjected to over and over.[20] Author Patricia Heberer presents examples of child victims of the

17 Candace Couse, 'Sick: Negotiating Body Trauma Through Visual Art Practice', in this volume.

18 Lenore Terr, *Too Scared to Cry: How Trauma Affects Children … and Ultimately Us All* (New York: Basic Books, 1990), see chapters 12 and 13.

19 Ibid., 244.

20 Ibid., 246.

concentration camps acting out their trauma in a harrowing 'gas chamber' game, in which they dug a trench and pushed stones into it, supplying the cries of the 'prisoners' with their own voices as the stone 'victims' fell.[21]

Then again, especially as children are still *learning* to know, we need to recognize the importance of their 'knowing-with', or co-knowing, in their ability to report on their experiences. Children's telling needs to be supported or aided by reliable third parties, perhaps family members in an informal setting, but often professionals in a more formal one. Part of the task for such helpers is to encourage children to express their experiences, and another is to help them put events in sequential and chronological order, which they may not be able to do for themselves. But another part is to assist them in actually understanding what the expression of that experience probably means, especially if they are not using words. However, according to Terr, even when expressions are quite literal, the child herself may not recognize the connection between the play or re-enactment and the events which led to it.[22]

C *Moral Challenges*

Children's testimony also challenges standard moral concepts, such as duty. In traditional western ethics, duty is associated with rules or principles which can or should be universalisable and objective, but this conception is probably untenable in regards to our moral responses to traumatized children. Rather than a universal rule, we probably will do morally better if we implement an ethic of caring, responding to the needs of the child rather than to any abstract sense of justice.[23] We clearly have a heightened duty to witness for/with children, but doing so relies on a similar duty not to ignore or avoid their pain.[24] Also, we must resist imposing on suffering children unreasonable duties to tell. Honesty too may be different in these circumstances; children may be unable to be fully honest about events, or to be honest in language, and as noted above, we must learn to read what is honest or authentic in their body language and acting out.

---

21 Patricia Heberer, *Children during the Holocaust* (Lanham: AltaMira Press, 2011), 300.

22 Terr, *Too Scared*, 241–245.

23 For the ethics of care see Virginia Held, *The Ethics of Care: Personal, Political and Global* (New York: Oxford University Press, 2007), Nel Noddings, *Caring: A Feminine Approach to Ethics and Moral Education* (Oakland, CA: University of California Press, 2003), and Joan Tronto, *Moral Boundaries: A Political Argument for an Ethic of Care* (New York: Routledge, 1993).

24 See Mary Louise Fellows and Beverly Balos, 'Guilty of the Crime of Trust: Nonstranger Rape', 75 *Minnesota Law Review* (1991): 605–609.

An important implication of this discussion is that many children's ability to sort the true from the false, an expectation or requirement of testimony that is both epistemological and moral, is either not fully developed or damaged in their traumatic experiences. What we recognize here is not only that the moral and the epistemological are inextricably intertwined, but that their interconnection should encourage us to understand that in effect it may not matter to children's witnessing *for recovery* whether they are 'telling' the 'truth' or not, if they are expressing the real effects of traumatic events. This is the importance of care ethics, in allowing us to privilege the needs of the testifiers, rather than focusing on what appears to be required for justice, but may not respond to those immediate needs. The interweaving of the moral and the epistemological in children's testimony points clearly to the fact that testimony does have multiple purposes, and that we must be careful about what we intend for and expect from children in the aftermath of trauma.

The point is that because in children's testimony we do recognize that we have a heightened duty to support and care for them, we *know* we need to be careful about all these things, but in particular it's easy to see how careful we need to be about *what the testimony is for*. In general, we want kids to tell their stories so that we can know how to help them make sense of and recover or heal from their experiences; issues of justice are to a certain extent a secondary matter. This is why in recent years the courts have initiated certain protections for child witnesses, such as closing the courtroom to observers, using video or closed circuit TV testimony, and preventing harassment and intimidation in cross-examination.[25] However, in the literature on adult testimony, this problem of purpose has been effaced. While we assume that adults are capable of presenting testimony perhaps with some difficulty but honestly and truthfully, we also have fascinating and somewhat perplexing theories about gaps and lacunae and impossibilities. My suspicion is that this kind of theorizing represents a tension between even the adult ability to cope with experiences of trauma and the requirement of justice that adults give testimony both for their own sake and the sake of others, including those who truly are unable to speak. That is, I believe there is a kind of slippage in the literature that does not fully recognize the different purposes of testimony, and that the one purpose may in fact be counterproductive for the other, especially if we are insensitive to the moral requirements of care, prioritizing justice over care in expecting people to testify at times and in ways they themselves are not ready or strong enough for.

25 Myers, 'Adjudication', 88–89.

3 Adults' Speaking: the Conventions of Justice

When adults give testimony in the standard ways and settings, they generally do so in a controlled manner, coherently, and even with a dignity in the face of atrocity that is very moving. One man's testimony of his experience being illegally arrested and severely beaten begins so very simply:

> Good morning. My name is Porfirio Domínguez Muñozcano. I am an architect. My professional credential is number 1379284. All of my life … for 16 years, I have been an architect, working in this profession.[26]

The testimony of Ali Abu-Shalal before a Commissioner of Oaths in Kuala Lumpur begins in essentially the same way, with a similar presentation of simple statements of identity and credentials.[27] Narration of the actual abuses in these cases was straightforward, orderly, following a linear chronological model. The narrators' use of language was moderate, given the events being described:

> I was electrocuted on three separate sessions … On the last session, as I was being electrocuted, I accidentally bit my tongue and was bleeding from the mouth. They stop [*sic*] the electrocution and a doctor was called to attend to me. I was lying down on the floor. The doctor poured some water into my mouth and used his feet to force open my mouth. He then remarked, "There is nothing serious, continue!" Then he left the room. However, the guard stopped the electrocution as I was bleeding profusely from my mouth and blood was all over my blanket and body. But they continued to beat me. After some time, they stopped beating me and took me back to my cell.[28]

For adults, there is no question that they are typically capable of presenting testimony according to the conventions that make it acceptable and credible. Adults are also usually capable of understanding the reasons for those

---

26 Porfirio Domínguez Muñozcano, 'Testimony of Torture Victim in Oaxaca', transcribed by Rights Action. *UpsideDownWorld*, January 8, 2007, viewed 22 January, 2015, http://upsidedownworld.org/main/mexico-archives-79/574-testimony-of-torture-victim-in-oaxaca.

27 Ali Abu-Shalal, 'Torture at Abu Graib: The Full Sworn Testimony of Ali Shalal' transcribed by *Global Research*, February 2007, viewed 22 January, 2015, http://www.globalresearch.ca/torture-at-abu-ghraib-the-full-sworn-testimony-of-ali-shalal/4865.

28 Abu-Shalal, 'Torture at Abu Graib', np.

conventions, which are connected to the goals of showing themselves as reasonable speakers, making compelling and believable statements, and asking for justice.

This last point helps in understanding why the conventions determining testimony emphasize the kind of speaking that they do. To ask for justice in such cases, when abuses or atrocities have been committed, is to ask that some official agency impose some sanction on the perpetrators, a penalty or punishment. In the literature on punishment, however, it is commonly acknowledged that punishments and penalties inflict harm, for example by restricting people's ordinary liberties. However, unless harms are legitimated by proper authority and procedures of justice, they must be considered wrong in exactly the same ways they would be if they resulted from crimes or abuses. Consequently, justice is a serious business, and must be conducted in ways and tones that reflect that seriousness, along with an understanding of and earnest appreciation of responsibilities, and chains of cause and effect. Although children are not always or perhaps even often expected to understand this, adults generally are, even after they have suffered atrocities and even regarding atrocities they have suffered.

A *The Impossible* Is *the Real*

Even for adults, however, we do in some ways recognize that testimony is problematic. One aspect of the difficulty of testimony that comes up again and again in different metaphors in the literature is the idea that trauma is simply unspeakable. Elaine Scarry draws this idea out of her study of torture and the ways that severe, prolonged pain reduces our use of language to mere animal sounds, taking away the capacity to conceptualize self and experience and make sense of them through speaking. In this way, speaking the pain, the trauma, is itself what becomes impossible, because the pain is overwhelmingly real. The pain becomes unspeakable precisely because it is also the experience that wipes away our ability to use sound coherently.[29]

On the other hand, Jacques Derrida puts the experience in terms of what he calls 'mythic violence', a violence that rips one away from one's sense of self, and the way that survival of such violence is itself not understandable. What is unspeakable here is not the inexpressible but the literally unknowable, as Derrida says we cannot even understand the fact of our own survival in the face of the traumatic event. If we can speak at all, we must do so from within the

29 Elaine Scarry, *The Body in Pain: The Making and Unmaking of the World* (New York: Oxford University Press, 1985), Introduction.

'lacuna' of our language, from within the gap between experience and knowing. But that gap itself appears to be a place without language, and so again there is an element of the inexpressible at work in his theorizing.[30]

Giorgio Agamben takes a slightly different tack, to put the issue in terms of 'a formulation of voice and identity within paradox'.[31] His account of what testimony is, and what it does, involves the idea that what is most human is so because of its ability to endure what is inhuman. Testimony is the giving of voice to that experience of surviving the inhuman, and in so doing becomes the hallmark of the human. So Agamben's picture of testimony involves a complex picture of what it means to be human, a speaking of that which is so alien to humanness that in experiencing it we in fact lose our humanity, but recover it again only through that speaking. He draws on the figure of the Muselmann, that character from the concentration camps who was emblematic of the living dead, the inhuman human body still apparently living, but whose humanity has been erased by what it has suffered. Because this character represents the enduring of inhuman treatment, Agamben refers to it as the real or total witness.

Of course this is far too brief a review to do justice to any of these complex articulations of testimony, but enough to make my point: that the literature on adults' witnessing is full of attempts to characterize the act of testifying as expressing what is inexpressible, unspeakable, unknowable, paradoxical and unintelligible. Yet, when we read accounts of (adult) testimony from court records and other types of deposition, what we see is entirely intelligible: in general, adults give exactly the kind of coherent autobiographical narrative that we expect.

I think this shows we really do have two sets of tasks and expectations for witnessing, which we take note of and separate in working with children, but one of which we seem to take for granted in working with adults. That is, we seem to take for granted that adults *will* be able to provide testimony for the purpose of seeking justice, the coherent narrative that is required by judicial process or by official review. And clearly this is necessary and important: we do need to be able to bring testimony to bear on human rights abuses as part of the ongoing effort to discourage them. But I think this confusing and paradoxical literature indicates that we also recognize at some level that the production of the coherent narrative, the ordered speaking of *'the real',* is only one piece of the work that needs to be done if we want to aid survivors as well as hold

30 Jacques Derrida, *Writing and Difference* (New York: Routledge, 1981).

31 Cubilié, *Women Witnessing Terror*, 3.

perpetrators accountable. The other piece is about aiding survivors in articulating not the events, but their effects and meaning; that is, it is about speaking *the impossible.*

B *Cross Purposes*

As these two purposes, reporting and recovery, are very different, we should not be surprised to realize that the modes of speaking in them are also very different, and perhaps work at cross purposes. But then the question is, why should it be the case that the kind of speaking used in official testimonial settings is not just inadequate to recovery, but also seems to sometimes work against it? An answer can be found in the literature on the use of narrative in trauma therapy. This literature is complex and extensive, so here I can only point to three features that have been identified as crucial for recovery, but which tend to be missing in official settings: emotional engagement, repetition of the right kind, and social reconnection.

As noted above, the narration of abuses in official settings is usually linear and coherent, but what is more, it is presented with detachment. One observer at the testimony of Abu-Shalal, quoted above, notes this feature of his speaking: 'he began to speak, albeit in a monotonous, emotionless tone. What can you expect from a person who went through hell several times'.[32] Roberta Culbertson describes this type of narrative as the recounting of the trauma by a 'survivor self', a self which in order to survive violation has separated from the events to the greatest extent possible, standing at a distance from them and speaking of them as though they had happened to someone else.[33] This emotionless, detached presentation is the result of a numbing that victims may experience as their nervous systems attempt to protect them from overwhelming realities as they happen. Afterward, the survivor may become stuck in this mode of speaking about their violation, which from a therapeutic perspective, is only a beginning in moving toward recovery, because 'the recitation of facts without the accompanying emotions is a sterile exercise, without therapeutic effect'.[34] Thus, whereas healing requires an integrated narrative, replete with the details of how it felt both bodily and emotionally, testimony in official settings encourages the kind of detached telling that represents only the earliest efforts of the survivor to communicate their experience.

---

32 Abu-Shalal, 'Torture at Abu Graib', np.

33 Culbertson, 'Embodied Memory', 172–173.

34 Judith Herman, *Trauma and Recovery: The Aftermath of Violence – from Domestic Abuse to Political Terror* (New York: Basic Books, 1992), 177.

Narrative therapy also requires that the survivor have the opportunity to repeat her story at relatively regular intervals (in sessions once a week, for example) in a safe and supportive atmosphere. Such repetition is crucial for the necessary transformation of the narrative from that of a detached 'survivor self' who cannot bear her own experience to that of an integrated, reconstructed self. This process of reconstructing the self is accomplished through a reconstructing of the story. Over time, as the survivor tells it again, she realizes increasingly that she is capable of telling without experiencing the disintegration the trauma caused. Each telling is an opportunity to add to the story those details that literally 'flesh it out', but as she does so, the survivor also gains control over the story and thus the events of it. In this way, through repetition of the story in the proper environment, a survivor transforms both the story and herself, not getting rid of the trauma, but reshaping it into an integrated part of her life, one which no longer has control over her.[35] Again, official testimony does not have a place for such transformative repetitions; where it does allow or ask for repetitions, the story is required to remain the same. Changes are seen as inconsistency, and as noted above, inconsistency is a property that invalidates official testimony.

Finally, a vital feature of recovery is social reconnection; Susan Brison explains this in terms of 'the fundamentally relational character of the self'.[36] This aspect begins with a survivor being aided in establishing a sense of safety, which is one of the aspects of ordinary life that trauma destroys. Without feeling safe, a survivor is unlikely to be able to access even those relational ties that were most important to her before; this is especially true, of course, for those whose abuse comes at the hands of someone previously trusted. But once safety is established, and the trauma story has undergone transformation, a survivor can begin reaching out once again to others in her world, and can once again create more ordinary social relations with people in general. Again, this goal is frustrated by the settings and practices of official testimony. Courtrooms and commissions are much more likely to be experienced as settings for an ordeal than for making meaningful connections. As noted above, commissions and juries are expected not to make too close a connection with those who testify, lest that connection impair their ability to properly assess and judge what they are hearing.

---

35 See, for example, Herman, *Trauma and Recovery*, 176–181, and Susan J. Brison, *Aftermath: Violence and the Remaking of a Self* (Princeton, NJ: Princeton University Press, 2002), 69.

36 Brison, *Aftermath*, 63.

4 Dissociating for Justice

One more perspective is extremely helpful in understanding how the requirements of official testimony can work against healing from trauma. In her book *Trauma, Torture and Dissociation: A Psychoanalytic View,* Aida Alayarian develops a theory of dissociation which differentiates between a healthy form and an unhealthy one. Dissociation, a phenomenon widely connected with traumatic experiences, both during and after, is described as a form of separation from self or of self from body that functions to insulate a person from the overwhelming experience of violence, helplessness and/or self-annihilation caused by severe abuses or violations. Says Alayarian,

> dissociation, especially from a relational perspective, is a form of psychical organization in which psychical conflicts and threats to self-preservation are regulated in the mind and can be considered as a mechanism of defence when the mind cannot cope any more.[37]

Although dissociation is generally understood as a defence mechanism preserving some part of the self, it also tends to be considered something unhealthy or maladaptive because that preservation often works at the cost of a splitting off, a 'taking away' of the person's sense of self.[38] When dissociation is very severe it can lead to a more or less permanent fragmentation of self, a literal multiplication of self which is referred to as dissociative identity disorder.

Alayarian argues, however, that it can also be a healthy coping mechanism under certain circumstances, as when 'the person consciously redirects attention away from something traumatic which might otherwise interfere with or overwhelm the psychic structure and functions'.[39] When dissociation is relatively deliberate in this way, it can actually help with the return to health that involves a re-integration of the self, a re-placing of the self within its own narrative on its own terms. This is because the healthy dissociation, by 'temporarily turning away from' the traumatic memory, opens up an inner, psychic space that enables the person to think about a traumatic experience and gain enough perspective on it to set it into the context of a whole, ongoing life. Because an unhealthy dissociation denies and disavows feeling and reality it is cut off from emotion, making it impossible for a full reintegration of the experience into

37 Alayarian, *Trauma, Torture and Dissociation,* 157.

38 Ibid., 103.

39 Ibid., 164.

the self.[40] An unhealthy dissociation, in keeping the overwhelming emotion of the experience at a distance, makes it 'possible to keep the person from feeling *anything*'.[41]

In articulating this theory of healthy dissociation, Alayarian's context is therapeutic practice, of course, rather than the discourse of justice. Further, she is explicitly talking about adults with some decent level of resilience, who can comparatively consciously dissociate specifically for the purpose of not being overwhelmed by their experience, but are not controlled by or submerged in the dissociation.[42] This leaves me with two concerns related to what I have argued about testimony: one is that children are not likely to be able to do this conscious, deliberate dissociation in the healthy way, and the other is that testimony for justice seems to *require* dissociation, of both adults, some of whom presumably can do it in the healthy way, and kids, most of whom presumably cannot.

Regarding children's dissociation under trauma, there is significant literature that makes two important points: first, that children are likely to be better at dissociating than adults are, and consequently are more likely to actually do it, and second, that they are unlikely to be able to exercise any control over it. According to Culbertson, children

> are suggestible ... their ability to enter a world that is separate from the one in which they reside, a world in which boxes become cars and carrots guns or knives, is significant.[43]

Along with this imaginative ability, children also are more likely to experience violence or a violation as self-annihilating because their sense of self is so unfinished, and they have much less understanding than adults do 'of what the body can take and what it cannot'.[44] This means they may achieve dissociation more easily than adults, both during the trauma, by 'going away' or entering a trance state, and in the aftermath, by forgetting or denying the events they cannot acknowledge as real.

Further, children will not be able to consciously direct or use dissociation in the ways that Alayarian says adults may do in their healthy recovery processes. 'The notion of healthy dissociation ... involves alterations in consciousness

40 Ibid., 166.

41 Ibid., 286, emphasis added.

42 Ibid., 58, 158, 160.

43 Culbertson, 'Embodied Memory', 181.

44 Ibid., 180.

in which the person becomes aware of being in a state of ailment, seeking help when there is need' but this is only possible because of 'the impact of healthy object relations in the developmental process and early personality formation'.[45] That is, healthy dissociation depends on the person's having had a healthy early life and development as a foundation for responding to traumatic events – but that is exactly what is missing from children whose early life is marred by severe trauma. Even if life is proceeding relatively typically for a child, severe trauma and/or prolonged trauma can derail that progress so significantly as to invalidate it. As Patricia Heberer puts it,

> While adults had known another life before the Holocaust and toiled to rebuild their lives in the postwar years on the memory of those former times, the children of the Shoah had no other chronology. The Holocaust was the indestructible present that shaped their lives, while their adult contemporaries could and often chose to exorcise such memories from their histories.[46]

This discussion indicates that even if there is a healthy form of dissociation, children are probably not the ones who will be able to manage it. They will probably experience dissociation as a defence, yes, but it will be the form that makes recovery more, not less, difficult. This leads to the second worry I have following Alayarian's theory: that justice appears to require dissociation. Such a requirement would be relatively unproblematic if it were the case that those giving testimony were reliably capable of dissociating in the healthy way, as a temporary measure enabling them to set aside the debilitating effects of the traumatic memory. However, if children are generally incapable of doing so, then in their cases justice may be imposing a re-traumatisation of the child in requiring testimony, especially under the standard conventions. At the very least, testifying may reinforce any dissociation a child has experienced, making therapeutic work even longer and more difficult than it otherwise might be. In cases where adults have not yet managed the work of recovery from trauma, and are not fortunate enough to have the ability to dissociate in the healthy way, they too, may experience testifying as increasing the burden of recovery. In this way, by requiring certain forms of discourse that 'distance' emotion and integration, justice works at cross purposes with the work of the abuse victim to recover, to build or re-build a healthy self.

---

45 Alayarian, *Trauma, Torture and Dissociation*, 158.

46 Heberer, *Children during the Holocaust*, 415.

5 Justice Is *Not* 'The Listening Other'

Witnessing for recovery has to be a doubled endeavour, a telling by the survivor but also a listening and validating, a second-order witnessing, on the part of others. Alayarian acknowledges this in her use of the term 'the listening other', referring to the role taken by the therapist in aiding the survivor in the task of reclaiming and recreating her life, her self.[47] Anne Cubilié articulates this second-order witnessing as a performative dynamic, an engaged, supportive enabling of the representation of the survivor's experience in whatever way she can manage.[48] Within this volume, Alison Atkinson-Phillips discusses in a similar way the importance of the engaged 'outsider-witness' whose important role is to reflect narrative back to the survivor, becoming a (limited) partner in the telling. Both the ethics and the epistemology of this witnessing for recovery are then complex and non-standard, because they will be about our obligations to support a representation of someone's experience as a truth *without challenge*.

Unfortunately, the more the witnessing is this performative dynamic, the more compromised it may be as a juridical tool, because it may be seen as 'contaminated' by that very engagement. This is what makes children's witnessing so very problematic in the courts, as it creates fears of 'leading' the witness, of 'supplying' a testimony that oversteps the reality of the experience and can then falsely incriminate. But it may be precisely this problem that makes it so necessary to recognize the different purposes of testimony, in that as second-order witnesses we need to make sure that we do engage, as recovery and healing cannot be done without support and acceptance. Ultimately, the goal of recovery is to successfully reintegrate into community; presumably doing so requires a community in which at least some members engage and support the survivor. Cubilié puts it more forcefully, but in a similar vein:

> Testimonial is more than a witnessing ... it is also a profoundly political act that demands a performative engagement with the witnessing by the spectator witness and in this way and others works to intervene in the culturally violent reconfigurations that the experience of [trauma] founds and marks.[49]

47 Alayarian *Trauma, Torture and Dissociation*, 73.

48 Cubilié, *Women Witnessing Terror*, 10.

49 Ibid., 4.

Clearly, this is an ethical engagement as well as a political one.

Ultimately, it seems to me that what is at issue in this paradoxical literature on testimony is something that we find much more easily and clearly in the literature on child sexual abuse/child trauma and recovery: the recognition that survivors need help to do more than survive. That need signals a moral obligation to care on the part of some, perhaps most, second-order witnesses. This is obvious when we consider the cases of children because we take for granted their inability to process and make sense of their experiences of violation, abuse and trauma. But what the literature of impossibility helps show is that adults have the same needs: not perhaps so much for the testimony of reporting, but for the kind of testimony that is crucial to their recovery. Essentially, the experiencing of atrocity reduces adults to the level of very young children, in its stripping away of adult abilities to understand and articulate the loss of self that atrocity inflicts. Adults as well as children must ask: why has this happened to me?, and must answer, must make some meaning of the events, in spite of the fact that the answer has nothing to do with what they may or may not have done to deserve such treatment. Ultimately, no one deserves such treatment, and this is what makes the task of recovery so difficult. Since adults as well as children cannot but flounder in the face of such a task, such impossibility and unintelligibility, they will need the same kind of engaged second-order witnessing children do; not simply spectators to reporting, but Alayarian's listening other, the performative dynamic of witnessing that Cubilié recommends when she says 'testimony and the responsibilities of justice and ethics are not just about an impossibility; they are also about what we are willing to do as witnesses to the witnesses'.[50]

However, this raises difficult questions: exactly what are 'we' willing to do as witnesses to the witnesses when the testimony is being presented as part of the process of seeking justice? What can we appropriately expect of second-order witnesses such as judges, members of juries, members of tribunals and commissions? The stumbling block is that our conceptions of justice include, fundamentally, the necessity of impartiality, of emotional disengagement. This is seen as crucial in order to be able properly to assess (the truth of) the testimony being presented, for conceptions of justice standardly entail that emotional connection with any parties involved in a dispute being considered under its aegis automatically contaminate the ability of hearers to participate appropriately. Is it possible that this stance can be changed without damaging (or at least changing) the processes, and results, of our justice?

50 Ibid., 3.

Perhaps not; at least, not in fundamental ways. We can, however, at the very least recognize what is being created by our justice systems and what effects it seems to have, not only on those giving testimony (and presumably those accused as well), but also those who function as the witnesses to the witnesses in this context. That is, the prerequisite of impartiality appears to impose on judges, juries, commissions, etc., a parallel obligation to dissociate. We expect such hearers to be able to 'set aside temporarily' their ordinary sympathetic responses to stories of abuse and atrocity so that they can function as disinterested observers, on the assumption that this is the only way to render an adequately even-handed, just outcome.

This requirement is, however, one of the conditions that makes it difficult for survivors to tell their stories in the first place: as noted in the literature on speaking atrocity for both children and adults, the fear of not being heard sympathetically and supportively is one of the major reasons for not telling. This fear functions in several ways, of course; it may be a fear of being misunderstood due to the impossibility of what must be said. It may stem from the seemingly instinctive recognition many survivors have that others simply do not want to hear, do not want to share the burden of their pain. Alternatively, survivors may fear the awful, unbearable response of being blamed by hearers for their own suffering, as is all too frequently the case for child and adult victims of rape, for example. From the position of the survivor, the obligation of neutrality on the part of official hearers creates one more circumstance in which the pain of their experiences is likely to be reinforced rather than relieved.

Again, if we are not willing or able to change our conception of justice, nor its procedures, we will not change this fundamental picture of what it means to witness, on the part of both those who give testimony of abuses and those who are charged with hearing it in an official capacity. Nevertheless, there are lessons to be learned once again from examining the testimony of children. Specifically, the accommodations that are made for children are also possible for adults. If we recognize that some adults who are traumatized are regressed in certain ways so that their needs are more like those of children, then we can also see that similar accommodations for them are not only possible, but in some cases may be the only humane option. If severely traumatized children should be protected by a simple screen from the fear, the mental and emotional disruption of being directly challenged in a public setting by those accused of their violation, why would we not think this could be appropriate for some adults as well? At the very least, it seems obvious that, as we have come to understand appropriate for some children, allowing the physical presence of a trusted, supportive advocate, a truly listening other for adult testifiers, is a change that could easily be made in our justice system without sacrificing anything we genuinely need.

6 Conclusion

It is a deeply distressing fact of the world that abuses and atrocities occur all too frequently. Their effects can be enormous: life-shattering, self-destroying, and reality-changing, for adults as well as for children. My argument here has been that there are lessons for us to take from work that has been done on understanding how to aid children in giving testimony, lessons that can be broadened to apply to traumatized persons of any chronological age. Grown-ups are not safe from any of these effects of trauma; they are not proof against the human body's and mind's frantic attempts to protect the self by insulating it from understanding what has been done. Consequently, it can be seen that the needs of some adults in response to trauma become like those of children; some adults lose their typical adult functioning in the face of assaults that no one should have to undergo.

Because we acknowledge a heightened responsibility to care for children due to the relatively uncontroversial assumption that they are not fully developed and thus not fully able to care for themselves, we find it comparatively easy to accept that for them, telling their stories as part of a therapeutic process is vastly different from giving official testimony. The idea that children need to be supported and aided through the process of testifying to their ordeals in a therapeutic setting is nearly self-evident (though not entirely so, as indicated by, for example, ongoing public reluctance to admit to the prevalence of child sexual abuse and the seriousness of its effects). As I have shown, children's inabilities to understand abuses against them, their difficulties in speaking clearly or coherently about those abuses, and their struggles in recovering, in re-constructing a healthy self, are well documented by those who work with them on these sometimes overwhelming tasks.

Further, I have argued that the term 'testimony' has very different meanings and discourses for different settings. On the one hand, when it is used in a therapeutic setting, it refers to the speaking survivors do in the attempt to re-construct their lives and re-order their reality; in short, to recover and heal. To be successful, this kind of speaking works to help survivors gain control over the traumatizing events and integrate them into their lives, repairing to whatever extent possible the damage done. This kind of telling cannot be successful, however, without the engaged participation of a listening other who responds and supports sympathetically, enabling 'healing through the communicative and distancing power of naming' the abuse, the pain, the wrongness, and helping to create a perspective that can encompass all of this within the context of a life, rather than allowing it to continue controlling that life.[51]

Testimony for justice, however, functions according to a very different set of criteria and expectations. Because justice is generally believed to rely on impartiality and neutrality, the telling that is considered appropriate for it must be straightforward, coherent, and non-metaphorical. It must need no interpretation; its meaning should be evident. For many survivors, this kind of testimony cannot be achieved without a dissociation from the experience that may well be unhealthy. That is, testimony for justice may work against the survivor's efforts at healing. Further, justice does not formally allow for a listening other; its hearers are also enjoined to dissociate in order to achieve the neutrality entailed in its conception.

Given these points, it is incumbent upon us to note two others: one, that if it becomes necessary for a child to give testimony in an official setting, that setting must be adjusted so as to make it as supportive as possible, and as little damaging as possible. Recent reforms in American and British courts, for example, indicate that this obligation is being taken seriously. The second point is, though, that if the experiences of adults and children in trauma are so very similar, then we must assume that their experiences of testifying to trauma may also be similar. If that is the case, then it appears fitting that we recognize for *all* trauma survivors a heightened duty to care, based not on age, but on what we know about how trauma is likely to affect those who suffer it.

I have not at any point intended to suggest that justice is a bad pursuit; quite to the contrary, given that abuses and atrocities are committed, we continue to need justice as a venue for seeking restoration from them and, hopefully, the cessation of future instances. I acknowledge as well that for some, testifying for justice creates a sense of closure or retribution that is gratifying and contributes to a stronger sense of self. What is indicated in my position is that the character of our conceptualization of justice means that testifying for its purposes can create a further ordeal for survivors, and that this may be counterproductive for their long-term projects of healing and recovery. I propose, then, that we take seriously what we have learned from our commitments to helping children and apply those lessons to the circumstances of testimony for traumatized persons of any age, should such support and assistance be called for.

51 Culbertson, 'Embodied Memory', 180.

Bibliography

Abu-Shalal, Ali. 'Torture at Abu Graib: The Full Sworn Testimony of Ali Shalal'. Transcribed by *Global Research*, February 2007. Viewed on 22 January 2015. http://www.globalresearch.ca/torture-at-abu-ghraib-the-full-sworn-testimony-of-ali-shalal/4865.

Agamben, Giorgio. *Remnants of Auschwitz: The Witness and the Archive*. New York: Zone Books, 1999.

Alayarian, Aida. *Trauma, Torture and Dissociation: A Psychoanalytic View*. London: Karnac Books, 2011.

Brison, Susan J. *Aftermath: Violence and the Remaking of a Self*. Princeton, NJ: Princeton University Press, 2002.

Corwin, David L. 'An Interview with Roland Summit'. *Critical Issues in Child Sexual Abuse: Historical, Legal and Psychological Perspectives*, ed. by Jon R. Conte, 1–26. Thousand Oaks, California: Sage Publications, 2002.

Cubilié, Anne. *Women Witnessing Terror: Testimony and the Cultural Politics of Human Rights*. New York: Fordham University Press, 2005.

Culbertson, Roberta. 'Embodied Memory, Transcendence and Telling: Recounting Trauma, Re-establishing the Self'. *New Literary History* 26.1 (1995) 169–195.

Derrida, Jacques. *Writing and Difference*. New York: Routledge, 1981.

Domínguez Muñozcano, Porfirio. 'Testimony of Torture Victim in Oaxaca'. Transcribed by Rights Action. *UpsideDownWorld*, January 8, 2007. Viewed on 22 January, 2015. http://upsidedownworld.org/main/mexico-archives-79/574-testimony-of-torture-victim-in-oaxaca.

Fellows, Mary Louise and Beverly Balos. 'Guilty of the Crime of Trust: Nonstranger Rape'. *Minnesota Law Review* 75 (1991). 599–617.

Freyd, Jennifer J. 'Memory and Dimensions of Trauma: Terror May Be "All-Too-Well Remembered" and Betrayal Buried'. *Critical Issues in Child Sexual Abuse: Historical, Legal and Psychological Perspectives*, edited by Jon R. Conte, 139–174. Thousand Oaks, California: Sage Publications, 2002.

Friedman, Richard D. and Stephen J. Ceci. 'The Child Quasi Witness'. *The University of Chicago Law Review* 82.1 (Winter 2015): 89–111.

Heberer, Patricia. *Children during the Holocaust*. Lanham: AltaMira Press, 2011.

Held, Virginia. *The Ethics of Care: Personal, Political and Global*. New York: Oxford University Press, 2007.

Herman, Judith. *Trauma and Recovery: The Aftermath of Violence – from Domestic Abuse to Political Terror*. New York: Basic Books, 1992.

Myers, John E. B. 'Adjudication of Child Sexual Abuse Cases'. *The Future of Children* 4(2), (Summer-Autumn 1994): 84–101.

Noddings, Nel. *Caring: A Feminine Approach to Ethics and Moral Education.* Oakland, CA: University of California Press, 2003.

Paz-Alonso, Pedro M., Christine M. Ogle, Gail S. Goodman. 'Children's Memory in "Scientific Case Studies" of Child Sexual Abuse: A Review'. *Applied Issues in Investigative Interviewing, Eyewitness Memory, and Credibility Assessment*, edited by Barry S. Cooper, Dorothee Griesel, and Marguerite Ternes, 143–171. New York: Springer, 2013.

Peterson, Carole and Brenda Parsons. 'Interviewing Former 1- and 2-Year Olds about Medical Emergencies 5 Years Later'. *Law and Human Behavior* 29.6 (Dec. 2005) 743–54.

Santos, Cristina, Adriana Spahr and Tracy Crowe Morey. '1st Global Conference – Testimony, Truth, Trauma, Memory, Engagement'. *Inter-Disciplinary.Net.* Viewed on 2 May 2016. https://www.facebook.com/events/475985079187816/. Conference announcement.

Scarry, Elaine. *The Body in Pain: The Making and Unmaking of the World.* New York: Oxford University Press, 1985.

Terr, Lenore. *Too Scared to Cry: How Trauma Affects Children … and Ultimately Us All.* New York: Basic Books, 1990.

Tronto, Joan. *Moral Boundaries: A Political Argument for an Ethic of Care.* New York: Routledge, 1993.

PART 3

Scripts and Performances of Testimony

CHAPTER 7

Trauma and Healing in Izzeldin Abuelaish's *I Shall Not Hate*

Marwa Sayed Hanafy

Abstract

The testimony *I Shall Not Hate* by Izzeldin Abuelaish, a Gazan doctor, published in 2010 can be read as an insight to his personal trauma losing three daughters and a niece in the Israeli incursion of Gaza Strip in 2009. It can also be read collectively as an insight to the Palestinian predicament under the Israeli occupation. But the true worth of the testimony, in my opinion, lies in the fact that it reflects the author's ways to continuously and relentlessly redeem his loss and recover from his personal trauma. Not only that, he also innovates modes of survival, adaptation and reconciliation that rendered him not immune to occurrences of trauma but less influenced by its devastating consequences. Recovering from trauma in the testimony represents a pattern that can be traced and analysed. The complexity of the testimony is revealed in the forward of the text written by an Israeli doctor, a dear friend and a colleague to the Palestinian author, and dedicated to his late three daughters killed by an Israeli tank. This chapter will focus on modes of healing and recovery from trauma adopted by the author in his testimony on the one hand and will focus on its value as a literary text on the other hand. The Gazan author uses his position as both a doctor and a trauma survivor in order to send a message of peace to the world that coexistence and reconciliation are possible only when Palestinian rights are recognized, respected and granted. The testimony stands on the border line between the author's two tendencies to remember and to forgive and offers the reader alternatives worthy of reconsideration.

Keywords

trauma – healing and recovery – testimony – survival – Palestinian – rights

 | DOI:10.1163/9789004391130_009

1 Questions of Trauma

Trauma is defined by Dena Rosenbloom and Mary Beth Williams as 'a bodily or mental injury usually caused by an external agent'[1] which means that it is an 'injury' that can either be physical or psychological or both interchangeably. The definition also refers to the idea of an 'external agent' which reveals the irresponsibility of the trauma subject to his/her present state of trauma. If seriously considered, the idea of 'external agent' refutes the sense of guilt transplanted in the psyche of the traumatized person and greatly obstructs ways to healing and recovery. A similar emphasis on the concept of 'injury' in Trauma Studies whether physical or psychological is stated as follows:

> Trauma, from the Greek word "wound," refers to the self-altering, even self-shattering experience of violence, injury, and harm. Crucial to the experience of trauma are the multiple difficulties that arise in trying to articulate it.[2]

The negativity of the trauma experience resides in its impact on the entity of the trauma subject which results in inherent feelings of imbalance. Accordingly, the person before trauma utterly differs from that after trauma. Relevant to the painful occurrences of trauma is the difficulty to retrospect and express feelings during or after trauma. Articulating the trauma necessitates the act of remembering which is equally painful to the occurrence of trauma. Accordingly, Judith Herman states in the introduction of her book, *Trauma and Recovery*, that '[r]emembering and telling the truth about terrible events are prerequisites both for the restoration of the social order and for the healing of individual victims'.[3] Consequently, though the trauma subject resorts to forgetting, as a way to protect him/herself from the painful experience of trauma, and believes in the productivity of that strategy, trauma studies assert the opposite: remembering becomes a strategy for both healing and recovery. This final point is what makes testimonial literature of great importance as it sheds light on the subjects of trauma who were able to surmount that difficulty of articulation to producing testimonies that contribute to the understanding of the trauma

1 Dena Rosenbloom and Mary Beth Williams, *Life after Trauma: A Workbook for Healing* (New York: Guilford Press, 1999), 17.

2 Leigh Gilmore, *The Limits of Autobiography: Trauma and Testimony* (Ithaca: Cornell University Press, 2001), 6.

3 Judith Herman, 'Introduction' to *Trauma and Recovery: The Aftermath of Violence – From Domestic Abuse to Political Terror* (New York: Basic Books, 1997), 1.

experience, whether to its subjects or scholars, from multiple disciplines or even the general public. Testimony is therefore defined by Herman as follows:

> Testimony names both a discursive demand in self-representation and the knot of resistance with which it contends: one is both abjured to speak and exposed to scrutiny, but the demand may be met with some degree of agency.[4]

Consequently testimonies act as the bridge between 'self-altering' and 'self-shattering' experiences resulting from trauma to an act of resistance that aims at 'self-representation' which most probably leads to a degree of balance if not to healing and recovery. According to Edward Said, Arabic literature always 'boasts a genre of Palestinian, so called "resistance" writing, which means a writing of self-assertion and of resistance to anonymity, political oppression, and so on'[5] and Arabic literature 'does not have an ample secular tradition of autobiographical or confessional writing'.[6] That statement has been altered thanks to a number of Palestinian writers who began the tradition of autobiographies and memoirs such as Mourid Barghouti's *I Saw Ramallah* (2002) and its sequel *I Was Born There I Was Born Here* (2012). Therefore, Abuelaish's testimony rises to occupy a prominent place in Palestinian literature written in English and when translated into Arabic adds to a tradition that is not primarily Arabic but rather western.

2 Analysis

The work of Izzeldin Abuelaish (1955-), *I Shall Not Hate*, is the author's testimony to what had occurred to him and his family during the Israeli incursion of Gaza Strip in 2009. Published one year after losing his three daughters and his niece, the testimony also brings into focus the life of Palestinians under the Israeli occupation from 1948 till 2009. The author is a Palestinian doctor and a loving father of eight children who managed to survive a sequence of traumatic events inflicted on him and his family primarily by Israeli occupation and managed to carve his own niche in how to face trauma on both the personal and collective levels. This chapter attempts to explore Abuelaish's testimony

4 Ibid., 43.
5 Edward W. Said, *The Question of Palestine* (New York: Vintage Books, 1992), 155.
6 Ibid., 155.

by answering two central questions: Why and how does the author surmount feelings of hatred assumed by his positionality as a Palestinian refugee living under occupation? Attempts to answer these questions mark the core of Abuelaish's journey from trauma to healing and recovery.

The analysis adopts a chronological order of investigating the various traumas faced by the author as a way to trace the development of his varying modes of dealing with trauma until he eventually achieves the conclusive stages of healing and recovery. However, this chronological order does not necessarily reflect the author's way of constructing his own narrative. In tracing trauma in the writing of Abuelaish, it is evident how historical trauma is intertwined with personal trauma. Leigh Gilmore points out that trauma:

> 'is never exclusively personal; it always exists within complicated histories that combine harm and pleasure, along with less inflected dimensions of everyday life. Remembering trauma entails contextualizing it with history'.[7]

To begin, the Israeli occupation of Palestine in 1948, or what is known as the *Nakba*/the Catastrophe, led to the displacement of Abuelaish's family from their native village, Houg.[8] The family's decision to leave was initiated by the news of massacres committed by forces of occupation in neighbouring villages and therefore the decision was meant to provide safety to the members of the family. This act of displacement is comprehensible taken into consideration that:

> [a]t the moment of trauma, the victim is rendered helpless by overwhelming force ... When the force is that of human beings, we speak of atrocities. Traumatic events overwhelm the ordinary systems of care that give people a sense of control, connection and meaning.[9]

The author never sees his native village and he only recollects its memory from childhood stories as he was born seven years after the family's displacement. The family members moved to Gaza city assuming their displacement to be temporary which proved to be a false assumption. A way to challenge amnesia, whether personal or collective, the author recounts that:

---

7 Gilmore, *The Limits of Autobiography*, 31.

8 Izzeldin Abuelaish, *I Shall Not Hate: A Gaza Doctor's Journey on the Road to Peace and Human Dignity* (New York: Walker & Company, 2011), 31.

9 Herman, *Trauma and Recovery*, 33.

> My father never gave up the ownership papers of his farm. Even today, though the land at Houg is known as the Sharon Farm and Ariel Sharon is listed as the owner, the deed and tax papers stay with me.[10]

The author still keeps official documents that confirm his rights to his father's lands defying the assumption of David Ben-Gurion (1886–1973), the first prime minister of Israel (1948), of Palestinians' short-term memory when he states that '[t]he old will die and the new generations will forget'[11]—yet, the new generation still fully remembers. Though the author was not an eye-witness to that first trauma in his family history, it holds a great significance as it introduced him to the initial familial trauma. Furthermore, he experienced its repercussions as he was born a refugee destined to suffer grinding poverty and inhuman conditions at the refugee camp. It is worth emphasizing that the trauma of Abuelaish's family holds a historical significance as it represents the trauma of millions of other Palestinian families that went through the same yet different experience of displacement:

> Yet as Tolstoy said about families, that happy ones were all the same and unhappy ones were each different in their unhappiness, the individual Palestinian trauma seems one out of 3 ½ million variations on the same theme.[12]

In other words, the trauma of *Nakba* becomes paradoxical in nature in so far as it groups all Palestinians together in one crucible of anguish and pain and different in so far as it shapes and reshapes the life of every individual.

The second trauma was instigated by the Arab Defeat in June 1967 known as *Naksah*/'setback'.[13] This time the author, who was only twelve years old, is an eye-witness and fully recollects scenes of invasion of his refugee camp:

> Israeli tanks rolled onto our street. The shelling, the shooting, and the fires breaking out all over the camp were utterly terrifying. Parents were fleeing, some leaving their children behind.[14]

---

10 Abuelaish, *I Shall Not Hate*, 32.

11 Ibid., 33.

12 Said, *The Question of Palestine*, 115.

13 Abuelaish, *I Shall Not Hate*, 53.

14 Ibid., 53.

The Israeli occupation of Gaza concretized for the author the meaning of trauma which according to Cathy Caruth 'describes an overwhelming experience of sudden or catastrophic events'.[15] This time the author fully grasps trauma first hand which 'inevitably brings loss' and which is concretized in the personal loss of his family's house that was demolished by forces of occupation.[16] Abuelaish's family was overcome by feelings of helplessness because now they are not only refugees but they were rendered homeless refugees: 'I had seen the destruction of my home, and to this day those images stay with me, but hate has never been part of my repertoire'.[17] For the second time, Ariel Sharon, who was the Israeli military commander of Gaza, ordered his forces to bulldoze hundreds of Palestinian houses as the roads were not wide enough for his tanks. The author recalls that: '[t]here wasn't a thing we could do. The level of inhumanity was astonishing, and it stayed with me to this day'.[18]

Instead of hate, survival and adaptation to the new reality imposed by trauma caused by 1967 *Naksah* obliged Abuelaish to redeem that personal loss by working for an Israeli family on a farm called Moshav Hodaia, near the town of Ashqelon. Therefore, at a young age (almost twelve years old), he was able to develop what Dena Rosenbloom and Mary Beth Williams call 'coping strategies'[19] which entail

> any effort that makes a hardship easier to bear … For trauma survivors, the hardships can extend beyond the event to the troubling reactions that follow. You may feel it is not possible to go on at times, yet you are finding ways to get through the day, the week, the months, and even the years.[20]

These 'coping strategies' enabled the author to shift his focus from subsequent traumas and obliged him to find a way to face them. He was able to earn enough money; when added to his mother's savings he was able to buy his family a new house and became a source of pride to his family.

The experience of working for an Israeli family was informative to the author in another way. Abuelaish expected the haughty attitude of the occupier he heard about and eye-witnessed during his life under occupation from the

15 Cathy Caruth, *Unclaimed Experience: Trauma, Narrative, and History* (Baltimore: John Hopkins University Press, 1996), 11.
16 Herman, *Trauma and Recovery*, 188.
17 Abuelaish, *I Shall Not Hate*, 62.
18 Ibid., 59.
19 Rosenbloom and Williams, *Life after Trauma*, 18.
20 Ibid., 33.

Israeli family. But contrary to his expectations, he found a fair treatment and 'so much kindness'.[21] He was able to draw a line between Israelis as human beings and Israelis as occupiers which he learned from the 'paradox between the warm hospitality of the Israeli family' and 'the brute force of Sharon's Israeli soldiers' and therefore 'made [him] recognize that [he] had to commit [himself] to finding a peaceful bridge between the divides'.[22] He remained grateful to that family even after becoming a well-known doctor and he even paid them a visit several years after to express his appreciation: 'I wanted to show them the affection, even love, I had for them'.[23] The love he deliberately shows the Israeli family manifests his utter rejection of feelings of hatred the subsequent traumatic occurrences might have placed in him.

However, the episode of working for an Israeli family is also revealing in so far as it shows how trauma of occupation exerted pressure on Palestinian children who were forced to work while they were supposed to be in schools. The author used to work and study simultaneously in order to create a balance between his rights as a child and what he is obliged to do as a Palestinian refugee. Although he shows a great deal of perseverance and patience in compromising his two roles, at certain points of his life he feels the futility of his endeavours at school:

> Why was I bothering with school when we were occupied and the future seemed so bleak? I was older now and better understood the consequences of occupation. My school grades notwithstanding, I began to question whether there really was a way out of this turmoil. Also, my family desperately needed any money I could earn, and I was good at finding jobs. Why shouldn't I just try to make life a little easier for my family? As the eldest boy, it was my job to provide. Perhaps I should give up on my dream of improving our lives through education.[24]

Consequently, Abuelaish decides to give up on his school education while only twelve years old and spend his time in finding jobs to be able to afford the essential needs of his family. It is important to take into consideration the 'age at the time of the trauma' as one of the decisive factors that influenced the author's decision to neglect his studies at that early stage of his life.[25] However,

---

21 Abuelaish, *I Shall Not Hate*, 58.

22 Ibid., 62.

23 Ibid., 88.

24 Ibid., 55.

25 Rosenbloom and Williams, *Life after Trauma*, 18.

other factors contributed to his retreat from that decision and these were the 'social and cultural relationships, previous coping strategies, availability of support before, during and following the traumatic experiences'.[26] At that crucial point, Abuelaish was grateful to his Palestinian teachers 'for being relentless in their encouragement to stay in school'.[27] Another incident that positively influenced his life was his stay as a patient suffering from arthritis in Al-Shifa hospital. There, he was introduced to the Palestinian medical community and how helpful they were to their patients. These two incidents in particular provided the author with an insight into how crucial his studies were and, most importantly, provided him with hope for a better future.

Through further developing his 'coping strategies' and through the continuous support he received from his Palestinian family, the author excelled in his studies at high school and became one of only four students in Jabalia refugee camp in Gaza to study medicine in Cairo University in Egypt. Later, he received a scholarship from the Ministry of Health in Saudi Arabia where he worked to get a diploma at the Institute of Obstetrics and Gynaecology at the University of London. He recalls:

> While studying at the University of London, I had noticed that most of the references I depended on for my thesis on fertility were by Israeli professors, so I decided to make a bold move and get in touch with the Israeli medical community to see what they were doing about infertility and to exchange ideas. Although the intifada continued apace, it didn't stop me from communicating with and eventually meeting my colleagues in Israel.[28]

Abuelaish finds no inconveniency to adhering to Israeli professors working on the same field of his specialization. He therefore was able to build on his past experience of working for an Israeli family and benefits from it in communicating with Israeli professors. Again he was able to differentiate between what is human and what is political. Abuelaish resumed his successful career in medicine as he also received a scholarship from Harvard to do a master's degree in health policy and management.[29] The above-mentioned 'bold move' acted by Abuelaish turns out to be one of his many initiatives bridging the divide between Palestinians and Israelis. He became the first

26 Ibid., 18.

27 Abuelaish, *I Shall Not Hate*, 56.

28 Ibid., 86.

29 Ibid., 105.

Palestinian doctor to study and work in a hospital in Israel. He always emphasized to his patients his identity as a Palestinian/Gazan doctor, not an Arab-Israeli one. He worked hard to earn the respect of his Israeli colleagues, professors and patients as he felt the burden of his responsibility as a representative of Palestinians in general and Gazans in particular. He patiently bore the hardships and humiliation he encountered while crossing borders between his refugee camp and Israel especially at the Erez checkpoint in order to achieve his goal. He says:

> People often tell me they admire my patience and ability to be calm and avoid rash and impulsive behaviour. I tell them I learned all of it while waiting in line at the Erez checkpoint.[30]

Moreover, he voluntarily developed his unofficial diplomatic role as a peace envoy between the two nations as he frequently invited his Israeli friends to his refugee camp to witness the injustices and humiliation suffered by the Palestinians and the inhuman conditions imposed on them by the occupation. He states:

> I did my share of pushing the envelope for coexistence even then by acting as an unofficial peace envoy for the region: I would host groups of Israelis at my home or in the homes of my friends one weekend every month. We toured the Jabalia refugee camp and Gaza City, showed them the conditions people live in, let them experience the overcrowding, and allowed plenty of time so they could talk to people, ask their own questions, and draw their own conclusions. Then we'd have coffee and sweets together – all of us, the Israelis and the Palestinians. We'd discuss, and we'd argue. These get-togethers brought home to me how similar we are when it comes to socializing.[31]

These get-togethers serve multiple purposes. First they offer the two parties the opportunity to deal with each other on a common ground of humanity separate from what is propagated by politicians. In doing so, the author offers a practical solution through face to face encounter that departs from ideal/idle talking. It is interesting how he bridged the divide even through language when he used 'we' and 'us' grouping Palestinians and Israelis together. To bring

30 Ibid., 103.

31 Ibid., 94.

Israelis to witness the suffering of the Palestinians is to bring into the Israeli focus the issue of Palestine.

The author offers to his Israeli friends the space to observe, think, question and come up with conclusions. In his interactive unique way, he casts light on the Palestinian cause and he asks for coexistence based on doing justice to Palestinians. He emphasizes:

> The thing is, you cannot ask people to coexist by having one side bow their heads and rely on a solution that is only good for the other side. What you can do is stop blaming each other and engage in dialogue with one person at a time. Everyone knows that violence begets violence and breeds more hatred. We need to find our way together.[32]

In recovering from the previous traumas caused by occupation, Izzeldin Abuelaish managed to successfully implement 'coping strategies' that enabled him to challenge not only his personal traumas (both caused by the *Nakba* and the *Naksah*) but those of Palestinians. In tracing and analysing the sincere efforts of the author, it is evident that he achieved many of the positive outcomes of a healing and recovery phase. These positive outcomes or 'benefits' of trauma as named by Dena Rosenbloom and Mary Beth Williams are best represented in the following: first 'recognizing your strengths'[33] which denotes that the trauma survivor: 'may find that [he/she] have gained new knowledge, insight, or wisdom from [his/her] experience'.[34] This is reflected in the author's unique insight into his ability to surmount the every-day obstacles imposed on him as a Palestinian refugee and his ability to achieve his dreams as a successful doctor. Second, there is this ability in 'bringing your life into focus'[35] which signifies how 'priorities in life can shift'[36] and proves to be true as Abuelaish shifts his focus from hate to efforts of reconciliation in one of the complicated conflicts in the world. Third, there is 'achieving emotional freedom'[37] which surmounts negative feelings to the positivity of self-expression and brings forth 'relief and allows more closeness in [...] relationships'[38] which is evident in

32 Ibid., 101.
33 Rosenbloom and Williams, *Life after Trauma*, 317.
34 Ibid., 317–318.
35 Ibid., 319.
36 Ibid.
37 Ibid.
38 Ibid.

the peacefulness the author enjoys with both Palestinians and Israelis. Finally there is the search for 'a greater meaning'[39] and in the case of Abuelaish, he managed to enjoy these benefits collectively. He stresses:

> As a physician who has practiced in Israel and Gaza, I see medicine as the bridge between us, just as education and friendship have been bridges. We all know what to do, so who is stopping us? Who is holding up the barrier between our two sides? We need to reach each other by embracing one another's realities, sending messages of tolerance rather than intolerance and healing instead of hate.[40]

In spite of all his sincere efforts and relentless endeavours, Abuelaish has to face the most harrowing tragedies of his life which is the shelling of his house during the Israeli incursion of Gaza Strip in 16 January 2009 and the killing of his three daughters, Bessan, Mayar, Aya, and his niece Noor. This same event fatally injured other members of his family including his daughter Shatha, his brother Shehab and his niece Ghaida. Abuelaish's instant feelings after this trauma were aired on the Israeli television after he called his Israeli friend Shlomi Eldar, a TV presenter, to stop the attack on Abuelaish's house. The author was able to instantly act in order to save other surviving members of his family and thus reduce the impact of trauma. That act of telephoning, whether conscious or unconscious is derived from the author's past experience of being exposed to a series of traumatic events. He is able to act in the moment of trauma with great efficiency instead of being obstructed by what had happened. This is how the author testifies his trauma directly after the moment of its occurrence:

> I wondered who could help us, who could get us out of this catastrophe. Then I realized I still had a connection to the outside world. I called Shlomi Eldar, but the call went to his voice mail. I left a message: "YaRabbi, YaRabbi – my God, my God – they shelled my house. They killed my daughters. What have we done?" all I could think was: This is the end. This is the end.[41]

39 Ibid., 320.

40 Abuelaish, *I Shall Not Hate*, 101.

41 Ibid., 177.

The author narrated how he performed all the necessary precautions during the Israeli war on Gaza by keeping his children together in a safe space inside their house, how he communicated with the outside Israeli mass media to report the massive destruction they were subjected to, how he tried his best to keep calm among his children who have recently lost their mother dying from acute leukaemia, how they tried to perform the daily chores including studying for exams, and how they planned to travel abroad to Toronto, Canada the moment the war ended. The author and his eight children were clinging to hope till the very last moment before the shelling of their house. Similar to witnessing the demolishing of his house as a young boy several years ago, he now witnesses the destruction of his house and the death of his daughters for no comprehensible reasons.

His voice in the Israeli television and the way he articulated his trauma can be interpreted in Trauma Studies as follows:

> Witnesses as well as victims are subject to the dialectic of trauma. It is difficult to remain clearheaded and calm, to see more than a few fragments of the picture at one time, to retain all the pieces, and to fit them together. It is even more difficult to find a language that conveys fully and persuasively what one has seen.[42]

The author's fragmented articulation of trauma reflects the complexity of orally testifying the trauma especially at the moment of its occurrence. Pertinent to the issue of articulating the trauma is the issue of faith in times of traumas. It is evident how the author named 'God' directly after the atrocity he witnessed which reflects that his deep faith in God was not at all shaken. It is presumed in Trauma Studies that trauma can also attack one's belief in God as:

> [t]raumatized people feel utterly abandoned, utterly alone, cast out of the human and divine systems of care and protection that sustain life. Thereafter, a sense of alienation, of disconnection, pervades every relationship, from the most intimate familial bonds to the most abstract affiliations of community and religion. When trust is lost, traumatized people feel that they belong more to the dead than to the living.[43]

42 Herman, 'Introduction' to *Trauma and Recovery*, 2.

43 Herman, *Trauma and Recovery*, 52.

Contrary to the assumptions mentioned above, the author's attachment to God is strengthened after the attack and it holds him together from falling apart. This was primarily because he is a strong believer as he repeatedly emphasized throughout the testimony and also through the faith of his son. He finds comfort in the words of his thirteen-year-old son who survived the brutal attack and saved his devastated father at that crucial moment: 'He told me not to be sad, that his sisters were happy and with their mother. He meant this; it came from the depths of his faith'.[44] The young boy succeeded to anchor his father at that peculiar time of desolation and despair. The son's sincere words rightly placed the devastated father on the road to healing and recovery. In addition, the author received the communal support from both the Palestinians and the Israelis at the moment of trauma (losing his three daughters and his niece and the injury of other members of his family). With the help of his Israeli friend Shlomi Eldar, the Israeli tank drove away from Abuelaish's house and instantly ceased fire. Eldar also managed to send ambulances to the nearest zone to Abuelaish's house to carry the injured to hospitals in Israel. The Palestinians in the neighbouring refugee camps hurried to reach Abuelaish's house with stretchers to carry the wounded to the awaiting ambulances while others kept the surviving children with them. All these factors contributed to relatively reduce the drastic consequences of the trauma caused by the Israeli's attack of the author's house in 2009. However, the author faced three main questions: 'Why did this happen to us? /And what am I going to do about it? / what am I to do to make sense of this?'[45]

In recovering from the 2009 trauma, Abuelaish was able to surmount the negativity of the tragic event and achieved its positive outcomes or what Rosenbloom and Williams call 'benefits' or 'gifts'[46] of the process of healing. He was thankful to the fact that he was with his children during the Israeli incursion of Gaza Strip and not working in the hospital in Tel Aviv. He was equally grateful to the fact that both his mother and his wife passed away before witnessing such a devastating trauma.[47] He also valued the notion that though he lost three children, he still enjoys the company of the other five.[48] He was satisfied that his children and he had previously decided to leave for Canada in order to hold the family together away from the political tension and recurrent wars. Moving to

44 Abuelaish, *I Shall Not Hate*, 178.

45 Ibid., 190–191.

46 Rosenbloom and Williams, *Life after Trauma*, 322.

47 Abuelaish, *I Shall Not Hate*, 192.

48 Ibid., 232.

Canada marked a new beginning to the author and his remaining children. He regarded Canada his 'new home' where he was welcomed together with his children in their neighbourhood, schools and universities.[49] In Canada, he found the communal support and psychological therapy he and his children needed. He was honoured worldwide as he received various prestigious awards and was even nominated for the Nobel Prize in 2010. He founded a philanthropic organization under the name 'Daughters for Life' to honour the memory of his daughters and to empower girls and women in the Middle East.[50]

However, the way to healing and recovery was incomplete as the author expected the Israeli government to apologize for the atrocities they have committed against his family by killing his three daughters and his niece and by destroying his house—but they did not. Neither did they offer any reparation to compensate his loss. The compensation Abuelaish asks for is intended to finance his philanthropic organization. To that end, the testimony of Desmond Tutu, the South African Noble Laureate and the peace activist, is found to be very helpful in grasping Abuelaish's request for apology and reparation. Tutu was part of the process of reconciliation in South Africa after the end of the apartheid. There were different ways to establish communal peace among South Africans and one of these ways was financial compensation. He says:

> The commissioners deliberately tried to avoid using the word "compensation." We agreed that there was no way in which anyone could claim to compensate, for instance, a family for the brutal murder of their beloved husband, father, and breadwinner. There is no way really of computing the devastation of such a loss. Moreover, if we were to try to compensate them, would victims be eligible for the same compensation for the kind of loss despite all kinds of difference in circumstances? There our recommendations to the President and Parliament provided that a sum of money reasonably significant in amount would be paid to those designated as victims, but that it would be acknowledged that it was really meant to be symbolic rather than substantial. It was a way the nation sought to say, in effect, to victims: We acknowledge that you suffered a gross violation of your rights. Nothing can ever replace your loved one. But as a nation we are saying, we are sorry, we have opened the wounds of your suffering and sought to cleanse them; this reparation is as balm, an ointment, being poured over the wounds to assist in their healing.[51]

49 Ibid., 208.

50 Ibid., 223.

51 Desmond Tutu, *No Future without Forgiveness* (New York: Doubleday, 2000), 61.

It is evident that the issue of compensation is problematic starting from its naming to its modes of implementation. However, it is a necessary prerequisite to redeem the loss and accomplish healing and recovery. Tutu's metaphoric use of medical constituents as 'balm,' 'ointment,' and the 'wound' directly intersects with Abuelaish's medical position as a doctor and gives more emphasis and credibility to the latter's call for reparation. It is clear that what is applicable in the case of South Africans is difficult to achieve in the case of Palestinians if not impossible.

The only Israeli apology Abuelaish received was an unofficial one and it was a poem written by Anael Harpaz, an Israeli woman who met three of the author's daughters at a peace camp they attended in the US several years ago. Harpaz wrote a poem in March 2009 entitled 'Where Love Resides ... in memory of Bessan'.[52] The poem is addressed not only to the late Bessan but also describes Harpaz's experience with the injured members of Abuelaish's family in an Israeli hospital after the attack and confirms the idea of the absence of feelings of revenge, hatred, or anger among its members. She writes:

> I heard no words of revenge
> nor hatred
> I heard no anger I heard the deep belief
> that peace is possible
> even with this enormous loss
> I have been strengthened
> from their strength
> I am more determined
> from their determination
> I am more at peace
> from their peacefulness[53]

It is not an easy task to prove Abuelaish's affirmation that he shall not hate after suffering the previously mentioned traumatic events and it requires a lot of effort to do so. But Harpaz's poem renders attempts of asserting the credibility of Abuelaish's testimony easier. Harpaz, in her poem, asks for forgiveness for what her people have done to the innocent family of Bessan and feels guilty for not being able to save the innocent child from that dreadful end.

52 Abuelaish, *I Shall Not Hate*, 199.

53 Ibid., 201.

The artistic expression of apology by Harpaz is part of *I Shall not Hate*, the artistic work of art written by Abuelaish which I regard as one of the outstanding 'benefits' of trauma. His testimony is written in English, in my opinion, to address a western and world-wide readership and is meant to 'inspire people' to act positively in order to promote world peace.[54] It is written with great passion reflecting Abuelaish's multiple voices as a loving father and husband, Palestinian refugee, peace envoy, and dedicated physician. The title of the testimony addresses the emotions and feelings of the readers and shatters any conceived pre-conceptions about the Palestinian-Israeli conflict and invites a new reading of its political and social contexts. The subject pronoun 'I' emphasizes the individuality and uniqueness of the author's positionality among both parties; whether Palestinians or Israelis. The pronoun 'I' also serves as the cry that has to be raised above persistent calls of wars and military excellence practiced by the occupier over the natives. The author is both the subject and survivor of subsequent traumas and meanwhile acts as the therapist to his wounded self and to these of his surviving children. The rest of the title 'Shall Not Hate' reveals a determinacy of the author to confront not only his feelings of rage, anger and hatred as a direct subject of a series of traumatic events caused primarily by the Israeli occupation but also serves as his message to both Palestinians and Israelis to control mutual feelings of hate that blind both parties' perception of the other on one hand and hinder possibilities of coexistence on the other hand. However, the title of the testimony can be misleading in so far as it can presumably suggest reconciliation based upon forgetfulness and amnesia and the book is replete with memories of the traumatic events suffered by the Palestinians throughout their history sending a message that to forgive is not necessarily to forget.

In scripting the trauma, the structure of the testimony is very important. It is divided into a dedication, a foreword, a map, nine chapters, an epilogue and acknowledgements. The dedication is for the memory of his parents, wife, and murdered daughters and to children everywhere. The foreword is by the author's Israeli friend and colleague, Dr. Marek Glezerman who adopts similar convictions as Abuelaish as he believes in the possibility of coexistence between Palestinians and Israelis. The foreword, moreover, gives additional truthfulness and credibility to Abuelaish's trauma as it occasionally faces Israeli attacks of falseness. The foreword is followed by a map of the Palestinian territories and Israel in order to help the reader visualize the difficulty of life under siege and complexity of moving back and forth between Gaza and Israel.

54 Ibid., 228.

The map is followed by nine chapters, among which the first chapter holds a great significance for its artistry. The chapter's title is 'Sand and Sky' and narrates the particularities of one specific day, 12 December 2008, that the author spent with his eight children before the trauma of losing three of them during the Israeli incursion of Gaza Strip in 2009. The chapter covers a large span of the author's life through quick flashbacks.[55] In addition, the author uncovers both the private and public spheres of the life of Palestinians in Gaza Strip till he briefly concludes his chapter with the trauma of losing his daughters. As for the other chapters, the author follows a chronological order in narrating previous traumas and the 'benefits' he gained from each one. Throughout his text, Abuelaish commemorates his late daughters by giving a repeated detailed account of their precious lives before their brutal murder. In this way, he establishes his own metaphorical monuments to honour them as sacrifices on the long road to peace and justice.[56]

In the heart of the testimony, the author dedicates a few pages that contained twenty-two photos that capture the different phases of his life and revolves around the author's private and public spheres. There is a photo of the author as a university student, another with his father and brothers, a third one with his mother, a wedding photo with his late wife Nadia. There are other photos of his wife Nadia and his daughters and sons. There is a photo of his niece, Noor and another of his apartment building in Jabalia refugee camp. There are other photos that document his role as a peace envoy between Palestinians and Israelis. All these photos document the author's life before the shelling of his house in 2009. Then follows a series of photos that capture the author's house after the Israeli brutal attack and depicts the pervasive destruction. Finally there are the photos of the graveyard in Gaza where the author's daughters were buried and the photo of the author looking at the graveyard. The placement of the photos in the middle of the testimony endows it with additional truthfulness on one hand and asserts the human element of the author's cause on the other hand. The photos played an influential role as visual aids that contributed to the overall powerful impact of the testimony.

The testimony is concluded with an epilogue which expresses its main objectives. The author wants his story to act as an inspiration to promote world justice, peace and human dignity. He ends his epilogue with conclusive, short and to the point remarks which reflect his precision as a physician and can be read as his prescription to feelings of hate which he differentiates from anger.

55 Ibid., 1.

56 Ibid., 217.

He describes hate as a 'chronic, severe, destructive sickness' while anger 'can be productive' as it 'propel[s] you toward necessary action for the betterment of yourself and others'.[57] Contrary to books which begin with acknowledgements, the author places his at the very end. This placement may be due to the fact that the author is mainly concerned with telling his story. He wants to build ties between the readers and himself as well as with the members of his family then pays tribute to those already familiar figures to the reader. He thanked his Palestinian family and friends as well as his Israeli friends especially Shlomi Eldar. He also thanked people from the international community who showed support to Abuelaish's cause. He expressed his indebtedness to Canadian friends who made the publication of the testimony possible. These feelings of indebtedness can be read as signs of surmounting the trauma and moving forward on the path of healing and recovery.

To conclude, Izzeldin Abuelaish's testimony is an exceptional work that calls for the Palestinian right in peace and human dignity derived from the author's traumatic experience; both personal and historical. As a physician, he prescribes the remedy for the Palestinian wound and invites the Israelis to hold their responsibility for causing that wound and subsequently share him his sincere efforts at healing and recovery.

Bibliography

Abuelaish, Izzeldin. *I Shall Not Hate: A Gaza Doctor's Journey on the Road to Peace and Human Dignity*. New York: Walker & Company, 2011.

Caruth, Cathy. *Unclaimed Experience: Trauma, Narrative, and History*. Baltimore: John Hopkins University Press, 1996.

Gilmore, Leigh. *The Limits of Autobiography: Trauma and Testimony*. Ithaca: Cornell University Press, 2001.

Herman, Judith. 'Introduction' to *Trauma and Recovery: The Aftermath of Violence – From Domestic Abuse to Political Terror*. New York: Basic Books, 1997.

Herman, Judith. *Trauma and Recovery: The Aftermath of Violence – From Domestic Abuse to Political Terror*. New York: Basic Books, 1997.

Rosenbloom, Dena and Mary Beth Williams. *Life after Trauma: A Workbook for Healing*. New York: Guilford Press, 1999.

Said, Edward, W. *The Question of Palestine*. New York: Vintage Books, 1992.

Tutu, Desmond. *No Future without Forgiveness*. New York: Doubleday, 2000.

57 Ibid., 233.

CHAPTER 8

The 'Piercing Breach of a Border': Irish Cinema as a Mediator of Modern Trauma

Emma Kelly

Abstract

From the box office successes of *Philomena* and *'71* to lesser-known, but critically acclaimed works such as *Calvary* and *Silent Grace*, Irish cinema's sustained interest in cultural and personal trauma indicates its popularity as a topic within both the Irish film industry and wider Irish society. Recent political, social, and legal changes have provided a new space in which the telling of stories on both a personal and societal level has become possible. Consequently, Irish cinema has become an important medium through which these previously marginalised and obscured voices may be heard. Engaging with Judith Herman's theory that the emergence of stories requires a specific context, my chapter examines social, legal, and political history to establish why previously unheard voices began to emerge in the Republic of Ireland in the late 20th and early 21st centuries. Concentrating on *The Magdalene Sisters* (2002), *Philomena* (2013), and *Calvary* (2014), my chapter examines cinematic representations of those 'othered' and abjected by a society enabled by what James M. Smith terms 'Ireland's Architecture of Containment': Magdalene Laundries, Mother and Baby Homes, Reformatory Schools, and Industrial Schools. This chapter explores how these representations enabled the disintegration of the division between the free self and the institutionalised other, and how this collapse triggered society's realisation that it, too, was responsible for this trauma. Through close examination of pivotal scenes from pre-report films such *The Magdalene Sisters* (2002), directed by Peter Mullan, and post-report films such as *Philomena* (2013), directed by Stephen Frears, and *Calvary* (2014), directed by John Michael McDonagh, my chapter also examines how, if at all, Irish cinema has explored possible paths in the journey from traumatic rupture to reconciliation.

Keywords

witness – clergy – identity – testimony – Ireland – abuse – rupture – reconciliation – popular culture – aesthetics – other – abject

 | DOI:10.1163/9789004391130_010

1 Introduction

Cinema has long been considered an important and influential tool for public mass-agitation. Due to its accessibility, popularity, and social connotations, film has often been regarded not only as a medium useful for entertainment, but also education, propaganda, indoctrination, and censorship. In an Irish context, cinema's importance was underscored on 19 February 2013 when Taoiseach Enda Kenny apologised on behalf of the Irish state to the victims and survivors of Ireland's Magdalene Laundries. This apology demonstrated the truth behind a hypothesis posed by artists, authors, and filmmakers in the years prior to this apology: that the Irish State and society as well as religious orders were culpable for the incarceration and abuse of vulnerable members of society. In revealing this cultural discrepancy, the public uproar caused by documentaries such as *Sex in a Cold Climate* (1998) and *States of Fear* (1999), and films such as *The Butcher Boy* (1997), *The Magdalene Sisters* (2002), and *Song for a Raggy Boy* (2003) prompted the initial steps taken to recognise the cultural trauma caused by years of institutional abuse: the provision of an official space in the form of a government enquiry in which survivors of Ireland's architecture of containment could testify about their time spent in institutions such as industrial and reformatory schools, Magdalene Laundries, and Mother and Baby Homes; institutions created to house abandoned, orphaned, and neglected children, juvenile delinquents, and 'fallen women'. This testimony formed a vital part of the reports published by both committees, namely *The Report of the Commission to Enquire into Child Abuse* (2009) and *Report of the Inter-Departmental Committee to establish the facts of State involvement with the Magdalen Laundries* (2013). Consequently, films released after the publication of these reports, such as *Philomena* (2013) and *Calvary* (2014), consider the impact that the enquiries and subsequent reports have had on mediating this cultural trauma, culminating in an exploration of forgiveness as a possible final step in the path from traumatic rupture to reconciliation.

The Irish Free State was established in 1922 on a nationalist bedrock of conservative political and Catholic views. For the first half-century of its existence, Ireland relied on strict censorship laws to maintain its political, economic, and cultural insularity. A direct result of this censorship was that cinema, viewed suspiciously as a foreign medium, was forced to adhere to the most severe censorship rules until liberalisation began to take hold in the 1970s. This liberalization allowed Ireland's film industry to examine previously unexplored topics in Irish history. Consequently, the cinema that emerged during this early period set the precedent for the Irish film industry's particular interest in becoming a cultural channel for portraying changes on the Irish cultural landscape. Moreover, the success of films such as *The Butcher Boy* (1997), *Song For A Raggy Boy* (2003), *The Magdalene Sisters* (2002), *Philomena* (2013), and *Calvary* (2014) indicates that Irish audiences hold a particular interest in films that challenge official narratives and seek to address complex cultural, social, and political realities. This interest is examined in Emilie Pine's *The Politics of Irish Memory: Performing Remembrance in Contemporary Irish Culture*, in which she argues that this obsessive return to the past is the legacy of the opening up of Ireland's recent history by Irish remembrance culture. A direct result of this revisiting is the creation of alternate narratives that take 'account of memories that were for too long "forgotten" or side lined by Irish history and culture', and the uncovering of subjects of national importance, specifically the trauma incurred by the abuse of women and children in Ireland's architecture of containment.[1] The recognition of these narratives is extremely important as they 'expand the traditionally narrow definition of Irish historical identity and reconfigure this identity through the framework of remembrance and trauma'; an action that thwarts cultural amnesia and addresses national guilt by providing a voice to those silenced by the past.[2]

2 Church-State Collusion and Its Legacy of Abuse

The clerical abuse scandals that came to light in Irish media in the late 1980s and early 1990s were not unique to Ireland, but the nature and number of reported cases were especially severe. In her chapter in this collection, Marwa Sayed Hanafy explores the theory that trauma is 'never exclusively personal; it always exists within complicated histories [...] Remembering trauma entails contextualising it with history'. In Ireland's case, this argument certainly rings true: one of the explanations as to why more cases came to light in Ireland than any other country is due to the fact that, in twentieth-century Ireland,, Catholicism came to be synonymous with national identity. Indeed, on 12 April 1951, at the height of the scandal surrounding the Church-State argument instigated by Dr. Noël Browne's 'Mother and Child Scheme', the then-Taoiseach John A. Costello stated 'I am an Irishman second: I am a Catholic first and I accept without qualification in all respects the teaching of the Hierarchy and

1 Emilie Pine, *The Politics of Irish Memory: Performing Remembrance in Contemporary Irish Culture* (Basingstoke: Palgrave Macmillan, 2011), 3.

2 Ibid.

the Church to which I belong'.[3] The fact that the leader of the Irish people saw himself first and foremost as a servant of Rome and not of the citizens of the Republic of Ireland illustrates the extent to which Catholic doctrine dictated public and personal life in Ireland, and may help explain as to why the government deferred to the Catholic hierarchy on social issues until as recently as the early 1980s. In order to understand how the Catholic Church came to be such a powerhouse in Irish life, one must return to the decades prior to independence and examine the founding reasons that led to the creation of this post-colonial Irish identity; an identity whose influence by the Catholic Church directly resulted in the creation of Ireland's architecture of containment. Ireland's architecture of containment was not solely restricted to Magdalene Laundries and reformatory schools. Rather, it encompassed a wide variety of social institutions such as the probation services, industrial schools, mother and baby homes, adoption agencies, and various asylums. Such institutions conspired to obscure from society citizens marginalized by the social and moral 'crimes' they had committed. These individuals posed a threat to the social order of the recently created Irish Free State and blemished the new, hyper-moral Irish identity prescribed to the State's society by governmental and religious factions. However, the conditions that led to the creation of an environment suited to facilitate this ostensibly seamless homogenous society began to form decades before the establishment of the Irish Free State. In her study, *Sex and Nation: Women in Irish Culture and Politics*, Gerardine Meaney examines how colonisation gave rise to the conditions responsible for the creation of a hyper-Catholic society in which perceived immorality was grievously punished. Engaging with Ashis Nandy's theory that 'a history of colonisation is a history of feminisation', Meaney puts forward the argument that colonised people aspire, through rebellion and the claiming of independence, to assert their masculinity though the exertion of what is considered to be the traditionally masculine entity of power.[4] These actions have an extremely detrimental effect on colonised females, as the colonised males tend to exert the power granted by their masculinity over females in order to prove their capability of self-governance. This demonstration of power does not typically cease at the end of colonisation; rather, through the imposition of strict gender roles and norms, this masculine domination tends to outlive colonisation by decades. Moreover, 'anxiety about fitness for a role of authority, deriving from a history

3 Basil Chubb, *The Government & Politics of Ireland, vol. 2* (Stanford: Stanford University Press, 1970), 103.

4 Geraldine Meaney, *Sex and Nation: Women in Irish Culture and Politics* (Dublin: Attic Press, 1992), 6.

of defeat or helplessness, is assuaged by the assumption of sexual dominance'.[5] As a result, women cease being autonomous entities and instead become desexualised symbols of the nation and its identity, therefore becoming much easier to control. Preoccupied with civil war and nation building, the government of the newly formed Irish Free State therefore responded to social, political, and economic instability in a manner typical of post-revolutionary societies: it 'compensated for its inability to control much of what was happening around it by asserting its power vis-à-vis restrictions against women'.[6] These restrictions largely took their form in conservative legislation that effectively removed Irish women from public life. Various legal documents from this period reflect and emphasise the shared agenda between the Catholic Church and the Irish Free State in the creation of institutional infrastructure. This deference to the Catholic Church had a two-pronged effect for the state: it failed to assert its independence and, in doing so, relinquished responsibility for the most vulnerable in its care. By authorising what was effectively the incarceration of women and children in Ireland's architecture of containment, the Irish State secured at least the façade of a morally pure country and society. The effects of such an effacement were endured by those who operated on the margins of society and were silenced and obscured, but even those who existed within society's boundaries were trapped within a specific national image and lived under the fear of punishment should they deviate from the prescribed ideals. The ideals prescribed to women were even enshrined in Bunreacht na hÉireann 1937, the Irish Constitution, which affirmed the State's recognition that 'by her life within the home, the woman gives to the State a support without which the common good cannot be achieved'.[7] This constitutional reinforcement of the belief that women belonged in the domestic sphere served to remove them from the public realm and strip away any public identity other than that of wife and mother; terms which were largely interchangeable in the Irish Constitution.

Two considerable articles of gendered legislation passed prior to 1937 helped create the conditions ripe for such a Constitution: the 1925 Civil Service Amendment Act and the 1927 Juries Bill. Though these acts seemingly concerned women's employment in the public sector and their right to participate as part of a jury in a court of law, in actuality they served to remove women from public, political and legal life. In doing so, these bills, and the government

5 Ibid, 7.

6 Maryann Gialanella Valiulis 'Power, Gender, and Identity in the Irish Free State', *Journal of Women's History* 4.4/7 (1995): 127.

7 Irish Const. art. 41.2.1.

that passed them, perpetuated the message that women were not to enter the public domain. Women were thus banished to the realm of the domestic, with their roles restricted to duties such as housekeeping and child rearing. The hypothesis that the government used legal means to control the lives of women is further evidenced after an examination of *The Carrigan Report* (1930) and the subsequent Criminal Law Amendment Act. *The Carrigan Report* (1930) was the result of the findings of a committee established to inquire into updating laws dating from the 1800s and to solve the problem of juvenile prostitution–parameters of enquiry that were later extended to include illegitimate pregnancies. Female doctors were among the witnesses called to testify in front of the committee members. The majority of practitioners voiced their concerns about the lack of sexual education available to Irish citizens, especially young females. They emphasised the importance of such an education in combatting unwanted pregnancy and venereal diseases, but their advice largely fell on deaf ears. The report failed to include this testimony; a concealment that repeatedly occurred in discussions concerning sexual matters. The findings and recommendations of *The Carrigan Report* (1930) were devastating in terms of providing support to women on the margins of society, as it recommended that the State defer to and aid the Catholic Church officials in the creation of institutions to house those who were found to be sexually immoral. In doing so, the report and the subsequent Criminal Law Act not only allowed for the enforcement of state policy 'with respect to institutional provision but also disembodied sexual practice, concealing sexual crime while simultaneously sexualizing the women and children unfortunate enough to fall victim to society's moral proscriptions'.[8] Moreover, these reports and acts conspired to create an environment in which it was almost impossible for a mother and her illegitimate child to survive. Under Irish law, those who became pregnant outside of marriage were not legally entitled to any social welfare and were further stigmatized by Acts such as the Illegitimate Children (Affiliation Orders) Act (1930). In a country with an overwhelmingly Catholic majority, it was often the case that the Catholic Church's view correlated with those of Irish society. In addition to facing legal stigmatization, local communities often conspired with Church and state to ostracise those who broke society's strictly implemented rules. Indeed, it was these entities that made available the confinement infrastructure that not only effectively incarcerated women occluded from society, but also normalised the disappearance from the community of

8 James M. Smith, 'The Politics of Sexual Knowledge: The Origins of Ireland's Containment Culture and the Carrigan Report (1930)', *Journal of the History of Sexuality* 13 (2004): 209.

those who did not ascribe to the Ireland's post-colonial identity. The normality of this disappearance in evident in both *The Magdalene Sisters* and *Philomena. The Magdalene Sisters'* Margaret, Patricia and Crispina arrive in a Magdalene Laundry as a result of a sexual experience: Patricia and Crispina gave birth to children outside of wedlock, whilst Margaret is the victim of an incestuous rape. Bernadette has not committed any sexual crime; she, like Crispina, has been placed in a Magdalene Laundry to safeguard her sexual purity and morality. What all four characters have in common with Philomena Lee, *Philomena*'s protagonist, is that they all vanished from their communities overnight with seemingly no alarm raised at their disappearance. Philomena recalls her father leaving her 'with the nuns, he was so ashamed he told everyone I was dead'.[9] Despite the lack of a wake or funeral for Philomena, these strange circumstances did not prompt the community into searching for her—they knew why and to where she had disappeared. In the eyes of the community and wider Irish society, Philomena has distorted her identity and could no longer exist within the margins of post-colonial Ireland—a transformation made explicit by the opening scenes of *Philomena*. Viewers of *Philomena* are introduced to the film's titular character during a flashback in which the adult Philomena re-experiences the event that led to her placement in Sean Ross Abbey mother and baby home: the conception of her son, Anthony. This scene opens on the reflected image of the adolescent Philomena in a house of mirrors at a funfair. The mirrors hold a deeply metaphorical and symbolic meaning, as their distorted images of Philomena are reflective of the way in which she will come to be seen by Irish society. The next scene, in which a bitten apple falls from Philomena's hand as she is being embraced by a man, explains why she will be viewed differently by society: interpreted metaphorically and viewed as a biblical reference, the apple is symbolic of Eve's sin and her status of as a fallen woman; a sin and status that resulted the expulsion of both Adam and Eve from the Garden of Eden. In twentieth-century Ireland, this biblical story was reimagined and reinterpreted so that only those guilty of Eve's sin —the women— were expelled from society. Anxious to prevent these 'crimes' from occurring, the State frequently intervened in cases in which they deemed a female's morality and purity to be at risk. This was often the case in instances in which girls were transferred to mother and baby homes and Magdalene Laundries from institutions such as industrial schools, reformatory schools, or orphanages. Whilst industrial and reformatory schools housed children who were abandoned, neglected, or juvenile delinquents, Magdalene Laundries

9 *Philomena*, dir. Steve Coogan, Stephen Frears. New York: The Weinstein Company, 2013, DVD.

and Mother and Baby homes typically housed 'fallen women': women who had committed 'immoral sins' such as pre-marital sexual intercourse, or were in danger of committing such sins. This situation was chronicled in a chapter in Halliday Sutherland's *Irish Journey* (1956), in which he held interviews with nuns from various Magdalene Laundries. His study found that if a girl received two confinements at the Children's Home in Tuam, an institution that catered solely for unmarried mothers and their children, she was sent to the Magdalene Laundry in Galway. Moreover, as many of the children born to unmarried mothers were often transferred from Magdalene Laundries and mother and baby homes to other institutional infrastructures such as orphanages, reformatory schools, and industrial schools, before being returned to a Magdalene Laundry or mother and baby home, this helped facilitate a collusion between Church and state that secured Ireland's architecture of containment.[10]

Like *The Magdalene Sisters'* Bernadette, who was transferred from St. Attracta's Orphanage to the Magdalene Laundry, those who came from industrial schools and orphanages had rarely committed any crime. Rather, their perceived naivety, caused by lack of experience in an environment other than an institutional one, created a need for the safeguarding of their morality; the very reason for Bernadette's transfer to a Magdalene Laundry. After seeing her talking to boys at the school gates, Bernadette's Principal contacted the religious order responsible for the local Magdalene Laundy and arranged for Bernadette's transfer to their facility. In actuality, Bernadette had behaved impeccably: when asked by one of the boys for a kiss, she refused him and replied that she is 'not that kinda girl'.[11] In an earlier scene she was also seen explaining sins to two younger girls. When asked 'Isn't it a sin to be beautiful?' Bernadette replied 'no, look at the Virgin Mary, she's beautiful, isn't she? It's a sin to be vain: vanity's a sin'.[12] Unfortunately for Bernadette, in the Irish Free State to be beautiful was to be a temptation, and to be a temptation was to be a threat.

Like Stephen Dedalus' assertion that history is a nightmare from which he is trying to awake, Ireland's institutional legacy continued to haunt it as it strove to establish itself as a modern and progressive society in the late twentieth century. A monumental event in this struggle was Ireland's joining of the European Economic Community in 1973—an occurrence that marked the end of the de Valera era of self-sufficiency, isolationism, and conservative economic and social policies. This cultural, economic, and social expansion also

10 James M. Smith, *Ireland's Magdalene Laundries and the Nation's Architecture of Containment* (South Bend: University of Notre Dame Press, 2007), 44.

11 *The Magdalene Sisters*, dir. Peter Mullan. Dumfries and Galloway: Miramax, 2004, DVD.

12 Ibid.

compelled Irish society to question the very foundations upon which its post-colonial identity was founded:

> this backward glance focuses both on the events of the past and on how the national story is told: what is slighted, what is stressed, and how narratives of history serve present attitudes and values.[13]

Crucially, this glance propelled State and society to acknowledge those in its history who had been silenced and occluded in the pursuit of a façade of perfection. This acknowledgement led to a study of forgotten Irish history that brought to light many cases previously hidden in the deep, dark depths of Ireland's architecture of containment: a discovery that has preoccupied literature and film as well as the media for the past quarter of a century.

3 Societal Culpability

The uncovering of clerical abuse scandals has led to the emergence of two radically different views of religious orders in Ireland throughout the twentieth century: the early to mid-1900s view of the clergy as educators, patriots, and caregivers or, following the media exposés of clerical abuses, as torturers, paedophiles, and sadists. The latter view has been strengthened by religious orders' refusal to release pertinent documents regarding institutions under its authority, and the securing of an indemnity clause that prevents abusers from being publically named; actions that have resulted in the placing of the blame firmly on the shoulders of the various orders implicated in the scandals. However, the journey undertaken by authors and filmmakers into Ireland's past has acknowledged the need to delve deeper into the narrative of the State and focus on a wider scope of enquiry in order to establish who did know, who must have known, and why those conscious of the abuse did not put an end to the maltreatment surrounding them. In analysing the past from multiple angles and ascertaining its implications on the present, film has cast a critical eye on twentieth-century Ireland, revealing a major discrepancy in Irish cultural memory: the culpability of State and society in the creation and facilitation of Ireland's architecture of containment.

13 Robert F. Garratt, *Trauma and History in the Irish Novel: The Return of the Dead* (Basingstoke: Palgrave Macmillan, 2010), 1.

In a country famed for its literature, the question of why is has been cinema that has most influenced public mind-set regarding this trauma may be posed. Unlike reading a book or watching television, activities in which the individual's attention can be easily distracted, a film's spectator is engaged with the story being portrayed on a screen larger than the spectator, with sound that drowns out human noises. This situation is exacerbated by the fact that whilst watching a film, especially in a cinema, one's actions are restricted to watching and listening. As a result, the audio-visual experience becomes intensified to the extent that the normal judgement functions of the mind become somewhat suspended. A direct consequence of this, and an important point to bear in mind when viewing traumatic narratives such as *The Magdalene Sisters*, *Philomena*, and *Calvary*, is that this environment encourages the spectator to form a series of identifications with the fictional characters. Rather than simply identifying with a particular character or situation, spectators frequently endorse the views and actions of a certain character or characters; an endorsement that solidifies the identification process and illustrates why cinema forms such a potent role in the influencing of public opinion. John Elis' *Visible Fictions: Cinema, Television, Video* argues that the identification process has two distinct phases. The first phase consists of 'identification with the cinematic apparatus itself', whilst the second involves 'narcissistic identification that can take place in relation to any human figure on the screen'.[14] Elis proposes that the second phase of identification is the outcome of cinema's parallels with psychic processes best described by psychoanalysis, and consists of two steps: the first is the perceiving of the projected image/character as an 'Other' rather than as the self, whilst the second consists of considering the character as being the desired self. Elis stresses that this identification process aligns itself with Lacan's theory that one of the crucial moments in the formation of a child's sense of self occurs when it becomes influenced by what it perceives to be a perfect human being.[15] Like the child, the spectator comes to view the character as being more co-ordinated than the viewer's own self. The spectator's opinions are thus influenced in favour of the character with whom they identify—an influence that colours their perceptions of other characters based on their interactions with the chosen individual. In terms of films such as *The Magdalene Sisters* whose plotlines contain images of clerical abuse, this process of identification with characters who suffered under the religious orders caused many spectators to react extremely harshly to portrayals of religious characters and

14 John A. Elis, *Visible Fictions: Cinema, Television, Video* (London: Routledge, 1992), 42.
15 Ibid.

therefore directly influenced attitudes towards religious figures in the wake of the abuse scandals.

Psychoanalysis is not the only frame of reference that proves useful to such a reading; cinematic and trauma theories overlap to illustrate how films with traumatic narratives are useful in terms of assimilating cultural trauma. An aim common to a multiplicity of trauma narratives is the endeavour to engage directly with audiences in order to make them aware of trauma; an endeavour made all the more pertinent by the assertion that, if left unexamined, trauma and traumatic memory can fester in the psyche of both individuals and larger bodies such as countries and cultures. Indeed, the fact that many similarities may be drawn between this chapter's examination of trauma testimony in a specifically Irish context and Sayed Hanafy's exploration in a Middle Eastern setting is proof of trauma's disregard for physical and mental boundaries. The articulation of trauma, be it in Western Europe or Palestine, requires the act of remembering; an act that may be as painful as the original trauma. This act of remembrance facilitates the endeavour of trauma texts to examine alternative narratives than the ones offered by official history. In doing so they attempt to alert the public to the discrepancies in official narratives and seek to reform cultural memory to include occluded and silenced accounts from the past. These are important endeavours when related to Ireland's hidden history of abuse and the films that seek to uncover this narrative. Laurie Vickroy's argument that 'traumatic narratives engage readers in a number of important social and psychological issues' is proof of this hypothesis.[16] Vickroy contends that trauma narratives attest to the fact that trauma often occurs both in the wake of colonisation and as a result of political ideologies; an argument that holds particular resonance in this case as the creation of Ireland's architecture of containment was a direct result of the post-colonial identity formed in Ireland during the early twentieth-century. Vickroy elaborates further on this theory by stating that in illuminating such aspects and forcing the public to confront their fears caused by a traumatic narrative, trauma texts 'elucidate the dilemma of the public's relationship to the traumatized, made problematic by the victims' painful experiences … and by the public's resistance'.[17] This theory is especially useful when considering *The Magdalene Sisters* and *Philomena*; films inspired by victim and witness testimony of their time spent in Ireland's Magdalene Laundries and Mother and Baby Homes.

16 Laurie Vickroy, *Trauma and Survival in Contemporary Fictions* (Charlottesville: University of Virginia Press, 2002), 2.

17 Ibid.

The Magdalene Sisters, based on the testimony of four former Magdalene penitents, and *Philomena*, based on the journey of Martin Sixsmith and Philomena Lee to find the son taken from Philomena in Sean Ross Abbey Mother and Baby Home, are strong examples of how witness testimony serves to expand traumatic texts. Indeed, trauma theorists such as Vickroy have posed that the reason why witness testimony broadcast through the medium of documentary and film is so powerful is due to the fact that features such as the tone of the characters' voices and their body language help viewers empathise to a higher degree.[18] Both narratives are further strengthened by the inclusion of a variety of diverse mediums: *The Magdalene Sisters* includes original film footage, photographs and a folk ballad, whilst *Philomena* contains photographs, newspaper articles, and home video. By presenting their viewers with these materials – evidence that had existed for decades – both directors compelled spectators to 'acknowledge what heretofore they had chosen to ignore but, invariably, always knew': that they too had been witnesses who had failed to question the events that took place right before their eyes.[19] In compelling spectators to bear witness to various forms of witness testimony, viewers carry out one of the main functions of witness-based trauma testimony: they 'unite around the re-experiencing of … woundedness'.[20] Though they are able to present their own personal and individual testimony, they also represent others who have been silenced. This is crucial as it creates and expands an established space in which other previously occluded voices may be heard. In the case of *The Magdalene Sisters* and *Philomena*, these narratives provided an environment that enabled survivors of Magdalene Laundries and Mother and Baby Homes to cast off the cultural stigma and silence and bring their stories on to the screens of the nation: a step vital to the healing process.

Regarding the inclusion of artefacts that highlight society's knowledge of Ireland's architecture of containment, *The Magdalene Sisters* includes a scene inspired by a photograph taken of penitents from Dublin's Gloucester Street Magdalene Laundry taking part in a Corpus Christi procession in the 1950s. The photograph consists of the image of a parade of Magdalene penitents, dressed in veils and cloaks, forming a procession in a street. Interestingly, members of An Garda Síochána, the State's police force, flank them on both sides. This photograph proves that there was significant Garda-State collusion in the operation and maintenance of Ireland's Magdalene Laundries and questions the

18 Ibid., 7.

19 James M. Smith, *Containment*, 140.

20 Roger Luckhurst, *The Trauma Question* (Routledge: London, 2013), 2.

State's argument that establishments such as Magdalen Laundries were religious facilities under the control of the Catholic Church, and therefore fell outside of State control. The scene involving the Corpus Christi procession opens on the image of laughing penitents wearing white veils, light blue cloaks, and miraculous medals walking in pairs towards the town where they join the Corpus Christi procession. However, their delight soon turns to embarrassment when they are shunned by the townspeople. Audio also plays a crucial role in this scene: the beginning of the procession is met with loud clapping that fades as soon as the penitents become the focal point of the procession. Moreover, though the pipers continue to perform the tune of 'Amazing Grace' in the absence of any clapping, very little grace is shown to the penitents as several townspeople cast their eyes downward or look away as they pass by. Therefore, the girls' temporary visibility serves only as a symbol of the nuns' service to the local community, and as a warning to younger members of society as to what will happen to them should they fall from grace.

The silence they are treated with continues throughout the scene, culminating in an event event that results in Crispina's sectioning in a psychiatric unit. At the sports day held prior to the procession, Margaret witnessed the sexual abuse of Crispina by the priest scheduled to celebrate the Corpus Christi mass. Determined to punish him, Margaret placed a poisonous plant in with his washing; an act of artistic license by Mullan as no such plant grows in Ireland. However, Margaret's plan backfires horribly as, in addition to causing grave irritation to the priest's skin, it causes Crispina to experience similar symptoms. The priest's skin becomes so irritated by the plant that, whilst celebrating Mass, he rips his vestments from his body before naked across the field away from the congregation. Whilst the community stared frozen and silent at the departing naked figure, Crispina rises to tell Sr. Bridget of her ailment before proceeding to yell 'You are not a man of God!' at the fleeing figure.[21] Crispina's loud protestations starkly contrast the silence of the congregation; a disparity that serves to symbolise the wider silence of the state.. However, it is Crispina who is ultimately silenced:, 'knowing that the local community and the state's police force have witnessed evidence of clerical sexual abuse and chosen to look the other way', Sr. Bridget chooses to guard against further scandal by immediately arranging for Crispina to be sectioned in Saint Vernon's psychiatric unit.[22] Sr. Bridget's actions also guarantee the silence of Margaret, whose fear of suffering a similar fate to Crispina prevents

21 *The Magdalene Sisters*, dir. Peter Mullan. Dumfries and Galloway: Miramax, 2004, DVD.

22 James M. Smith, '*The Magdalene Sisters*: Evidence, Testimony ... Action?' *Signs* 32 (2007): 444.

her from disclosing the abuse she witnessed. Margaret is therefore rendered complicit in the occlusion and silencing of a victim of clerical abuse; complicity shared by members of wider Irish society who also remained silent when faced with evidence of clerical abuse.

4 'I want you to know that I forgive you': Post-Report Films and Forgiveness

By inspiring acts of international remembrance and commemoration, films such as *The Magdalene Sisters* aided in the creation of an environment in which the once-silenced voices of victims and survivors of institutional abuse could be heard and led to the establishment of the Commission to Inquire into Child Abuse (1999) and the Inter-Departmental Committee to Establish the Facts of the State Involvement with the Magdalen Laundries. The culmination of both committees was the publication of two reports, commonly called The Ryan Report (2009) and The McAleese Report (2013). Both reports echoed what Irish films had depicted for years: the culpability of State and society in the creation and maintenance of Ireland's architecture of containment. Though the Irish government had quickly admitted accountability for the abuse of children in industrial and reformatory schools, it was not until after the publication of *The McAleese Report* (2013) that Taoiseach Enda Kenny finally admitted responsibility and 'apologise[d] unreservedly to all those women for the hurt that was done to them … as a result of the time they spent in a Magdalene Laundry'; an action that acknowledged the truth behind the message of state and societal culpability carried by pre-Report films such as *The Magdalene Sisters*.[23] Despite the success of such films, it may be argued that some of their aspects, such as the subjectivity of character representation, placed limitations on them that served to hinder, to a certain extent, their reliability. Influenced by the findings of *The Ryan Report* and *The McAleese Report* and wary of placing limitations upon themselves in a manner similar to pre-Report films, post-Report films such as *Philomena* and *Calvary* sought to continue the work of pre-Report films in a more objective manner.

The publication of the government reports was a monumental event in the history of the Republic of Ireland. For the first time, the public was granted

23 'In Full: Enda Kenny's State Apology to the Magdalen Women', *The Journal*, February 28, 2013, viewed on 10 December 2013, http://www.thejournal.ie/full-text-enda-kenny-magdalene-apology-801132-Feb2013/.

access to previously secure official records of assorted religious orders and various government bodies. *The Ryan Report* was compiled largely based on witness testimony and investigated several industrial and reformatory schools, analyzing instances of physical, sexual, mental, and emotional abuse as well as neglect. Its findings correlated with several cinematic depictions, notably that the abuse that was rife in the industrial and reformatory school system did not go unnoticed:

> Parents, relatives, and others knew that the children were being abused as a result of disclosures and their observation of marks and injuries. Witnesses believed that awareness of the abuse of children in schools and institutions existed within society at both official and unofficial levels.[24]

This evidence of official collusion was not solely confined to the investigation surrounding child abuse in Irish industrial and reformatory schools. Rather, as depicted in *The Magdalene Sisters*, the subsequent McAleese Report also established that there was official and unofficial state collusion in the maintenance of both Magdalene Laundries and Mother and Baby Homes. In order to determine whether collusion between successive Irish governments and the religious orders responsible for the management of Magdalene Laundries and Mother and Baby Homes had taken place, the commission analysed admissions to Magdalene Laundries. This examination provided substantial proof of collusion between Magdalene Laundries and various State services, and established the probability that a significant percentage of referrals were either ‘a *compelled* act [by the State], a *legal* condition agreed to by the women in question, or a voluntary move *facilitated* by the State’.[25] Crucially in regards to the aim of *The Magdalene Sisters* to illustrate Garda collusion, the findings of the Report also established that ‘referrals by members of An Garda Síochána occurred in a range of occurrences’ and that they also facilitated Ireland’s architecture of containment by transporting women to Magdalene Laundries ‘on

---

24 Republic of Ireland. Dept. of Children and Youth Affairs, *The Ryan Report: Commission to Inquire into Child Abuse*, vol. 1 Dept. of Children and Youth Affairs, 2009, viewed on 23 May 2014, http://www.childabusecommission.ie/rpt/pdfs/

25 Republic of Ireland. Dept. of Justice and Equality. *Report of the Inter-Departmental Committee to Establish the Facts of State Involvement with the Magdalen Laundries*. Dept. of Justice and Equality, 2013, viewed on 6 May 2014, http://www.justice.ie/en/JELR/Pages/MagdalenRpt2013.

a more ad hoc or informal basis'.[26] Like The Ryan Report, The McAleese Report also proves that that there was official knowledge about occurrences within the walls of Magdalene Laundries. However, these reports also established that not all of society ignored the abuse in their midst. Some voices did speak out against the abuses they witnessed in the state; The Kennedy Report (1970) is proof of this. In an endeavour to create a dichotomy of good versus evil, pre-report films such as *The Magdalene Sisters* neglected to include this aspect of Irish history: an omission that lessens the objectivity of their narratives and provided Post-Report films with a new direction in which to take films centring on narratives of clerical abuse.

A central flaw of films such as *The Magdalene Sisters* is that the religious figures featured within their narratives are frequently reduced to stereotypical villains. The films do not shed any light on their life, character, and personality outside of their religious vocation. As a result, such characters serve to exist as merely two-dimensional representations of pure evil created solely to emphasise a dichotomy of good versus bad. One of the strongest examples of this type of character is *The Magdalene* Sisters' Sr. Bridget, who is physically, emotionally, and mentally abusive, and is portrayed as a cold, calculating individual whose only concern is money. The audience's first encounter with Sr. Bridget is a close-up shot of her fingers counting through rolls of pound notes whilst she simultaneously lectures the newly-arrived penitents about the institution's rules. Though these girls have been placed under her care, she does not lift her eyes from the pound notes to welcome them. Rather, she chastises Margaret, a victim of rape, for talking: 'Did no one ever tell you that it's bad manners to interrupt, or were you too busy whoring it with the boys to listen?'. She then strips Rose of her identity by renaming her Patricia, and emphasises her absolute authority by informing the girls, 'I decide when and if you're allowed to leave, and I think I can safely say it could be quite some time'.[27] Her physical punishments are extremely severe; in one scene she beats Bernadette and cuts her hair so viciously that Bernadette's eyes and eyelashes become encrusted in blood. Sr. Bridget's final scene further emphasises her view of the girls as commodities rather than individuals. Realising that Bernadette and Patricia are attempting to escape, Sr. Bridget tries to physically restrain them. However, once they hand over the missing key to the safe she lets them go, thus illustrating that her capitalistic concerns were of greater importance than her duty of care.

26 Ibid.

27 *The Magdalene Sisters.*

The religious figures portrayed in post-report films such as *Philomena* and *Calvary* contrast those featured within pre-report narratives. Indeed, the creation of 'evil' characters to fulfil a narrative purpose is even referenced in *Philomena* as Martin, tasked with writing Philomena's story, confirms that 'evil's good. Story-wise, I mean'.[28] Though some of the characters depicted in post-report films do possess traits akin to those represented in *The Magdalene Sisters*, the inclusion of religious characters with positive attributes as well as flaws succeeds in creating more three-dimensional and realistic characters. This concern is also reflected in *Calvary* through the characterisation of the protagonist, Fr. James Lavelle. Though he did not enter the priesthood in the usual manner —he was ordained after the death of his wife with whom he had a daughter— Fr. Lavelle carries out his parochial and clerical duties with as much fervour as the traditional priests featured in *The Magdalene Sisters*. He treats his parishioners with kindness and compassion even though they regard him with disdain, disrespect and, on occasion, disgust. Though his daughter Fiona has committed a mortal sin by attempting suicide, he does not treat her like a sinner. Rather, he comforts her and when pressed to answer her question of whether or not she would 'have suffered eternal damnation' had her attempt succeeded, replies 'God is great. The limits of His mercy have not been set'.[29] He treats another of his parishioners, Veronica, an adulteress who would have traditionally been considered a sinner, in a similar manner. Rather than judge Veronica for her actions, Fr. Lavelle actively seeks to establish the facts surrounding her domestic abuse and to put an end to the violence. However, Fr. Lavelle is not depicted as a being a flawless human being. It is evident that he has a troubled relationship with both his daughter and alcohol, and is prone to sarcastic and ill-tempered outbursts; imperfections that illustrate his humanity and prevent his character from becoming reductive and two-dimensional.

Philomena also contains individuals who emphasise the misconceptions surrounding members of religious orders. Though Sister Hildegarde is depicted as a callous person who believes that penitents in her care must endure penance in order to atone their sins, the behaviour of the majority of the nuns featured is unremarkable. That of Sr. Annunciata, however, is notable. In addition to treating Philomena with kindness and compassion, she also views her as a friend. She does not appear to judge Philomena for having a child outside of wedlock, but rather converses with Philomena in a light-hearted, friendly, and conspiratorial manner: 'I bet the father was handsome.'[30] She also performs an

28 *Philomena*.

29 *Calvary*, dir. John Michael McDonagh. Sligo: Reprisal Films, 2014, DVD.

30 *Philomena*.

act of kindness for Philomena. Realising that Anthony would likely be adopted out of Sean Ross Abbey without Philomena's prior knowledge, Sr. Annunciata borrowed a camera and took a photo of Anthony. She then later presented the photo to Philomena, knowing that it would be the only memento Philomena would had of him. Decades later, Philomena still cherishes that one act of kindness: 'Whenever I look at the picture of Anthony I say a little prayer for Annunciata ... if she hadn't taken that I'd have nothing'.[31] In a narrative where Martin constantly criticizes the nuns and clergy, Philomena's recollections of memories of both kindness and cruelty persistently remind the viewer that the situation did not and does not continue to be as definite a dichotomy of good and evil as some people, such as Martin, believe. By the end of the film, Martin has also come to understand and empathise with Philomena's views, and shows an acceptance of them by placing holy water on Anthony's grave. It is this realisation and action that allows Martin and Philomena to leave Sean Ross Abbey having 'come full circle'..[32] The inclusion of characters such as Fr. Lavelle and Sr. Annunciata therefore serve to illustrate that whilst society continues to perpetrate a blanket cycle of judgement and blame against all members of religious orders, it is destined to remain trapped *in* and *by* this cultural trauma. Both *Philomena* and *Calvary* meditate on this, ultimately imploring viewers to consider how forgiveness – an act unimaginable at the time of the release of *The Magdalene Sisters* – may impact the healing process.

Unlike Jack Brennan, the man behind *Calvary*'s opening death threat, Philomena actively undertakes a process of working through her trauma. The audience's first encounter with Philomena takes place in a church, where she is lighting a candle. Through the intermingling of present day scenes with those from the night on which she met Anthony's father it is evident that she is lighting the candle on behalf of her son. Despite the abuse suffered by Philomena at the hands of the nuns, and unlike Martin who treats religion and religious beliefs with disdain, Philomena remains devout in her religious convictions. The only time in which her faith falters is as she is attending confession immediately after Martin has expressed his incredulity at her decision to confess:

> What sins? The Catholic Church should go to confession, not you: "Forgive me Father for I have sinned, I have incarcerated a load of young women against their will, used them as slave labour, and then sold their babies to the highest bidder."[33]

31 *Calvary*.

32 *Philomena*.

33 Ibid.

Philomena becomes agitated and asks Martin what he is trying to prove by constantly complaining about the Catholic Church. Martin responds by belittling her faith: 'We don't believe something just because we're told it's the truth … Hooray for blind faith and ignorance'.[34] Martin's words obviously affect Philomena, as she exits the confessional before giving her confession and fails to bless herself with holy water upon exiting the church. Though Martin may have thought he was providing Philomena with clarity about her situation, his comments cause Philomena to experience further pain.

Calvary also explores the ways in which unmediated trauma lends itself to cycles of re-traumatisation. As per the details of the death threat, Fr. Lavelle journeys to the beach on the date and time given to him by the speaker. Upon his arrival he is approached by the local butcher, Jack Brennan., who brandishes a handgun.. In the ensuing conversation, it becomes apparent that Jack's behaviour is heavily influenced by the effects of what he terms 'a hell of a lot of physical and psychological torture': the sexual abuse he was subjected to as a child in a reformatory school.[35] He applies this belief to all priests, even those such as Fr. Lavelle, whom he deems 'a good priest'.[36] Though he admits to burning down the church and abusing his wife, he vehemently denies slitting the throat of Fr. Lavelle's dog. This denial then leads Jack on to the topic of clerical abuse. Jack asks Fr. Lavelle if he cried when his dog died, Fr. Lavelle answers that he did, to which Jack replies: 'And when you read about what your fellow priests did to all those poor children down all those years, did you cry then?'.[37] Fr. Lavelle replies that he did now, but his attempts to explain his answer are cut short by Jack, who shoots him in the abdomen. Unlike the inquiries that permitted both victims of abuse and members of religious orders to give testimony, Jack refuses to listen to Fr. Lavelle, and cuts short Fr. Lavelle's attempts to reason with him by fatally wounding him. The montage that follows this frame suggests that Jacks actions have not altered anything in his community: the writer eats an ice cream; Veronica carries on cheating on her husband; Michael Fitzgerald remains lonely in the Big House; Detective Stanton examines counterfeit money; the serial killer Freddie Joyce remains tortured by his thoughts; the ex-priest Fr. Leary reads *The God Delusion*; Leo, a male sex worker, sits contemplatively on the edge of an unmade bed; Milo joins the army; Dr. Harte continues to treat the dead in a disrespectful manner; Brendan Lynch drinks in his pub; and the French widow returns home.

34 *Calvary*.
35 Ibid.
36 Ibid.
37 Ibid.

Ultimately, the consequences of Fr. Lavelle's death are detrimental. Fr. Lavelle's death causes pain to his daughter Fiona and results in Jack's imprisonment; an imprisonment that emphasises the cyclical nature of unresolved trauma, as it was Jack's childhood incarceration in a reformatory school that drove him to commit murder. *Calvary*'s final scene occurs immediately after this montage. This scene is set in the visiting room of the prison in which Jack is incarcerated and features Fiona and Jack. Though no words are spoken, the similarities between this scene and that of the final interaction between Fiona and Fr. Lavelle pose the possibility that Fiona is visiting Jack with the intention of forgiving him. The final interaction scene occurs shortly before Fr. Lavelle's death and concentrates on a phone conversation between Fiona and her father. In the course of the conversation, Fiona enquires as to Fr. Lavelle's opinion on sins and sinning,. Fr. Lavelle pauses before replying, 'I think there's too much talk about sins, to be honest, and not enough talk about virtues'.[38] When encouraged to share his 'number one' virtue, Fr. Lavelle replies: 'I think forgiveness has been highly underrated'.[39] With this exchange resting on her mind, it is likely that Fiona visited Jack in prison in order to offer her forgiveness. In the same way she instigated the conversation about sins and forgiveness with her father, she initiates the conversation with Jack by being the first person to pick up the phone in the visiting room; a move which prompts the end of the film as the end credits roll after Jack mirrors her by picking up his connecting phone. *Philomena*'s final scene, which takes place in of Sean Ross Abbey, also touches upon the topic of forgiveness. Upon realising that Anthony is interred in the ground of Sean Ross Abbey, Philomena and Martin return to the abbey. Martin confronts Sr. Hildegarde, demanding an apology and explanation as to why Philomena was not informed of her son's final resting place. Sr. Hildegarde quickly defends her actions: 'those girls have nobody to blame but themselves and their carnal incontinence. What's done is done, what do you expect us to do about it now?'[40] Philomena, who has remained unnoticed by both Martin and Sr. Hildegarde throughout this altercation, enters the room and replies to Sr. Hildegarde's: 'nothing, there's nothing that can be done or said. I found my son, that's what I came here for'.[41] Martin then becomes extremely agitated, swearing at Sr. Hildegarde and questioning Philomena's decision to 'do nothing about the situation'.[42] Philomena silences Martin by stating, 'but it

38 Ibid.

39 Ibid.

40 *Philomena.*

41 Ibid.

42 Ibid.

happened to me, not you. It's up to me what I do about it. It's my choice', and taking the final step in her own healing process: 'Sister Hildegarde, I want you to know that I forgive you'.[43] Though she acknowledges that 'it's hard for me', Philomena realises that, for her, performing forgiveness is necessary in order to work through her trauma and escape from the traumatic cycle synonymous with unexamined traumatic experience.[44]

5 Conclusion

The 1990s was a monumental decade in terms of changes to the Irish cultural, political, and social landscape. Not only did this decade see the closure of the last Magdalene Laundry in 1996, the implementation of the recommendations of *The Kennedy Report* (1970) to modernise and deinstitutionalise reformatory establishments, and the replacing of the Child Care Act (1908) with the Child Care Act (1991), it also saw the explosion of a media exposés and memoirs that brought to light Ireland's hidden litany of abuse. The cultural significance of these events and their ensuing literary and cinematic representations cannot be underestimated: they forced Ireland and Irish society to acknowledge a previously hidden history whilst simultaneously destroying the culture of shame and silence surrounding female sexuality, abuse, illegitimacy, and sexual crimes. These stories and representations not only forced the nation to finally acknowledge and reimagine its own role in the maintenance of Ireland's architecture of containment, society was also obliged to examine the implications of the trauma incurred by this litany of abuse and its effacement from the history of the state. However, this Irish cultural obsession with remembering the past has had a twofold effect: though this preoccupation has succeeded in encouraging the re-imagination of the past and has therefore pluralised Irish historical narratives and identity, the fixation on traumatic aspects of history has led to an anti-nostalgic viewing of the past that limits the benefits of ethical remembering. Should this anti-nostalgic view continue, the benefits reaped from the recovery process thus far will be endangered as the entire point of the exercise, to 'remember the past and to perform that remembrance, but to do so in order to create a more just future', will be forgotten.[45] Thus, the act of ethical remembrance is not only an action; it is a duty. By remembering both

43 Ibid.

44 Ibid.

45 Emilie Pine, *Politics of Irish Memory*, 7.

the victims and the victors of the past, and bearing in mind the lessons learned from past traumas, memory not only brings justice to the past and the present, but also offers the hope of recovery in the future. Should this duty be forgotten or misinterpreted, a risk of returning to the cycle of trauma remains.

Faced with the cinematic portrayal of the litany of abuses synonymous with Ireland's architecture of containment and the trauma that incurred as a result of both the abuse and its discrepancy in Irish cultural memory, Irish society became faced with two choices: to ostensibly forgive and forget with the intention of covering up the revelation, or to delve into the past, ascertain its role in the abuse, and seek to make amends for its actions. Ireland chose the latter option; the creation of the tribunals of enquiry and their subsequent reports is proof of this. Moreover, the monuments that now dot the Irish physical landscape, such as that dedicated 'to the women who worked in Ireland's Magdalene Laundry institutions and the children born to some members of those communities' are shrines of remembrance and physical reminders that serve to correct years of silence and secrecy. This process of ethical remembering constantly evolves and progresses in line with the needs of society to secure a more just past, present, and future for all involved. This progression ensures their legacy will outlive the generations that made recovery possible and positively influence those to come.

Bibliography

Bunreacht na hÉireann. Article 41. 1937. Viewed 2 June 2014. https://www.constitution.ie/Documents/Bhunreacht_na_hEireann_web.pdf

Calvary. Directed by John Michael McDonagh. Sligo: Reprisal Films, 2014. DVD.

Chubb, Basil. *The Government & Politics of Ireland*. Vol. 2. Stanford: Stanford University Press, 1970.

Elis, John A. *Visible Fictions: Cinema, Television, Video*. London: Routledge, 1992.

Garratt, Robert F. *Trauma and History in the Irish Novel: The Return of the Dead* Basingstoke: Palgrave Macmillan, 2010.

Gialanella Valiulis, Maryann. 'Power, Gender, and Identity in the Irish Free State'. *Journal of Women's History* 4.4/7 (1995): 117–136.

'In Full: Enda Kenny's State Apology to the Magdalen Women'. *The Journal*, 28 February 2013. Viewed 10 December 2013. http://www.thejournal.ie/full-text-enda-kenny-magdalene-apology-801132-Feb2013/.

Luckhurst, Roger. *The Trauma Question*. London: Routledge, 2013.

Meaney, Gerardine. *Sex and Nation: Women in Irish Culture and Politics*. Dublin: Attic Press, 1992.

Philomena. Dir. Stephen Frears. New York: The Weinstein Company, 2013. DVD.

Pine, Emilie. *The Politics of Irish Memory: Performing Remembrance in Contemporary Irish Culture*. Basingstoke: Palgrave Macmillan, 2011.

Republic of Ireland. Department of Children and Youth Affairs. *The Ryan Report: Commission to Inquire into Child Abuse*. Vol 1. Dublin: Department of Children and Youth Affairs, 2009. Viewed 23 May 2014. http://www.childabusecommission.ie/rpt/pdfs/

Republic of Ireland. Dept. of Justice and Equality. *Report of the Inter-Departmental Committee to Establish the Facts of State Involvement with the Magdalene Laundries*. Dublin: Dept. of Justice and Equality, 2013. Viewed 6 May 2014. http://www.justice.ie/en/JELR/Pages/MagdalenRpt2013.

Smith, James M. 'The Politics of Sexual Knowledge: The Origins of Ireland's Containment Culture and the Carrigan Report (1930)'. *Journal of the History of Sexuality* 13.2 (2004): 208–233.

Smith, James M. *Ireland's Magdalene Laundries and the Nation's Architecture of Containment*. South Bend: University of Notre Dame Press, 2007.

Smith, James M. '*The Magdalene Sisters*: Evidence, Testimony ... Action?' *Signs* 32:2 (2007): 431–458.

Song For A Raggy Boy. Directed by Aisling Walsh. Ireland: Subotica Entertainment, 2003. DVD.

The Butcher Boy. Directed by Neil Jordan. Ireland: The Geffen Film Company, 1997. DVD.

The Magdalene Sisters. Dir. Peter Mullan. Dumfries and Galloway: Miramax, 2004. DVD.

Vickroy, Laurie. *Trauma and Survival in Contemporary Fictions*. Charlottesville: University of Virginia Press, 2002.

CHAPTER 9

Performing Witnesses: Frameworks of Memory in Contemporary Performing Arts

Mateusz Chaberski

Abstract

The aim of this chapter is to discuss the performative potential of testimony in the context of contemporary performing arts employing different technologies of media representation. The author introduces a concept of the performing witness referring to the artistic practice of contemporary practitioners who invite actual amateurs to participate in artistic projects in order to make their intimate, often traumatic testimony experienced by a larger public. Thus, witnesses are allowed to enter both the stage of the theatre and the stage of history hitherto occupied by dominant narratives about the past. On the other hand, however, witnesses not only perform but they are constantly being performed as credible witnessing beings. In other words, the ontological status of the witness within a performance event always depends upon a plethora of performative strategies employed by artists which are crucial for the emergence of a particular testimony. Firstly, the author critically examines Jan Assmann's theory of cultural memory of the 1990s by returning to the concept of the frameworks of memory formulated by the French sociologist Maurice Halbwachs. Secondly, the author applies Halbwachs's concept to the analysis of two contemporary performances: Rimini Protokoll's *Mnemopark* (2008) and Jan Klata's *Transfer!* (2006) in order to show performative aspects of the Halbwachsian frameworks of memory. What is of particular interest here is the production of 'the authentic' by the use of media technologies and the physical presence of performing witnesses.[1]

Keywords

witness – performativity – memory – studies – frameworks of memory – performing – arts

1 Supported by the Foundation for Polish Science (FNP).

 | DOI:10.1163/9789004391130_011

The widespread use of digital technologies across contemporary performing arts necessitates radical methodological modifications within the definition of testimony as a performative phenomenon. As Christine Ramsay comments on the testimonial production of Atom Egoyan, his multimedia work relies on '[h]is fascination with the malleability of the moving image, our experience of the world as mediated "screen subjects" and our immersion in the image.'[2] In other words, Ramsay seems to suggest that the position of the witness in the highly mediatised culture of today is not firmly grounded in his or her essentialist presence but it is subject to negotiation between the material and the digital image. I would like to take Ramsay's remark as a point of entry into the intricate nexus of processes lying behind performing witnesses in contemporary performance art. The expression 'performing witnesses' employed here is clearly intended to be ambiguous. On the one hand, it refers to the artistic practice of contemporary practitioners inviting actual amateurs to participate in artistic projects in order to make their intimate, often traumatic testimony experienced by a larger public. Thus, witnesses are allowed to enter both the stage of the theatre and the stage of history hitherto occupied by dominant narratives about the past. On the other hand, however, witnesses not only perform but they are constantly being performed as credible witnessing beings. In other words, the ontological status of the witness within a performative event *always* depends upon a multitude of performative strategies employed by artists which are crucial for the emergence of a particular testimony. I believe that testimony in performance is never purely discursive in nature as it functions at an intersection of the material presence of the witness and different frameworks of memory in which his or her testimony emerges. This challenges the hitherto accepted binary of individual vs. cultural memory permeating contemporary memory studies influenced by Jan Assmann's seminal work *Cultural Memory and Early Civilization*.[3]

In order to scrutinise diverse effects achieved by performing witnesses in contemporary performance, in my chapter I adopt a trajectory based on three movements. The first movement is a backward one: I critically examine Assmann's dichotomous theory of cultural memory of the 1990s by returning to the concept of the frameworks of memory formulated by the French sociologist Maurice Halbwachs in the early 1920s. The second movement aims at

2 Christine Ramsay, 'Atom Egoyan and the Place of the Witness' in this volume.

3 Jan Assmann's work was first published in German in 1992 under the title *Das kulturelle Gedächtnis: Schrift, Erinnerung und politische Identität in frühen Hochkulturen*. In this chapter I refer to its English translation. Jan Assmann, *Cultural Memory and Early Civilization* (Cambridge: Cambridge University Press, 2011).

applying Halbwachs's concept to the analysis of contemporary performance *Mnemopark* (2008) by the German company Rimini Protokoll. Performative potential of the Halbwachsian frameworks of memory may elucidate the process of combining live witnesses' testimonies with a plethora of media technologies. Finally, in the third movement, from the perspective of *Mnemopark*, I scrutinise the Polish theatrical performance *Transfer!* (2006) by Jan Klata in order to prove that frameworks of memory are in operation even if hardly any digital media are employed by the artist who attempts to stress the 'authentic' physicality of the performing witnesses.

1 First Movement: from Cultural Memory to Frameworks of Memory

In his influential work *Cultural Memory and Early Civilization*, the German sociologist and Egyptologist Jan Assmann laid the foundation for what we presently refer to as memory studies. Assmann's academic feat consists of providing a clear and precise classification of memory processes according to the categories of cultural and communicative memory. According to Assmann, '[c]ultural memory is a matter of institutionalized mnemotechnics'[4] which means that a particular institutionally accepted version of the past is passed from generation to generation by means of different cultural forms of expression. Thereby a version of the past becomes the official history of a society while the other mode of remembering refers to the transfer of memories which occurs on the level of smaller communities and usually relies on the oral testimony of the witnesses of the past. It is crucial that the testimony they pass on to their descendants is their own version of the past which often runs counter to the dominant historical narratives. Assmann fetishises oral testimony of the witness as a uniquely subversive means of talking about the past. Thus, he artificially dissects two modes of remembering which are in fact inextricably linked. For, it may easily be proved that individual memories of the witnesses and the process of their transmission are as culturally influenced as the dominant version of the past formed by institutions of power. Let us then examine Assmann's theory in order to find a link between the two modes of memory which, as he claims, are 'two ends without a middle.'[5]

As Assmann's theory is clearly sociological in nature, cultural memory is prioritised over communicative memory since it becomes a historical narrative

4 Ibid., 37.

5 Ibid., 35.

constructed in order to meet particular political ends. Thus, cultural memories may be relatively easy to grasp in the analysis of cultural artefacts and practices. From this perspective, communicative memory becomes an idealised mechanism of remembering free from any cultural influences whose forms, Assmann claims, are 'informal, without much form, [characterised by] natural growth, arising from interaction and everyday.'[6] The author's use of the adjective *natural* indicates that his theory is based in the traditional nature/culture binary.

In fact, however, the boundary between the Assmannian modes of remembering is extremely thin, which may be shown as we scrutinise Assmann's theory in a broader socio-political context. *Cultural Memory and Early Civilization* was in fact a fierce reaction of the German academic against the oppressive and intensive policy of commemorating the Holocaust led by the unified Germany in the 1990s. As more and more eyewitnesses of the Holocaust passed away, the German state felt an urge to record and interpret their testimony. For Assmann this was the last moment when the memory of the tragic past could be transmitted by 'the generation that experienced the traumatic horrors of Hitler's persecution and the annihilation of the Jews.'[7] Assmann believes that their communicative memory was natural only because they often defied the dominant discourse about the Second World War and they did not contribute to maintaining the official version of the bad Germans versus the good Jews. However, suffice it to invoke the analysis of Primo Levi's work *If This is a Man* conducted by Hayden White in his essay 'Figural Realism in Witness Literature'.[8] White convincingly argues that Levi's testimony of his survival in Auschwitz is not an account of events free from cultural influence but is 'presented in [literary] figures and tropes which give them their concreteness and their power to convince us of the sincerity of the author.'[9] This means that every witness attempting to articulate the most individual and traumatic testimony inevitable employs different culturally influenced strategies of narrating the past.

Moreover, the individual-cultural aspect of testimony postulated by White is pertinent to the testimonial works of contemporary art. For example, in Atom Egoyan's installation *Auroras* (2007) a single traumatic testimony of a woman who survived the Armenian genocide is re-enacted in a series of short

6 Ibid., 44.

7 Assmann, *Cultural Memory*, 36.

8 Hayden White, 'Figural Realism in Witness Literature,' *Parallax: Witnessing Theory* 30 (2004): 132–145.

9 Ibid., 145.

films screened one alongside another in a gallery space. Each of the films represents a different actress retelling the testimony of Aurora Mardiganian. Thus, the viewers may experience the testimony performed not only by different subjects but also by means of different modes of filming. Assmann would definitely argue that Egoyan's installation is an exponent of cultural memory as it utilises an individual testimony of the witness as a means of creating a particular version of the past to be imposed on the viewers. Conversely, as Timothy Long succinctly observes in his article 'Chorus: Positioning the Witness in Atom Egoyan's *Auroras*', Egoyan's artistic strategy 'brings into question the filmic conventions by which victims are framed as sacred subjects and held at a safe remove from the viewer's life world.'[10] In other words, each convention employed by the artist slightly modifies the testimony, which paradoxically makes her memories more vivid for the audience instigating their extremely affective experience. Thus, due to different media employed by the artist, Aurora's testimony is not petrified in a single interpretation but may undergo various reconfigurations and thus be still alive. This short example of contemporary artistic practice indicates the inadequacies of Assmann's theoretical system and his clear-cut division between communicative and culture memory. We should rather formulate a theoretical model of memory encompassing different possible (re)configurations of the individual and the cultural that form a given performed testimony.

In order to forge a new theory of memory that avoids the Assmannian communicative/cultural memory binary, it is worth invoking the theoretical considerations of the early 20th century French sociologist Maurice Halbwachs. In his inquiry the two modes of remembering, so carefully separated by Assmann, are interdependent and influence one another. Halbwachs's considerations revolve around a complex question: to what extent are my memories really mine and to what extent are they influenced by the social group of which I am a member? With great precision he outlines the problematic status of memory in the preface to his book *La mémoire collective*, published posthumously in 1968 in which Halbwachs analyses his own memories of visiting London for the first time.[11] He was strolling through the city accompanied by two of his friends, an architect and a painter, who told him stories about the city. The former drew his attention to the architectural details of the Westminster Abbey whereas the latter took him to the most important galleries and talked about the rules of perspective which were used in planning the city. When several

10 Timothy Long, 'Chorus: Positioning the Witness in Atom Egoyan's *Auroras*' in this volume.

11 Maurice Halbwachs, *The Collective Memory* (New York: Harper & Row, 1980): 22–24.

years later Halbwachs returned to London, he soon realised that his memories of the city are not based on his own past experiences but that they mainly comprise of the stories told by his friends. Moreover, a walk he took in one of the boroughs of the city instigated memories of one of Dickens's novels he read as a child. Attempting to explain the mechanisms of memory exemplified by this anecdotal story, Halbwachs claims that

> Our memories remain collective, however, and are recalled to us through others even though only we were participants in the events or saw the things concerned. In reality, we are never alone. Other men need not be physically present, since we always carry with us and in us a number of distinct persons.[12]

Thus, Halbwachs's memories of London were not only his own but they were significantly influenced by the stories of his guides which then triggered his personal childhood memories. Let us now scrutinise in more detail the consequences of the Halbwachsian thinking about memory and its pertinence to the question of testimony in contemporary performance.

In his work *Les cadres sociaux de la mémoire*, Halbwachs claims that the boundary between individual and collective memory is extremely fluid.[13] This is because he combines sociological thinking about the social reality with the findings of early 20th century psychology with regards to memory processes. On the one hand, individual memories are determined by the social frameworks in which they emerge. On the other hand, Halbwachs refers to a psychological model of memory which is selective in nature in order to elucidate processes of collective memory whereby a social group assigns meaning only to carefully selected events and collective experiences from the past. The common ground for the social and the psychological aspect of Halbwachs's theory is the concept of the social frameworks of memory. The frameworks are ideas, values and social conventions that a particular group in a given moment imposes on its members and considers crucial for their identity. Social frameworks of memory are also tangible as they also comprise physical locales in which a social group functions. The frameworks serve as points of reference for the individual memories of the group members. Therefore, Halbwachs claims that '[t]he frameworks that could enable us to reconstruct our memories before

12 Ibid., 23.

13 Maurice Halbwachs, *Les cadres sociaux de la mèmoire* (Chicoutimi: Cégep de Chicoutimi, 2002).

they vanish are not purely individual but are common to all people belonging to a certain social group.'[14] We can see that the French philosopher, contrary to Jan Assmann, perceives memory as an individual-collective phenomenon. In order to elucidate the Halbwachsian thinking about memory, we should refer to the very definition of the frameworks which is quite unique. Halbwachs does not perceive the frameworks as merely static picture frames which firmly determine the shape of particular memories and testimonies, but rather reinforces their being in a constant state of flux.

To analyse what a social framework of memory might be, let us quote *in extenso* from *Les cadres sociaux de la mémoire*:

> Each time we put our memories in different frameworks of our actual ideas, the frameworks transform the memories and they, on their part, modify the frameworks. This new moment, this new place contributes our perception of time and space, which sheds a new light on our social group. Thus, we might talk about a perpetual process of re-adaptation whereby a particular event forces us to modify the notions we inherited from the past. If it was merely a linear transition from one fact to another our existence would be constrained to living in a singular present moment. In reality, however, we must incessantly switch frameworks which are slightly different every time. Therefore, we must always present all the elements of the frameworks to ourselves anew as any change, even the most inconspicuous one, modifies all the relations between the elements transformed with any other elements of the framework. Thus, a visit, a walk, a book we are reading changes my memory of a given morning from the past or even my memory of yesterday. I constantly strive to find their position in time. I recall the places I recently visited in order to situate them in reference to the place I head for or visit right now. I recall my friends, people I ever came across and issues I discussed with different groups of people ... I recall all this to recreate the sense of the conversations I am having today or articles and books I am currently reading.[15]

14 Ibid., 98, my own translation. 'Les cadres dont nous parlons, et qui nous permettraient de reconstruire nos souvenirs après qu'ils ont disparu, ne sont pa, nous l'avons dit, purement individuels: ils sont communs aux hommes d'un même groupe.'

15 Ibid., 101, my own translation. 'Chaque fois que nous replaçons une de nos impressions dans le cadre de nos idées actuelles, le cadre transforme l'impression, mais l'impression, à son tour, modifie le cadre. C'est un moment nouveau, c'est un lieu nouveau, qui s'ajoute à notre temps, à notre espace, c'est un aspect nouveau de notre groupe, qui nous le fait voir sous un autre jour. D'où un travail de réadaptation perpétuel, qui nous oblige, à l'occasion de chaque événement, à revenir sur l'ensemble de notions élaborées à l'occasion

We can see that according to Halbwachs, memory is not only in a constant state of becoming between the individual and the collective but it is performative in the sense that there is an interaction between personal memories and socio-political and cultural contexts in which they emerge. Consequently, any modification either in a memory or in its framework results in a completely new interpretation of the past and the present. Thus, Halbwachs's concept of frameworks of memory bypasses the binary thinking about memory being purely individual or cultural in nature. Using Manuel DeLanda's terms, we should rather think about memories as assemblages of components pertaining to different scales of social organization which may enter into relations, which every time transforms their status.[16] Thus, memories must be scrutinised not as essentialist entities but rather as relational beings emerging in a specific context. Let us now apply Halbwachs's theoretical findings to performing witnesses in contemporary performance art which may be perceived as a rich field of relations between personal testimonies and different frameworks of memory—be it socio-political contexts or performative strategies employed by the artists.

2 Second Movement: *Mnemopark* and Frameworks of Memory

The performative potential of the Halbwachsian frameworks of memory may be illustrated by referring to *Mnemopark*, a performance devised in 2008 by the Berlin-based company Rimini Protokoll. I choose this example because

des événements antérieurs. S'il s'agissait de passer simplement d'un fait antécédent à un fait conséquent, nous pourrions être perpétuellement dans le moment présent, et en lui seul. Mais il faut en réalité passer sans cesse d'un cadre à un autre, qui diffère sang doute très peu du précédent, mais qui en diffère: c'est pourquoi nous devons sans cesse nous représenter à nouveau presque tous les éléments de ce cadre, puisque tout changement, si léger soit-il, modifie les rapports de l'élément transformé avec tous les autres. C'est ainsi qu'à l'occasion d'une visite, d'une promenade, d'une lecture que je fais aujourd'hui, je repense à ce matin, à hier, pour fixer leur place dans le temps; je repense à d'autres endroits où j'ai été ces derniers jours, pour situer par rapport à eux ceux où je me rends, ou bien où je demeure, aujourd'hui; et je me représente les amis que j'ai vus, les gens que j'ai rencontrés dans les rues, et les questions qui intéressent des groupes plus ou moins étendus, dont nous avons parlé, dont j'ai su ou vu qu'on s'occupait, ces derniers temps, pour me faire une idée plus précise de la portée actuelle des propos que nous allons tenir, de l'article ou du livre que j'ai sous les yeux.'

16 See Manuel DeLanda, *A New Philiosophy of Society. Assemblage Theory and Social Complexity* (New York: Bloomsbury, 2006), 18–19.

the work of Rimini Protokoll is characterised by combining testimonies of witnesses (whom they often refer to as 'experts-actors') physically present on stage with numerous technologies of digital representation. As Kara McKechnie points out, Rimini Protokoll creates a 'reality [that] is scripted and overtly mediated for performance.'[17] The blend of the real and the mediated in their performances inevitably challenges the received notion of the 'authentic' status of witnesses' personal testimony opening space for numerous frameworks of memory. In *Mnemopark,* the space takes a tangible form of a railway model. As the company explains on their website:

> [t]he world of *Mnemopark* is based upon an actual railway model – 1:87. What does society look like in its industrially manufactured reduplication? By means of minicameras *Mnemopark* advances into a model of the Alps, into the zones of a mysterious land. Thus a landscape simulation becomes film set. Meadows, forests, and barns are really faked up, though that only leads to a higher degree of their fictive reality.[18]

Rimini Protokoll invites four experts-actors – old members of a Swiss railway model club – to interact with the space and share their testimony with the audience. Each of them is given a solo performance in which they talk about their past using the technological means of representation to recreate their memories in front of the spectators. In order to scrutinise the strategies of performing witnesses in *Mnemopark* let me situate their testimony in two concurrent frameworks of memory: technology of mediatised image employed by Rimini Protokoll and the socio-political discourse introduced by the artists. How does the switch between the two frameworks modify the status of the individual testimonies of the experts-actors?

In order to analyse the function of media as a framework of memory, it is crucial to first describe the apparatus employed by Rimini Protokoll. In *Mnemopark,* the artists use real-time film image from three cameras: one is applied to the model train which travels through the landscape; the other camera is embedded in the glasses that the witnesses wear for most of the performance; finally, another camera captures the witnesses as they react with a greenbox situated next to the railway model. Rimini Protokoll utilises this tripartite apparatus in order to superimpose different camera images on a screen situated

---

17 Kara McKechnie, 'Instance: Rimini Protokoll, Mnemopark (2005)' *Mapping Intermediality in Performance,* edited by Sarah Bay-Cheng, Chiel Kattenbelt, Andy Lavender, and Robin Nelson (Amsterdam: Amsterdam University Press, 2010), 75.

18 Ibid., 76.

behind the railway model. Thus, spectators not only observe the outcome of technological manipulation, but they are constantly aware of the whole process of manufacturing media images. For example, at one point the expert-actor Hermann Löhle talks about his house and family in Switzerland. In order to do so, he enters the greenbox space and sits on a high stool while the other experts-actors set the model train in motion. The screen shows the view from the slow-moving locomotive. Gradually, the colours become more vivid and suddenly the image of Hermann filmed from the back is inserted into the locomotive view. The experts-actor performs a series of movements in the greenbox which are translated into his journey through the landscape on screen. The other experts-actors follow the model train and animate the elements of the landscape in order to illustrate Hermann's testimony. At one point of Hermann's performance, they place a model of his house on the landscape. Hermann waves to the small figurines situated in front of the house and the audience sees them filmed from the camera placed in Hermann's glasses. As Hermann comes near the house, the image of the landscape model dissolves into a pre-filmed footage showing Hermann giving a tour around his actual house talking about his family. What is the effect of this complicated technological apparatus on the witness's testimony?

Hermann's sequence clearly shows that media technology is used by Rimini Protokoll to reveal different conventions of traditional documentary theatre lending credibility to the witness's testimony. In this respect, Rimini Protokoll creatively explores the potential of cinema as a metaphor of memory. As the Dutch cultural historian Douve Draaisma explains, the Lumière brothers' invention was instantly interpreted as a model of human memory. As Draaisma rhetorically asks, 'isn't human memory just like cinematography, a combination of movement and stasis, a magic marriage of camera obscura and photography?'[19] Hermann's solo performance critically examines this magical thinking about memory as a film being a mere record of human memories. As Kara McKechnie comments upon *Mnemopark*,

> [t]he fact that we can see the storyteller's point of view, along with a seemingly convincing insertion of them interacting with the model landscape, does not entirely make for make-believe, but is pleasurable for an audience prepared to indulge in knowing illusion.[20]

19 Douve Draaisma, *Metaphors of Memory: A History of Ideas about the Mind* (Cambridge: Cambridge University Press, 2000), 134.

20 McKechnie, 'Instance.', 79.

In other words, Hermann's testimony may turn out to be interpreted by the audience as a personal believable story, and thus gain affective potential, due to the disillusionment strategies employed by the artists who constantly raise the spectator's awareness of media involved in the transmission of memories. Therefore, Hermann as a performing witness is in possession of his own testimony but the status of his memories as his own must be reinforced by appropriate technological operations.

However, if we place *Mnemopark* in a different framework of memory, experts-actors' memories perform yet another function. This may be exemplified by the presence of a professional actress throughout the performance. Not only does she provide links between individual performances of the experts-actors but also she situates their testimonies in a broader socio-political context of contemporary Switzerland. For example, in the opening section of the performance, she describes the landscape model using geographical terms pertaining to the actual properties of the Swiss landscape. Thus, the landscape model constructed by Rimini Protokoll becomes both the landscape of witnesses' memory and a metonymy of the Swiss society. In this context, the testimonies of experts-actors inevitably exemplify particular social problems. For instance, at one point of *Mnemopark*, the only female expert-actor Heidi Mühlthaner talks about the moment in the past when her interest in nature motivated her passion for creating landscape models. She recreates her memory by painting actual figurines of animals and people in front of the audience, which is projected onto the screen. The intimate aspect of her testimony is reinforced by a gentle background music. However, as the sequence unfolds, the music turns out to be a linking device merging the testimony with the film sequence introduced by the actress. The sequence that appears on the screen is a fragment of a Bollywood film shot in Switzerland. In a matter-of-fact voice, the actress informs the audience about the number of Bollywood movies produced in the country as well as the potential damages filmmakers may do to the pristine natural landscape. Meanwhile, experts-actors burst into a quasi-dance routine throwing colourful scarves in the air, which clearly parodies the Bollywood style.

The overt strategies of comedy used by Rimini Protokoll in this sequence introduce elements of social criticism of the Swiss preoccupation with preserving the 'natural' landscape as the hallmark of their notorious neutrality. In fact, the alpine landscape epitomises Switzerland's entanglement in the assemblage of capitalist processes, which means everything but being neutral. For the Alps have always been part of the global tourism providing scenic views for the richest who found refuge in the pristine landscape. Think of the Polish director Roman Polanski's house arrest in his Gstaad villa which saved him from being deported to the US to face the sexual abuse charges. In the context of Mnemopark, however, the juxtaposition of the personal testimony and a kitschy Bollywood movie may be interpreted as a means of raising the audiences' awareness of the ongoing commercialisation of Swiss natural landscape. Heidi's intimate memories are involved in a particular debate about the mechanisms of contemporary capitalism which affect natural environment. Thus, the testimony becomes an exponent of sentimentalist thinking about 'invaluable' nature which is to be cherished only by individuals who should prevent its commodification. Consequently, it is virtually impossible to distinguish the expert-actor's personal testimony from its status as an argument put forward by the artist.

The analysis of the performative potential of the frameworks of memory in *Mnemopark* proves that the status of performing witnesses not only emerges at the intersection of different modes of media representation but also is a result of particular socio-political discourses introduced by artists. However, it would be inadequate to claim that the mechanisms are pertinent solely to performances employing state-of-the-art technologies of media representation, as in the case of Rimini Protokoll. Thus, let us scrutinise an example of a more traditional theatrical performance in order to show that frameworks of memory influence the testimony even if there is seemingly no technology involved in the artistic process.

3 Third Movement: *Transfer!* and Performing Witnesses

In order to show the influence of frameworks of memory on performing witnesses in a theatrical performance, let us focus on the production *Transfer!* (2006) by the Polish young director Jan Klata. The production is based on memories of Polish and German citizens who were expulsed from their houses in the course of the resettlement programme enacted in the aftermath of the Second World War. The cast combines actors with amateurs who are the witnesses of the event. In order to distinguish them from Rimini Protokoll's experts-actors, I will refer to them as amateurs-actors to reinforce their lack of professional training, as highlighted by Klata. To understand the place of *Transfer!* in Polish contemporary theatre, it is indispensable to mention the context in which it was created. *Transfer!* was first staged during a time of an intensive conflict between Polish and German cultural memories of World War II. For the German part, there was the action of Erica Steinbach, a right-wing activist who has campaigned for the privileged status of memories of the Germans expelled from their country, now Western Poland. While for the Polish side the conflict, has revolved around the sense of injustice stemming from the mass resettlement project carried out after the war. In this context, Klata aims at confronting the actual actors of the events so that post-war resettlements cease to be an area of institutional remembrance. However, in order to establish credibility of the amateurs-actors' testimonial, the director employs a number of strategies that may be perceived as frameworks of memory. Let us examine the consequences of employing the frameworks for establishing the status of witnesses entering the stage.

To show the function of theatrical techniques as frameworks of memory in *Transfer!*, it its crucial to focus on the very set design of the piece which is organised around two spaces: the mobile platform placed over the stage where the actual actors playing Churchill, Roosevelt and Stalin are placed and the stage itself covered in soil which becomes the space of the amateurs. This spatial configuration may be interpreted in Hayden White's terms as a division between those who write history and those who are excluded from the process.[21] The juxtaposition necessarily affects the status of the witnesses. Churchill, Roosevelt and Stalin are depicted in a manifestly farcical convention as characters who are merely playing with history in disregard of its consequences. In this context, the spectator tends to empathise with the amateurs-actors whose emotional engagement in the stories they tell reinforces their reliability as witnesses. Therefore, the set design provides an environment for constituting the witness of history.

The problematic aspect of performing witnesses in Klata's production, may be illustrated by the strategies of post-dramatic theatre employed in *Transfer!* which revolves around the material presence of the actor's body. The tangible nature of the body serves as a framework of memory operating beyond intellectual perception of the audience. Klata exploits the tension between the semiotic and the phenomenal aspects of theatrical reality. The first example of the post-dramatic strategy to be discussed in reference to *Transfer!* is the relation between the body of amateurs-actors and the character they perform. The script of the production was written by two dramaturges Sebastian Majewski who worked with the Polish participants and Dunia Funke who recorded the testimonials of the German amateurs-actors. What is important, is that there is a difference in dramaturgical techniques employed by the artists. The lines spoken by German amateurs-actors were the unabridged version of their memories recorded by the dramaturge. As for the Polish members of the

21 Hayden White, 'The Historical Event,' *Differences: A Journal of Feminist Cultural Studies* 19.2 (2008): 10.

cast, their parts were merely inspired by their testimonial and entirely written by Majewski. As a result the amateurs-actors are clearly uttering lines written for them by someone else—and their delivery evokes children reciting poems in school. This momentarily engages the audience who often encourages the amateurs-actors to continue their performance. Thus, two questions arise: to what extent is the testimonial manipulated by the artists and how authentic are they in the audience's reception?

Writing about amateurs in theatre, a Polish theatre scholar Artur Duda claims that 'performing oneself is a particular form of being.'[22] Klata appears to exploit this form of being on stage to legitimise the status of amateurs-actors as witnesses of history. Their blatantly untheatrical behaviour paradoxically contributes to strengthening of their position as witnesses. The elderly people forget their lines and the work of the prompter during the production is vital. In other words, in performance, heavily scripted testimonials become believable as the process of remembering onstage resembles the work of memory which comprises moments of hesitation and uncertainty about the correct version of the past. The effect is further reinforced by different reactions of the amateurs-actors to their mistakes and slips of memory ranging from nervous laughter to gestures of resignation. In other words, as Erika Fischer-Lichte puts it, contemporary performance constantly 'switches focus between the actor's phenomenal and semiotic body, thus transferring the perceiving subject into a state of betwixt and between.'[23] Thus, one can say that there are two modes of experiencing performance: the order of representation which focuses on the fictional entities on stage and the order of the presence which concentrates the spectator's attention on the actor's physicality. The two experiential modes are coexistent within a production which aims at maintaining a balance between them. However, the borders between representation and presence are extremely fluid and the actor is constantly situated in the liminal space between himself or herself and the character he or she performs. Consequently, both modes of experiencing theatre influence the audience's perception of the performance.

In *Transfer!* the balance between the two orders of perception is severely uneven. Intuitively, we know that the amateurs are bodies placed on the stage rather than semiotic figures they enact. In consequence, it is important to analyse their physicality as a framework of memory. The most conspicuous physical aspect of the amateurs-actors is their advanced age. The spectator instantly

22 Artur Duda, *Teatr realności* (Gdańsk: Słowo/Obraz/Terytoria, 2006), 170, my own translation. 'Granie siebie z pewnością stanowi szczególną formę bycia sobą.'

23 Erika Fischer-Lichte, *The Transformative Power of Performance* (New York: Routledge, 2008), 89.

notices their impaired movement: some of them are crippled, the others use crutches. Therefore, the audience becomes emotionally engaged in the performance being anxious about the health condition of the amateurs-actors. Moreover, putting the aging body in the theatrical space stresses the typical physical features associated with old age. The monochromatic light employed by the artists stresses their wrinkles and physical exhaustion during about two-hour long show. As a result of this performative strategy, the body becomes a means of memory which records the actual passing of time and in the process of giving testimonial, the disabled aging body becomes a time machine which transfers the spectators into the past. This effect manifests itself in the scene where one of the German amateurs-actors covers her ears hearing one of Hitler's speeches. The gesture directs the audience to the time of war when the woman as a young girl feared the aggressive voice of the Führer, which generates a huge affective reception among the audience.

The strategy of accentuating the physicality of the witnesses is most efficient in situations where the amateurs-actors step outside the carefully crafted script. There are two groups of scenes in which their material presence is the overriding factor in authenticating their testimonial. The first one is comprised of songs and nursery rhymes from the amateurs-actors childhood whereas the other one is based on memorabilia the participants of Klata's artistic project carry with them onto the stage. In both cases they are objects of memory that work, as it were, as *objets trouvés* which are introduced into the reality of theatrical illusion. Thus, the stage functions as a medium of conveying the re-enacted memories of the witnesses of history. This authenticating strategy of exploiting the voice and object belonging to amateurs-actors may be exemplified by one of the final scenes of *Transfer!* in which an elderly lady reads out the list of people who lived in her home village before the resettlement. She made the list as a sort of mnemonic exercise after having arrived in Wrocław (Western Poland). The woman has noted down the name, surname and the nationality of the inhabitants. Subsequently, the order of names matches the topography of the village, thus resembling Frances the ancient loci mnemotechnic system described by Frances Yates in her *The Art of Memory*.[24] Thus, the scene aims at engaging the spectators' sensory perception in the process of remembering and names enable them to recreate an intimate and intricate map of the woman's memory. The spatial and temporal dimension of the testimony converges in a highly affective performance of the witness. Moreover, the scene generates a huge subversive potential as in the official narrative

24 Frances Yates, *The Art of Memory* (New York: Routledge, 1999), 1–26.

the space would be represented as merely a point on the map of the pre-war Poland whereas in *Transfer!* it becomes a space of diverse ethnicities viewed through the subjective lens of the witness.

To conclude, the concept of the Halbwachsian frameworks of memory enable us to investigate different strategies of performing witnesses in contemporary performing art, especially those employing various technologies of media representation. On the one hand, the analysis of *Mnemopark* has indicated that witnesses testimony changes its status depending on the framework in which it functions, be it media technology used or socio-political context in which it is situated. However, on the other hand, the study of theatrical strategies used in the production of *Transfer!* by Jan Klata has proved that frameworks of memory operate even if the artist employs scarce media technologies reinforcing the witness's physicality. Therefore, performing witnesses are always dependent on the various intricate processes merging the individual and the collective which are responsible for the status of their testimony.

Bibliography

Assmann, Jan. *Cultural Memory and Early Civilization*. Cambridge: Cambridge University Press, 2011

DeLanda, Manuel. *A New Philiosophy of Society. Assemblage Theory and Social Complexity*. New York: Bloomsbury, 2006.

Draaisma, Douve. *Metaphors of Memory: A History of Ideas about the Mind*. Translated by Paul Vincent. Cambridge: Cambridge University Press, 2000.

Duda, Artur. *Teatr realności*. Gdańsk: Słowo/Obraz/Terytoria. 2006.

Fischer-Lichte, Erika. *The Transformative Power of Performance*. Translated by Saskya Iris Jain. New York: Routledge. 2008.

Halbwachs, Maurice. *Les cadres sociaux de la mémoire*. Chicoutimi: Cégep de Chicoutimi, 2002.

Halbwachs, Maurice. *The Collective Memory*. Translated by Francis J. Ditter and Vida Yazdi Ditter. New York: Harper & Row, 1980.

McKechnie, Kara. 'Instance: Rimini Protokoll, Mnemopark (2005),' *Mapping Intermediality in Performance*. Edited by Sarah Bay-Cheng, Andy Levender, Chiel Kattenbelt and Robin Nelson. 75–84. Amsterdam: Amsterdam University Press, 2010.

White, Hayden. 'Figural Realism in Witness Literature,' *Parallax: Witnessing Theory* 30 (2004): 132–145.

White, Hayden. 'The Historical Event.' *Differences: A Journal of Feminist Cultural Studies* 19.2 (2008): 9–34.

Yates, Frances. *The Art of Memory*. New York: Routledge. 1999.

PART 4

Testimonial Embodiments

CHAPTER 10

Sick: Negotiating Body Trauma through Visual Art Practice

Candace Couse

Abstract

Recognizing the sick body as both the abuser and the object of abuse, I argue that in sickness the body is doubly mastered. Through a first-hand testimonial, I consider the role that art production plays on an artist undergoing body trauma. Through a visual account—an installation—I ask how art production at this precipice may contribute to reorientation after sizeable shifts in understanding. I examine the role of the artist in achieving new understandings of the sick body through the analysis of a body of work that offers a physical, dynamic access point for empathetic relations between bodies, exchanging ideas and experiences that may occur through the viewing experience. Through affect theory and the notion of affective art, this chapter examines how body trauma is something not only experienced inside a body but also something that that can be projected into objects and space. Understanding visual art as an object ripe for this form of projection, the viewer is unbound and able to meet an extra-subjective aspect of pain memory in encountering art. In this affective encounter, the artist's preceding intentions fade and what is left is a cry in the dark: a sensuous quality of trauma that might be isolated and taken up by the artwork, allowing for a new site for a sensuous experience that extends temporally and spatially to engage the viewer in a lived experience.

Keywords

anatomical – body – embodiment – identity – illness – self – trauma – visual accounts – visual art – sick

The *Testimony: Memory, Trauma, Truth, Engagement Project: 2nd Global Meeting* conference brought up truly rich ideas around autoethnographic modes of trauma testimony. Self-reflective writing and artistic production that explore

 | DOI:10.1163/9789004391130_012

personal experience connect deeply private stories to the public domain and all the cultural, political, and social understandings that intersect both spheres. The isolating territory of pain is a place where experience cannot be easily shared or comprehended. Through the act of self-reflective production, aspects of illness, emotional trauma and pain memory can be given a home outside of the body, propelled outward onto the page or objects in space, and there it can wait, readily available for an encounter with another. In this encounter, an experience is made accessible around the subject of trauma and pain that demands no exact interpretation but fosters an affective encounter between the one who suffers and the one who bears witness. This mode of relating, often unattainable in everyday encounters with others, is here driven by the pre-set systems of the creative object and how it is grappled with. Visual art and poetry are two artistic endeavours that are a particularly good fit for the language of trauma; fractured and unfettered, they leave room for their reader and the marks of their author.

Heather Taylor Johnson's *Testimony: Memory, Trauma, Truth, Engagement* conference presentation, "Illness Narratives: A Poetry Reading" on the topic of pain and poetry is a key analysis that illustrates the problematic nature of encounters that attempt to interpret pain and illness by clinging to linear narratives. Undoubtedly, these liner systems are pursued because they have a temporal trajectory. In resolving trauma's beginning, middle and end we hope that we have unlocked the formula on how cruelties come to pass and hope we can somehow prevent them. With trauma and illness, as Taylor Johnson knowingly points out, there is no resolution because there cannot truly be a time before or after, only a 'somewhere-in-between'. We can, then, appeal to foster a compassionate and affective encounter in hopes of counteracting the same narratives of pain and suffering that repeat again and again through cycles of psychic and physical violence between bodies over time and across space. Because the sick body is as much a social being as it is a physical one, violence is performed in the social and biological space. Taylor Johnson's writing and the ideas around trauma testimony explored in the *Testimony: Memory, Trauma, Truth, Engagement Project* have invigorated my interest in how we might change our thinking in a way that disrupts a tendency for cyclical repetition of violence between bodies. In considering this, I wish to centre my analysis on the violence and trauma unique to the sick body as it is produced and reproduced both bodily and socially.

In 1951, the term, 'sick role' was coined by functionalist sociologist Talcott Parsons and subsequently entered into in the lexicon of medical sociology. The sick role encapsulated the rights and obligations of the sick body. The argument specified that being sick signifies that the body enters a role of 'sanctioned deviance', which occupies a space away from the public sphere that requires policing by the medical profession. The sick role understands illness and body trauma as a form of aberration that interrupts social functionality.[1] Many decades later, upon reading this, one might recoil at the severity of this definition. One perhaps may take comfort in the idea that we do not currently view sick bodies in such a way, but I would caution the reader not to make that assumption. I contend that the sick body is at once physically ill and ascribed the social position of 'sick', which moves beyond a physical condition to contain altered rights and obligations within its social environment. There is much ground that may be covered through the lens of body trauma. Illness is only one expression of many, but one that deserves attention for its unique position of holding a body in a strange, exclusionary state of physical powerlessness.

This chapter presents a feminist, autobiographical reading of the sick body by looking at the status and treatment it contracts under existing patriarchal institutions. Reflecting on personal, traumatic sick-bodied experience, I ask: how can we escape the snare of knowledge produced under the corporeal universal?; how can more just ways of knowing be inserted into existing conditions?; and how can this insertion create radical transformation? To answer these questions, I turn to the theme of testimony in visual art. Asserting that art has the capacity to become a site for radical transformation, I connect Affect Theory—with its emphasis on bodily experience—to the concept of affective art. Affective art, as I frame it, has strong roots in Theodor Adorno's theory of 'authentic art', which understands works of modern art as 'social monads' that are 'societally mediated' and have 'socially significant meaning'.[2] Affective art can be described as a theorization of the condition in which the work of art is both produced and received, allowing for alternative expressions—in this case, of trauma—and the radical transformation of systems of knowledge in which we find ourselves encased. Moreover, in drawing the idea of affective art from affect theory, I can explore the politics of thinking through the body. By thinking through the body, I refer to the ways in which the body can be reconsidered as a site of knowledge rather than an obstacle to transcend or to dominate. In this way of relating to the world, the felt comes first, leading one into thought. As an artist and scholar, I put forward a personal account of my sick body and the corresponding moment in my own artistic practice. In doing so, I will make myself the 'rabbit in the

1 Millon Blaney and Roger D. Davis, *Oxford Textbook of Psychopathology* (New York: Oxford University Press, 1999), 446.

2 Theodore Adorno, *Aesthetic Theory*, translated by R. Hullot-Kentor (Minneapolis: University of Minnesota Press, 1997), 9.

laboratory' while also noting, at this juncture, the limits of my ability to assess the success of my particular work in terms of the emancipatory qualities art may possess as discussed in this chapter. In keeping with Adorno, it must be stated that this 'rabbit' could be replaced by another, as what matters here is the 'single relationship between the subject who confers meaning and the meaningless object, between rational significance and its accidental bearer'.[3] There exist works (like Roland Barthes' *Roland Barthes par Roland Barthes*, or Adrienne Rich's *Of Woman Born*) that take the unusual step of combining autobiography and scholarly work.[4] Here, I am endeavouring to do this as well. My hope in following suit is to dispense similarly with the traditional knowledge bracketing and to connect my ideas to the physical happenings and history of my body. In short, what follows is an examination of how meaning is ascribed to bodies, how these meanings cause harm, and how art creates affective connections that provide opportunities for thinking through the body towards radical transformation.

1 Putting a Voice to Body Trauma

In Western culture, we readily and unfairly equate the refusal to speak of trauma with the refusal to deal with trauma. The idea of 'dealing' through 'speaking' suggests a cultural understanding that trauma necessarily must be mitigated by one's relationship to others: *your trauma must become our trauma, or at the very least, we must understand your trauma if we cannot have it.* However, this exchange so often ends before it begins as words cannot always be found, pointing to a failure of the rationalistic approach. The idea that physical pain does not simply resist language but actively destroys it is shared by Virginia Woolf and Elaine Scarry. For Woolf, we simply do not have the words to adequately embody pain and everything must follow 'as if'.[5] For Scarry, pain is inward, often without an external object with which to relate.[6] Pain heightens the divide between self and other; it is that which can be effortlessly grasped

3 Max Horkheimer, Theodor Adorno and Gunzelin Schmid Noerr, *Dialectic of Enlightenment: Philosophical Fragments*, translated by Edmond Jephcott (Stanford: Stanford University Press, 2002), 7.

4 Jane Gallop, *Thinking through the Body* (New York: Columbia University Press, 1988), 6.

5 Virginia Woolf, 'On Being Ill', *Collected Essays*. Vol. 4 (New York: Harcourt, 1967), 194.

6 Elaine Scarry, *The Body in Pain: The Making and Unmaking of the World* (New York: Oxford University Press, 1985), 5.

by one, yet so easily oblivious to another. This gap leaves a space where the body in pain can face doubt about its existence or may encounter the other's freedom to deny its existence altogether. Furthermore, when pain robs the body of a voice, the task of articulating the hidden pain is taken up by medical professionals who seek to use their knowledge to speak for the sick body and elevate the discourse into the public realm. Here, in the public sphere of political action, the patient's voice is met with misgivings while the doctor's words embody authority and trustworthiness, enabling the 'deviant' pain of the sick body to enter the social sphere on the physician's terms. This means that there are political consequences to the expressibility of the sick body: silenced or misrepresented, the self becomes confined to the body—like pain—without an external object with which to relate.[7] In its 'deviant' state, the sick body is without an acknowledged voice and is permitted only obligations. These obligations are to submit to and cooperate with the medical professional who is tasked with returning the body to the fold.

There are, of course, ways in which medicine knows its objects. There is not the needed space in this chapter to fully delve into the trap that is post-enlightenment thinking with its Instrumental means that prescribe the limited ways a thing might be talked about, calculated, measured, or incised. If I had room, I could speak more to the fluidity of the body: the ambiguous congress of the tumour that grows inside the body and the body that holds it or the body as an object and the experience of pain the patient senses. Pluralities like this protest against the rigid classifications of how bodies are shaped and sources of knowledge are realized in current medical understandings. The desire to understand the sick body, historically, has been less about wanting to know the fractured, nuanced gradation in the appearance that body trauma so frequently exhibits, and more to classify, to inscribe constrained meaning to and to categorize the body in ways that erase critical nuance: the raped person becomes 'negligent', the tortured person becomes 'hero', and the person in pain becomes 'dying'. In *The Second Sex*, Simone de Beauvoir writes, '[a]n object that men have already mastered becomes a tool; cut off from its natural bonds, it loses its deepest attributes'.[8] Through the act of instrumentalizing the body, medical and social institutions have bound it up in reductive classifications. These labels create an inherent danger in trauma testimony, regardless of who is doing the speaking; when one seeks to escape the overwhelming trap the

7 Scarry, *The Body in Pain*, 4–33.

8 Simone de Beauvoir, *The Second Sex*, translated by Constance Borde and Sheila Malovany-Chevallier, (New York: Vintage, 2011) 173–174.

classification of victimhood provides and explores the richly nuanced world of experience. This becomes a demanding task. Still, as we will come to see, particular expressions of trauma and testimony have the potential to be actualized through a form of empathy that is more complex, and further still, potentially become a site of radical transformation.

Trauma is multifaceted, and one could not truly understand the trauma of another even if it could be described with exactitude in available language or visual representations. In the essay, 'Projected Memory', Marianne Hirsch seeks to redeem hidden suffering and interpret contemporary instances of testimony. Hirsch describes an affective encounter to the experience of others grounded in both difference and identification: '[feeling and suffering with the others] means ... the ability to say, It could have been me; it was me, also, and at the same time, but it was not me'.[9] In this method of relating, one may have hope to free the subsumed particular out from under the universal, which is to say one can observe, and indeed participate in, a particularity of a traumatic memory without characterizing those who give testimony, or stripping them of their subjectivity. 'It could have been me; it was me, also, and at the same time, but it was not me', can offer a critical alternative to the oversimplification and entitlement that lie at the heart of medical and social institutions. Ambiguity, nuance, and fluidity can be privileged in the affective relationship to others. Elizabeth Grosz notes that the politics of difference demands the existence of an ethics of difference, 'an ethics of the ongoing negotiations between beings whose differences, whose alterities, are left intact but with whom some kind of exchange is nonetheless possible'.[10] One space that is conducive to this type of exchange is art because art is richly multifaceted, borrowing methods, modes, and genres, and as it traverses the boundaries of academic disciplines, it can provide indispensable alternatives to fixed understandings. Art becomes a site for cries in the dark from pain that has been concretized as irregular by pervasive cultural myths. As a sensory impression, art may function in a way that is beyond the illustration of a happening (an answer offered by the artist), and, rather, engender a manner of thinking through this encounter between artist, art, viewer, and world.

9 Marianne Hirsch, 'Projected Memory: Holocaust Photographs in Personal and Private Fantasy', *Acts of Memory: Cultural Recall in the Present*, edited by Mieke Bal, Jonathan Crewe, and Leo Spitzer, (London: University Press of New England, 1999), 9; her emphasis.

10 Elizabeth A. Grosz, 'Sexed Bodies', *Volatile Bodies: Toward a Corporeal Feminism* (Bloomington: Indiana University Press, 1994), 192.

2 The Sick Artist

In February of 2009, I found out that I had an abnormal growth on my spine. I had been suffering from back pain, yet I was nevertheless quite surprised to find out the source of my pain. For some time, there could be no definitive diagnosis due to the location of the mass and troubles with imaging. I was scheduled for surgery and told they would do a biopsy once they had removed it. It was believed that I had a rare germ cell tumour. I was entirely alarmed by the idea that my body could be in possession of such a thing without me being conscious of its existence, without my hand in its making. What amplified this feeling was the realization that if I did indeed have a tumour filled with germ cells it could, in theory, be reproducing any part of me inside it. It could be growing miniature versions of my organs, replicated with precision, if not with permission. I spent a significant amount of the year following my operation lying in bed with an open wound and the help of a home-care nurse. I had some time on my hands and during this juncture, some significant thoughts occurred to me. I was horrified that I could be so unacquainted with something that was going on within my own body, and I was surprised by how different I became to others and others to me. I felt I had become a separate thing: a thing that was in the world, yet somehow set apart from it. My body no longer felt like my mind, but nor was it something that I could control if I were to treat it as a vehicle that I had acquired through some strange birth right. If I perceived a barrier between myself and the external, would this separation not allow for governance on some level? Evidently, not entirely. The sick body becomes alien to consciousness, revealing our illusion of control. One is othered in this betrayal of the body: an act that rips identity from the ties that keep it embodied, while simultaneously using those ties to fasten the mind to immotility, like a prisoner bound to the mast of a sinking ship. 'The feeling of pain entails the feeling of being acted upon',[11] writes Scarry. Here, the assailant is my body. However, there were other aggressors, too. When hands and tools penetrate in scheduled intrusions, the sick body throws open the distinction between the public and the private in the closest possible way. This medical treatment—this science—I received had a flavour to it that I only began to recognize as all too familiar the longer the treatment continued. It smacked of domination: of power and submission, of knowledge and ignorance, of mattering and not mattering. It is disingenuous to think of science as outside of culture, even as it probes ever deeper for the truth about nature. It operates as

11 Hirsch, 'Projected Memory', 16.

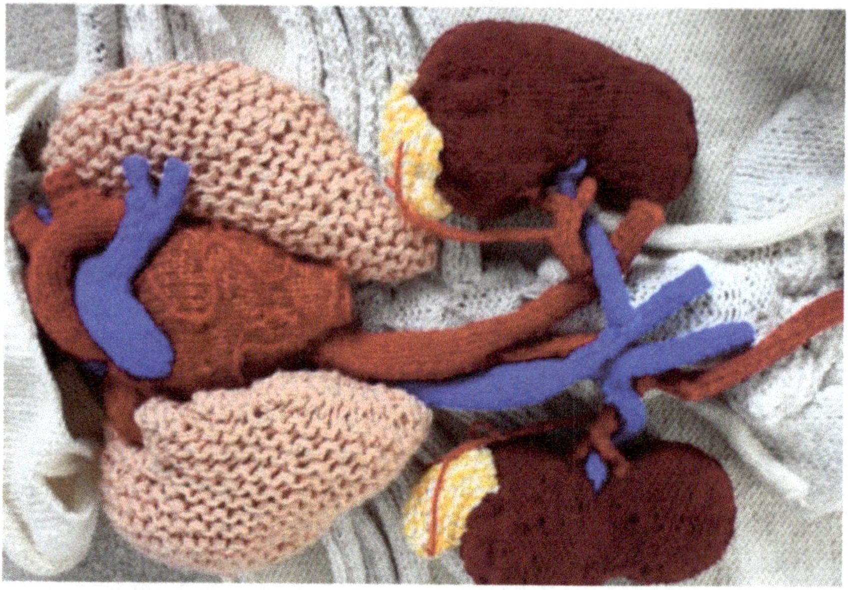

FIGURE 10.1 Detail of the knitted body in progress

a hegemonic system. Emily Martin takes this up in, 'The Woman in the Body: A Cultural Analysis of Reproduction', she writes,

> [T]he content of science presents a male-biased model of human nature and social reality. We find that the attributes of science are the attributes of males; the objectivity said to be characteristic of the production of scientific knowledge is specifically identified as a male way of relating to the world. Science is cold, hard, impersonal, "objective" women, by contrast, are warm, soft, emotional, "subjective."[12]

In science, the feminine voice is concealed in the wound and the masculine in the explanation of it. This is true of all sick bodies, not just female ones. Indeed, doctors neither trusted nor heard my voice. They sought to circumvent my requests in favour of a teaching opportunity, and my rare status made a spectacle of me. My insights about my body—what little faith I still have in them—are undoubtedly not preferred to ultrasounds, MRIs, and more blood work. These results will determine how much pain I am in, if at all.

12 Emily Martin, *The Woman in the Body: A Cultural Analysis of Reproduction* (Boston: Beacon, 2001), 21.

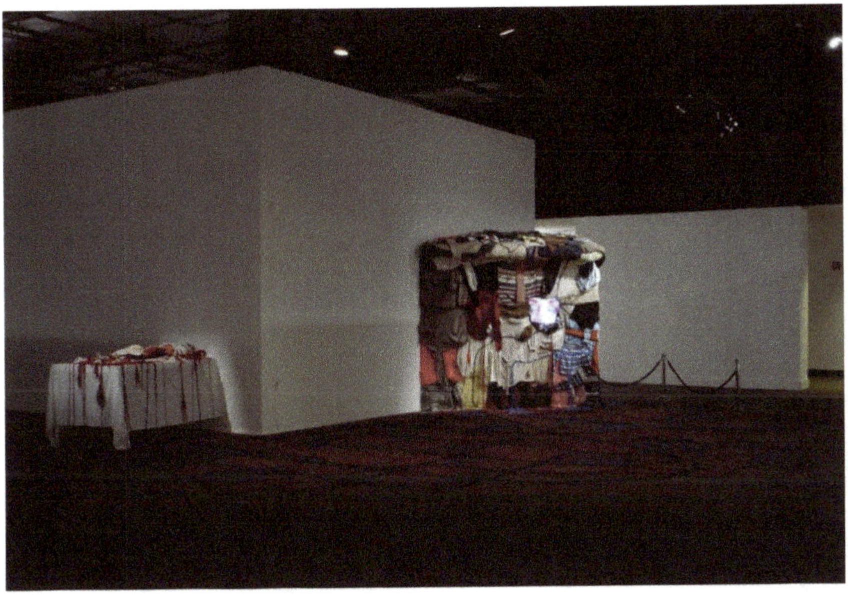

FIGURE 10.2 Detail of *Landlocked*
© 2009. PHOTOGRAPHER CANDACE COUSE. USED WITH PERMISSION.

The critique here is not that medical professionals may be right or wrong in their assumptions; it is that their assumptions are deeply cultural and speak to so much more than what they appear to say. They speak to the perceived nature of women, of men, of the sick body and indeed of the purpose of existence. To overcome my fear of vanishing and to attempt motility in what little ways I could, I fabricated a replica of my body out of yarn. I wanted to make a tangible and fully dissectible stand-in for my body so that I could come to know it through the act of exploration and the gathering of sensory information. Perhaps, in this way, I felt I could salvage my world order and gain back control. I chose to knit the body entirely, including skeletal structure, organs, blood vessels and skin. I experimented. I filmed the dissection of my body, attempting to map, or peg down that which necessarily belongs to me. I planned out large-scale installations where my body could reach outside of itself and sprawl across the floor in a tangled map of viscera.

This project exemplifies how body trauma is something experienced inside me, but also something that I can project into objects and space. Jill Bennett proposes that in, 'giving trauma extension in space or lived place, it invites awareness of different modes of inhabitation'.[13] In encountering the work, the

13 Jill Bennett, *Empathic Vision: Affect, Trauma, and Contemporary Art* (Stanford: Stanford University Press, 2005), 12; her emphasis.

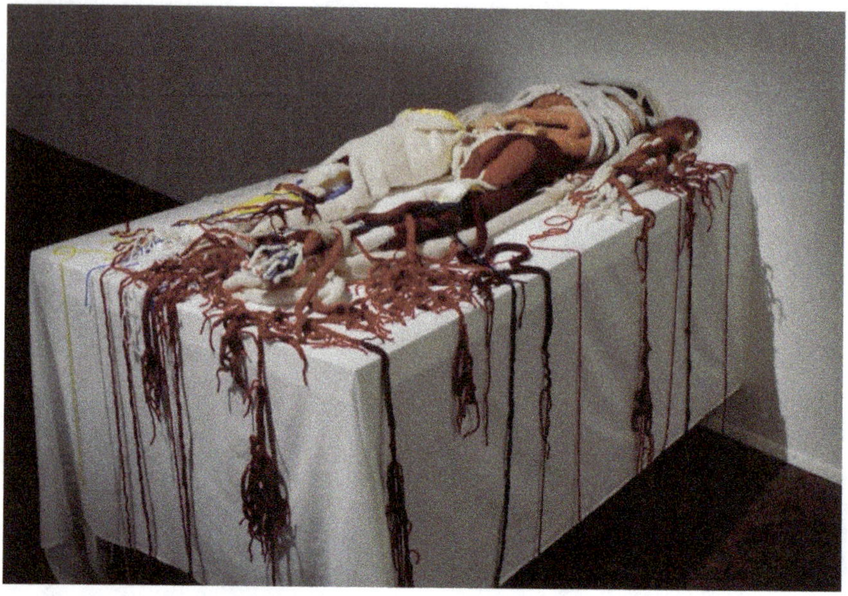

FIGURE 10.3 Detail of *Landlocked*

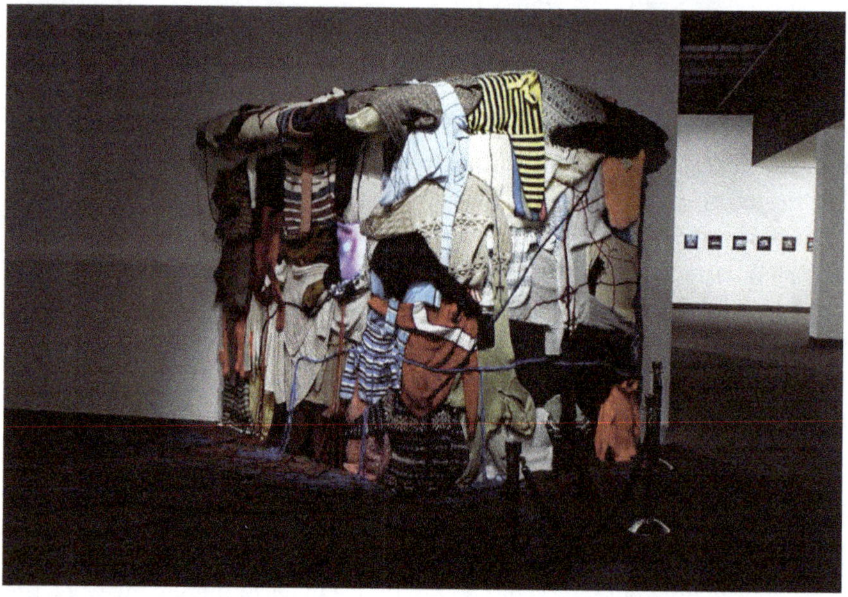

FIGURE 10.4 Detail of *Landlocked*

viewer could meet an extra-subjective aspect of my pain memory. In the affective art encounter, works of art are material reflections on the order of the world, societally mediated, and have socially significant meaning. Recalling that affective art is a theorization of the condition in which the work of art is both produced and received, the role of the artist, artwork, viewer, and world are all, undoubtedly, particular experiences, but they also meet in synthesis through the affective art encounter that allows for the radical transformation of systems of knowledge in which we find ourselves encased. As the artist, my motivations and intentions fade away as the viewer encounters the work, and what is left is a cry in the dark; a sensuous quality of trauma that might be isolated and taken up by the artwork, allowing for a new site for sensuous experience that extends temporally and spatially to engage the viewer in a lived experience. The body is turned inside out, anatomized and the border of facial likeness that personifies so many particular social, political, moral, and aesthetic codes melts away, along with the distance between the viewer and artwork, allowing bodies and their differences to meet without tight, ensnaring limitations. Disruptions of the inscribed, socially embedded meanings the body bears may crumble through cultivating self-reflexive encounters when bodies are brought into relation.[14]

For the viewer, envisioning the mechanics of death unfolding in a space they inhabit, sensuously experienced through the art object and acted upon—not the artist—but the viewer, circumvents the moral line. No overlay of a moral narrative is possible. Therefore, the mediating role of language or moral judgment is removed. One does not feel pity when one views this knitted body, but a more immediate, more carnal connection. One might see a sick body as vulgar, or venerate the sick person for their courage or tenacity from a hospital bedside, but in the exhibition, the viewer is at once the sick body and the witness and these reductions seem absurd. Such an experience would in no concrete way illustrate my particular experience of body trauma, brought on by illness, for the viewer. However, it would engender a relational language of trauma that advances from sensuously encountering my testimony in its affective expression, what Adorno would call authentic art.

Adorno's understanding of authentic art, taken into my larger understanding of affective art, is that art is still inherently a social construct, but it is 'both an artefact and a social fact', allowing it to be assembled 'in and against society'

14 Heidi Kellett, 'Skin Portraiture: Relational Embodiment and Contemporary Art', *Probing the Skin Cultural Representations of Our Contact Zone* (Newcastle upon Tyne: Cambridge Scholars Lady Stephenson Library, 2015), 239.

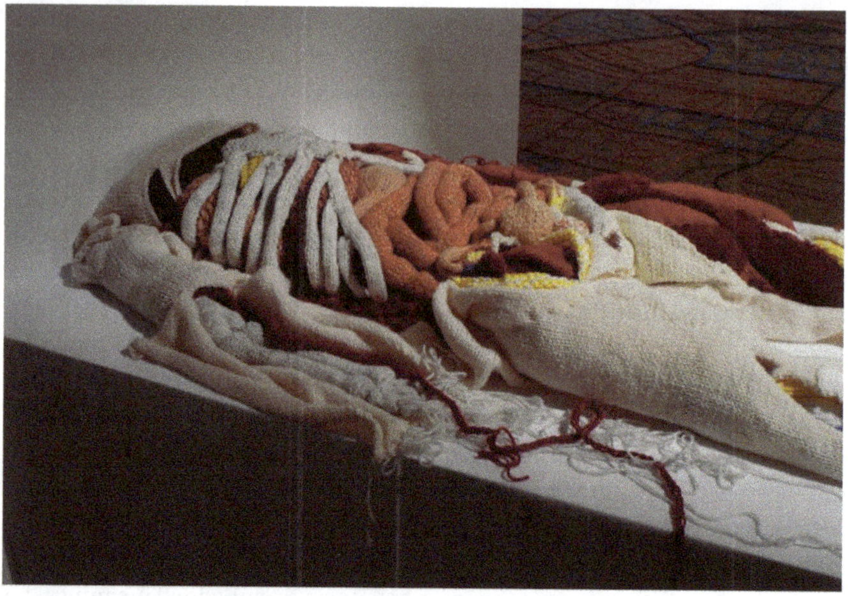

FIGURE 10.5 Detail of *Landlocked*

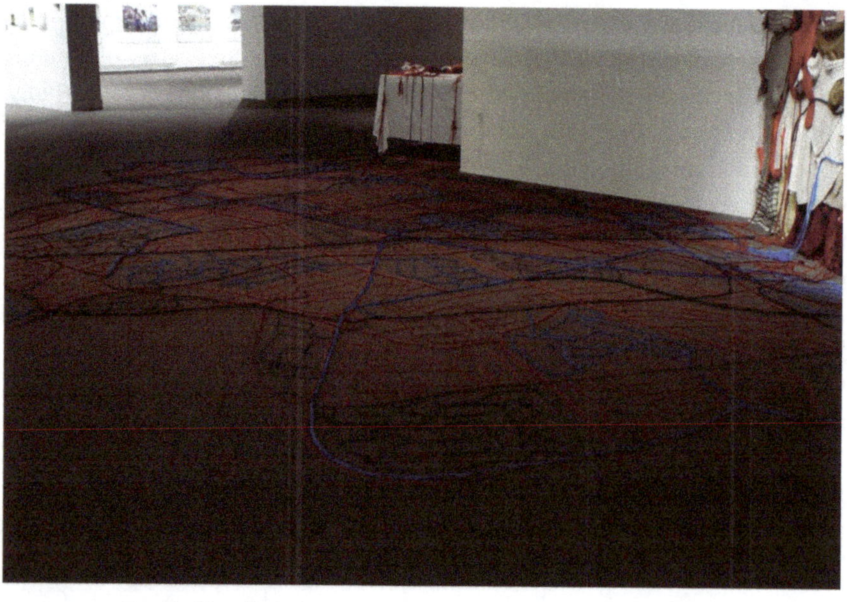

FIGURE 10.6 Detail of *Landlocked*

and be immediately a critical theory of society and a point of departure for radical politics.[15] It is, in fact, these very remnants of social production that become the letters that the viewer might take up and reassemble into the vocabulary of transformation. Affective art offers feeling and reflection, but not answers. An artwork exists in reference to what has preceded it: it is an ambivalent shadow, a trace. It resists precision and cannot answer what is, or what is not. It avoids the mere imitation of what already is. In this way, it bucks the system. It offers moments of reflection that can bring about changes in the general consciousness and thus also in social reality. However, just as an artist cannot control the response to her work, affective art cannot pledge change. The inability of affective art to act, declare or assert is that which allows it to oppose instrumental rationalization. Adorno's autonomous art has a disengaged, non-participatory, existence, and it is both complex and arbitrary. When successful, its messages are ambiguous. Adorno writes, 'only those artworks are enlightened that, vigilantly distant from the empirical, evince true consciousness'.[16] Adorno suggests that 'ultimately, aesthetic comportment is to be defined as the capacity to shudder', and here, the obligation falls to the viewer to foster openness to authentic art so as to provide the opportunity—through the actions of the viewer—for art to revitalize life. Hellings writes,

> Life must be lived as art must be entered, both freely and with discipline, both lightheartedly and deadly serious—subjectivity could learn a lot from the objectivity of art if only it opened itself up to all the grit and splinters facing it.[17]

We need moments that have the capacity to upset both mind and matter; moments that allow us to think through the body. Affective art has a distancing effect (an intimacy with, yet inevitably detached relationship to the artist and her experience) and it puts forward a great refusal through modernist strategies: it confronts society through its otherness; it critiques society, and can transform it; it inhabits a space of theoretical inquiry and is the site from which a politics of empathy emerges, free from our everyday, entrenched ways of thinking about the world. Through these opportunities, it provides us with glimpses of alternatives that we may have assumed were beyond us. This is to

15 James Hellings, *Adorno and Art: Aesthetic Theory Contra Critical Theory* (Basingstoke: Palgrave Macmillan, 2014), 3.

16 Theodor Adorno, Rolf Tiedemann and Robert Hullot-Kentor, *Aesthetic Theory* (London: Continuum, 2002), 86.

17 Hellings, *Adorno and Art,* 109.

say, under the right conditions a viewer who is open to this participatory act can engage with it. Through this engagement, it may come to enter the social consciousness and lead to practical change. Resistance and emancipation can be realized.

3 Baring Witness

We are perhaps all too familiar with the problems of bearing witness as contained in documentaries, literature and all media at large. The framing of the 'good' and 'bad'[18] creates moral interpretations that readily see us jumping to venerate the protagonist and demonize the antagonist. This tendency to subsume particulars under such universals is a symptom of domination under prevailing power structures. Presumptuous characterizations, dehumanization, and classification are all familiar by-products of a sick body witnessed. Like the raped body, the sick body often lacks the real-estate to contain blame to the topography of their body alone. Yes, they are told that their body has betrayed them, but they are also told that their clothing, lifestyle choices, and attitudes have brought them their pain and caused their body to betray them. Questions are even asked about the state of their mother's womb, what she put in her mouth and swallowed down by the directions of her doctor and what she did not. Beauvoir writes about man's horror in the face of the stain of biological functions: birth, life, and the female body shock him back to the recognition that he is of nature and therefore in the grip of death.[19] His reaction to his loathed dependence is to transfer the stain onto the bodies of women, and all those whose bodies betray them as unlike the universal. If death is the work of women, no body is more instrumentalized that the sick woman's body: this body is the battleground where man's mastery over nature rages and the subjecthood of the body, here, is without value beyond cause and cure. This domination is taken up so wholly in behaviour and language that medical professionals must undergo coaching to mask it with recitals on bedside manner. Indeed, I would go so far as to say that the sick body, itself, is feminized, which is to say that even sick male bodies are feminized. The male body turned deviant has been reclassified by its new placement in relationship to death. In

18 Susannah Radstone, 'Social Bonds and Psychical Orders: Testimonies', *Traumatizing Theory: The Cultural Politics of Affect in and beyond Psychoanalysis*, edited by Karyn Ball (New York: Other Press, 2007), 104.

19 De Beauvoir, *The Second Sex*, 165.

classing the sick body, pain is a symbolic substitute for death. Scarry notes the intuitive human recognition that,

> Pain is the equivalent in felt experience of what is unfeelable in death. Each only happens because of the body. In each, the contents of consciousness are destroyed. The two are the most intense forms of negation, the purest expressions of the anti-human, of annihilation, of total averseness though one is an absence and the other a felt presence, one occurring in the cessation of sentience, the other expressing itself in grotesque overload. Regardless, then, of context in which it occurs, physical pain always mimes death, and the infliction of physical pain is always a mock execution.[20]

The man, regularly free to enjoy his transcendence, seemingly unencumbered by his body, often abhors his new connection to nature and to the feminine. His repulsion commonly moves quite beyond the physical ailment and sits almost entirely on the feminized, social positioning of 'sick', to which he is now a member. Men speak of their illnesses as misogynists speak of their wives: they scorn their vulnerability, leakiness, helplessness, and dependence; they are disgusted by their inability to contribute meaningfully to the world, their station and often their failure to think rationally. This stylization of the body is sustained and regulated by social means that see this behaviour as belonging to a natural order as opposed to the rational or scientific. The sick person is tied to the feminine because they are 'bodily' and subject to nature, the medical practitioner is 'cultural' and 'mental' and, therefore, higher functions are presumed to occur. While social stratification based on gender performs in this space, such treatment of this positioning is seen as ethical because its projection of what is natural works in harmony with the directives of the universal male: it operates through the self-elaborating mechanisms mirroring the myth of the feminized, sick body. The continuation of this myth of the naturalization (feminization) of the sick body means that the conversation of male and female healthcare workers, and the ways in which medicine 'knows' its objects are reified in their unfolding from a point of patriarchy. This myth of the feminized sick body, produced and circulated by the behaviours and choices of individuals, possesses space where radical transformation may occur. Undeniably, an institution contingent on the practices of individuals can be undermined by the collective actions of choosing individuals. In affective artwork,

20 Scarry, *The Body in Pain*, 31.

a language of sensation replaces a language of words. Communicable affect enables us to see the attributes of pain and thus, seizes on something unspeakable in a language which is so often coded by domination masquerading as reality.

Affective art, as discussed here, gives weight to bodily experience, to the ways in which the body can be reconsidered as a site of knowledge rather than an obstacle to transcend or to dominate. Carrying ideas forward from Adorno's authentic art, there arise some potential points of criticism that should be addressed on the subject of dominance. For example, what can be questioned is whether the freedom to make artwork is inherently tied to some degree of socio-economic privilege. Is it characteristically bourgeois? While this certainly may be the case (and almost exclusively so in Adorno's time and much of Western history) we have reached a point in our contemporary, globalized state where the idea of who is recognized as an art maker, and what is recognized as art in terms of material and concept, has expanded tremendously. Art is encountered and produced by the child street-artist in the slums of Brazil to the renowned artist and his retrospective in the Guggenheim. The 'hung' authority, previously essential for the display of art, has been coaxed from the white cube and thrust into the ghetto, the war zone, the coffee shop or onto the internet. I shall not argue that elitism or significant disparities in market value do not exist (they do!) but they are relegated to the marketplace and are not commensurable to the affective encounter with the work. One is equally able (or unable) to connect with the work of the street artist or the renowned artist, and in the ever more technology-rich world where we live the accessibility of the artwork is increasingly less limited by one's proximity or socio-economic class. If there exists the impression that because artists effectively express body trauma they may come to be thought of as the authentic class of sufferers, and, therefore, seize concern away from others,[21] I rebut this as well. In the production of affective art, the artist offers the cry in the dark, the sensuous quality of human trauma that may be isolated and taken up by the artwork allowing for a new site for a sensuous experience that extends temporally and spatially to engage the viewer in a lived experience. The work invites awareness of different modes of inhabitation.[22] When bodies are brought into relation in this encounter, it is the viewer's body that does the work of feeling, relating, thinking and changing. As stated in the introduction, the 'rabbit' (artist) could be replaced by another, as

21 Ibid., 11.

22 Bennett, *Empathic Vision,* 12; her emphasis.

what matters here is the 'single relationship between the subject who confers meaning and the meaningless object, between rational significance and its accidental bearer'.[23]

To be clear: art is not superior to language in its ability to faithfully translate the experience of trauma. However, it does achieve its own distinct capacity to contribute actively to this politic. Art can register and embody affect in its arena. Art resists testimony presented in a didactic sense, for art is a vehicle for the relational transmission of experience that may lead us to conceptual engagement. It does this in its capacity to sensuously seize us and involuntarily engage us affectively while disengaging us from socially embedded paradigms of alterity: reductive characterizations. Art expands our capacity for sympathetic understanding while remaining critical of the limits of empathy: 'It could have been me; it was me, also, and at the same time, but it was not me'. For Adorno, art does not shock us with a new truth, but rather thrusts us into a stripped down mode of critical inquiry. We think through the body. Art presents the traumatic memory of the sick body as that which is beyond representation, but that which may find expression. Scarry's work on the Holocaust uncovered the need to recognize not just that pain and trauma can be apprehended in the image of the wound, but that it may not be possible to apprehend pain and trauma without it.[24] Without the cry in the dark, our contextualizations of pain become once more the realm of the inadequate 'feels as if' and the threat history provides is the ever growing distance between a temporal frame. The immediacy of both the body and trauma cannot be sustained in these realms. Affective expressions of testimony exceed both language and history in that they are ready at hand and have political significance as they enter public consciousness. We might look to the Holocaust or rape culture to see how this plays out. Adorno affirms, 'aesthetic fictions speak' while 'communicative speech merely conceals'.[25] Through the artwork, the felt characteristics of pain, its certainty, can be transposed onto the world. In affective work the encounter with affect becomes the object of analysis and in our critical discourse we are allied neither with 'good' or 'bad' characterizations of body trauma. In fact, we have seen how one may even dismantle how such characterizations come to pass and how meaning is inscribed onto bodies through their relationship to what Elizabeth Grosz calls 'a corporeal universal', a projection of an able-bodied,

23 Horkheimer, Adorno and Gunzelin Schmid Noerr, *Dialectic of Enlightenment*, 7.

24 Scarry, *The Body in Pain*, 16.

25 Theodor Adorno, 'The George-Hofmannstahl Correspondence, 1891–1906', *Prisms* (Cambridge: MIT, 1981), 224.

healthy, white, heterosexual, middle-class male that, 'takes itself as the unquestioned norm', and sees all others reduced to the role of mutations.[26]

Historically, we have largely taken the body for granted in our search for the soul and in singularly valuing transcendence over immanence. By knowing one universal model for this transcendence we have created a world filled with traps chock-full of all those who cannot reflect the universal model and, therefore, must only fuel it. The feminization of body trauma plainly reveals the ways in which transcendence and immanence are still being unequally valued, illustrating how the use of bodies deviant from the universal model is still deeply rooted in our cultural perception (visible or invisible) as instruments necessary for the transcendence of the universal body. For the sick body, this means the designation of the 'sick role' (a social positioning bracketed off with nature, death, and therefore in the grip of the feminine) which liberates, by the contrast it provides, the medical professional in their task of inquiry, knowledge, domination of nature and their utter difference. The masculinized bodies (both male and female) of medical professionals have the authority and privilege to 'venture into the realm of the body without being trapped there'[27] and in this peripheral exchange with the 'realm of the body' their status as intellectuals and authorities on the body can be fully explored with the object on hand for their knowledge to act upon. This is domination hidden under a white coat. This position of mastery, with its reappropriations of the numerous productions of history, subsumes the particular under the universal, disbelieves the body as a critical aspect of our humanity, as the necessary instrument of all human action—our tool of tools—a prerequisite for all our perception, action, and even thought. To think through the body is 'to connect with what has been so cruelly disorganized'[28] in the mind-body split. We need moments like those brought forward by affective artworks that cause a shuddering because thinking through the body is a challenging task as modern thought is schematized by the universal male perspective and the universal male gains status by way of estrangement from the body through dominating the bodies of others.

Thinking through the body is a philosophical act that steps away from post-enlightenment, universal subject thinking. We cannot equally value immanence and transcendence and think through the body while we strive to

26 Elizabeth Grosz, 'Sexed Bodies', *Volatile Bodies: Toward a Corporeal Feminism* (Bloomington: Indiana University Press, 1994), 188.

27 Gallop, *Thinking through the Body*, 7.

28 Adrienne Rich, *Of Woman Born: Motherhood as Experience and Institution* (New York: Bantam, 1977), 7.

master it intellectually, for this is a surplus of such patriarchal thinking.[29] We require the kinds of encounters found in affective art to reopen what Irigaray calls 'the figures of philosophical discourse-idea, substance, subject, transcendental subjectivity, absolute knowledge'[30] so that we may reimagine them and find freedom. Affective art is one such political phenomenon that may make room for concrete change.

Bibliography

Adorno, Theodore. *Aesthetic Theory*. Translated by R. Hullot-Kentor. Minneapolis: University of Minnesota Press, 1997[1970].

Adorno, Theodore. *The George-Hofmannstahl Correspondence, 1891–1906*. Translated by Samuel Weber and Shierry Weber-Nicholsen. Cambridge: MIT Press, 1981.

Adorno, Theodore, Gretel Adorno, Rolf Tiedemann and Robert Hullot-Kentor. *Aesthetic Theory*. London: Continuum, 2002.

Adorno, Theodore, and Robert Hullot-Kentor. *Philosophy of New Music*. Minneapolis: University of Minnesota Press, 2006.

Bennett, Jill. *Empathic Vision: Affect, Trauma, and Contemporary Art*. Palo Alto: Stanford University Press, 2005.

de Beauvoir, Simone. *The Second Sex*. Translated by Constance Borde and Sheila Malovany-Chevallier. New York: Vintage, 2011.

Gallop, Jane. *Thinking through the Body*. New York: Columbia, Columbia University Press, 1988.

Grosz, Elizabeth A. *Volatile Bodies: Toward a Corporeal Feminism*. Bloomington: Indiana University Press, 1994.

Hellings, James. *Adorno and Art: Aesthetic Theory Contra Critical Theory*. London: Palgrave Macmillan UK, 2014.

Hirsh, Marianne. 'Projected Memory: Holocaust Photographs in Personal and Private Fantasy', *Acts of Memory: Cultural Recall in the Present*, edited by Mieke Bal, Jonathan Crewe, and Leo Spitzer. London: University Press of New England, 1999, 3–23.

Horkheimer, Max, Theodor W. Adorno, and Gunzelin Schmid Noerr. *Dialectic of Enlightenment: Philosophical Fragments*. Stanford: Stanford University Press, 2002.

Irigaray, Luce. *This Sex Which Is Not One*. Ithaca: Cornell University Press, 1985.

Kellett, Heidi. 'Skin Portraiture: Relational Embodiment and Contemporary Art'. *Probing the Skin Cultural Representations of Our Contact Zone*, edited by Caroline

29 Gallop, *Thinking through the Body*, 4.

30 Luce Irigaray, *This Sex Which Is Not One* (Ithaca: Cornell University Press), 74.

Rosenthal and Dirk Vanderbeke, 239–270. Newcastle upon Tyne: Cambridge Scholars Lady Stephenson Library, 2015.

Martin, Emily. *The Woman in the Body: A Cultural Analysis of Reproduction.* Boston: Beacon, 1987.

Millon, Theodore, Paul H. Blaney and Roger D. Davis. *Oxford Textbook of Psychopathology.* Oxford: Oxford University Press, 1999.

Radstone, Susannah. 'Social Bonds and Psychical Orders: Testimonies'. *Traumatizing Theory: The Cultural Politics of Affect in and beyond Psychoanalysis,* edited by Karyn Ball, 101–126. New York: Other Press, 2007.

Rich, Adrienne. *Of Woman Born: Motherhood as Experience and Institution.* New York: Bantam, 1977.

Scarry, Elaine. *The Body in Pain: The Making and Unmaking of the World.* Oxford: Oxford University Press, 1985.

Taylor Johnson, Heather. "Illness Narratives: A Poetry Reading." *Testimony: Memory, Trauma, Truth, Engagement Conference,* July 31, 2014, Mansfield College, Oxford University, UK.

Woolf, Virginia. 'On Being Ill'. *Collected Essays.* Vol. 4. New York: Harcourt, 1967.

CHAPTER 11

Very Becoming: Transforming Our Settler Selves in Occupied Australia

Rachel Joy

Abstract

In Australia the ontological position of the Occupier has rendered the collective memory of invasion and occupation faulty or forgotten. Today it manifests in a lack of will by Settler Australians to engage with the devastating effects of our denial of Indigenous sovereignty upon Indigenous communities. In re-thinking a way to be non-Indigenous Australians that has integrity and rejects an Occupier subject position unconditionally, questions of ontology must be addressed. We must ask ourselves about the very nature of our Being, in relation to the land we claim as ours and we must wonder that we have few troubling thoughts or memories nor memorials to tweak our consciences. What strategies can we employ to open up such questions? As an artist of white Settler origins I suggest that the sensory and emotional experience rendered through visual art can create a space to bring into existence new ways of thinking and of being in Australia. Critically engaged non-Indigenous artists have the opportunity to make a cultural space, through their art practices, for robust public discourse acknowledging Indigenous sovereignty and the promise it holds for all of us.

Keywords

visual art – whiteness – occupier – settler – indigenous sovereignty – Australia – identity – memory – being – place – materiality – affect

As a cultural product art tells our stories; it can tell us who we have been, who we are and most importantly, who it is we might yet become. But what is it that makes visual art different from literature in this respect? In making artworks, artists allow us to *see* differently, visual art is a method, not necessarily for making sense of the world, but for making meaning, and it gives that attempt a physical form. It is the visual language of the artist that conveys so much for

 | DOI:10.1163/9789004391130_013

which there are no words. It is the consideration and employment of space, place, scale and the relationships of objects, materials, light and darkness, colour and texture, to convey meaning and evoke emotion. Such approaches are used by artists to ask questions of our selves but not necessarily to provide the comfort of answers. To this end political art relies on ambivalence and subversion to destabilise our preconceptions and opens up spaces for discussion, for new ways of understanding, thinking and allowing for the possibility of mystery; that there may be some things we cannot know.

As an artist my research largely happens in my studio. What I'm trying to do is to find a way to express through my art what it is to be an Occupier Australian and how we might become something better. I'm primarily a sculptor and printmaker so materials and processes are my language, my lexicon. My practice has a grammar to it, if you like, there are rules to be learned but as is true for all good novelists or poets, once learned, the rules can to a certain extent be broken or bent for effect. If I take this verb and I use it in its gerund form how does it alter the meaning of a sentence? What happens if I change its position in the sentence? Likewise, what are the properties of a material? How will it behave when it interacts with X? What is its language, what can it say?

Because my concern is to pose questions not necessarily to answer them, my work is always propositional; I am interested in asking, *what if* ...? But I am not flippant, rather I think very deeply about the ideas, the proposals, the processes I use and why I make the decisions I do. All art is political because it involves aesthetic choices that are inherently cultural, and thus politically loaded, including and perhaps especially, the decision *not* to recognise our actions or our work as political. So one could claim there is in fact no abstract art because it always involves the artist herself. Art is about decisions, about problem solving and relationships: relationships between maker and materials, art and viewer, artist and world. Many people, when they think of art, think of art objects, a painting or a sculpture, as something finite, closed and complete. My practice is less about the object produced than the process of producing it. Whatever emerges will speak of the process that produced it and what emerges will have veracity so long as the process has integrity and this is further complicated by ideas. Yes, what's it all about?

Broadly speaking my art is about searching for justice. Currently I'm making art about genocide. I make genocide art in an Australian context, not art about The Holocaust, but art about the invasion and occupation and on-going colonial violence that shape relationships in contemporary Australia. This is a difficult thing to make art about because apparently it doesn't exist. If one speaks of genocide with most non-Indigenous Australians the conversation will shift towards discussions of The Shoah. If one attempts to steer the conversation back towards contemporary or even historical Australia and government sponsored or occluded attacks on the country's First Peoples one will be met with looks of incredulity and likely branded a *black armband*[1] extremist. It is equally difficult to move people towards taking responsibility for what has happened or for what continues to take place today. As far as most Occupier Australians are concerned, it didn't happen, or not like that, it wasn't that bad, it certainly wasn't genocide and we're not Nazi's, we're nice. The 2008 Apology by then Prime Minister Kevin Rudd to the Stolen Generations has in fact made it more difficult to discuss notions of Indigenous sovereignty or a treaty in Australia because the Apology was seen as a form of closure rather than an opportunity to begin a healing process. Instead, Aboriginal Australians continue to be positioned as a problem to be solved rather than a sovereign people whose humanity and claims to land must be recognised if we are not all to be diminished. The need for Occupier Australians to transform our selves is nowhere heard on the national agenda. Yes it's rather tricky to make art about something that doesn't exist, but to use the vernacular; I'm giving it a go.

So how do you make genocide art and can art make a space for the becoming of something better? The profound impact of the Holocaust on cultural production, especially in post-war Europe, is well illustrated by Elizabeth Matheson in her chapter "Immersive Space and the Place of the Witness". In making this kind of art one must be concerned with trauma and testimony, silence and speaking, listening, witnessing. One confronts truth and truths, memories, fragments, non-linear narratives, catharsis and closure, pain and suffering; red raw or lumpy old memories like scar tissue traces. So what can art do? It can witness. And through witnessing it can make a space for new relationships to develop between Indigenous and non-Indigenous Australians. My hope is that as a pre-condition of such a process, art can be part of a movement towards making a new way to be non-indigenous in Australia that has integrity.

Firstly we must acknowledge whose land it is and that it has been stolen. Some stories can only be told by Indigenous peoples, others perhaps cannot be told at all, yet there are stories occupiers *can* tell about frontier history and about contemporary iterations of colonial violence because they are not only indigenous stories. Some of these stories are ours also and we must take responsibility for our part in them; Indigenous peoples didn't do colonialism and genocide to themselves; it was Settler Australians who invaded, stole the land,

1 This term was coined during the 'History Wars' of late 90's early 2000's Australia as a pejorative adjective used to describe historians or cultural commentators who recognised the invasion, dispossession and occupation of Australia's First Nations peoples by the British.

occupied it, murdered people who resisted and continue to do so today. The burden of the trauma of colonialism has rested with the Indigenous community for too long. This is not a burden they should have to shoulder for it is of our making and thus it is the Settler community who must make it our responsibility to see the Occupation as a Settler problem.

How does one then move to a place of becoming something better? What would that look like? Once we acknowledge that we are Occupiers, how do we live with that reality and is there any way that we can become anything else? Surely the Occupier being is not the best that we can be? But how do we initiate a process of becoming ourselves anew? How do we speak the unspeakable; represent the un-representable?[2] How might we move beyond a Coloniser mind-set of 'friends and enemies' towards a place of thinking and questioning? Perhaps one way is through a language of artistic processes and materials that enables witnessing

When artists place a work of art in a public place we are making a space for self reflexivity, for memory work, we are offering people an opportunity to be involved in the artwork as witnesses; but more than this, through the process of witnessing they are themselves transformed, if only momentarily. An act of witnessing can be a kind of speech act, an action, and in engaging in witnessing our own identity changes. In this way, sincere acts of witnessing wear a Janus head; they look back to the past in acknowledgement but also orient us into the future suggesting who it is we might yet become. What constitutes a speech act and why is it useful for our purposes? Hannah Arendt states that speech is the medium through which humans become equal because through it we recognise and understand each other as equal members of a human community.[3] She considers speech acts to be revelatory because they are the means by which actors are revealed to the world in their true nature as subjects with unique identities.[4] Works of art that aim to work as acts of witnessing have the potential to be speech acts of considerable power. Power as considered by Arendt,

---

2 Since Theodore Adorno first wrote of the impossibility of writing poetry after the Holocaust in his 1949 essay, 'Cultural Criticism and Society' in Theodore Adorno *Prisms,* Cambridge MA: MIT Press, 1997, commentators have continued to grapple with the problems of representing trauma including Dori Laub, James E. Young and Andreas Huyssen among many others.

3 Patrick Hayden, ed., *Hannah Arendt Key Concepts* (Durham, UK: Acumen Publishing, 2014), 14.

4 Hannah Arendt, *The Human Condition* (Chicago: University of Chicago Press, 1958), 150.

> … is contrary to domination and violence in that it is the result of participatory interaction between unique individuals who reciprocally affirm their equality. It is actualized by collective action and speech intended to create or locate shared interests and a relatively stable space where freedom may be revealed.[5]

Works of art that engage a public and require them to reflect or make meaning can be seen as collective actions intended to create a space of shared interests, so perhaps in this sense they can be a path towards real shared power as opposed to the violence of liberal democracy where the political class rules largely because of its ability to impose it's own 'will against the resistance of others'.[6]

Speech acts are not limited to the spoken word and may take many forms. It is illustrative of the limits of the spoken word that most important spoken word speech acts are accompanied by spectacle, large or small. Visual gestures add an important element to the speech act that cannot be affectively conveyed through spoken words alone. Political figures present their speech acts in front of a wall of books (so they appear erudite), flanked by national flags (to impart status and nationalism), they are perhaps clad in military uniforms (for violence and action) and in this era of a visually literate public, if the message is important it will be simulcast, on all networks and on screens in public places, a la Orwell's *1984*. Long after the nuances of words have faded from our collective memory a catchphrase and the gestures will live on as significant elements in the construction of spectacle.

Let us consider for a moment the way that spoken word speech acts have been bastardised by what Ghassan Hage calls 'warring' or Settler colonial societies.[7] In such societies freedom of speech becomes a void. There may be words but they have no content. In Australia there currently exists a state of freedom of speech yet speech is so undervalued that what we are left with is the ability to freely speak only those words that carry no meaning. As we have seen in the culture wars of 1990s and early 2000s Australia, attempts to make speech acts containing any ethical content and thus posing a challenge to the dominant order were shut down and labelled un-Australian. In the name of 'democracy' our Settler nation attempts to deny freedom of speech to those

5 Hayden, *Hannah Arendt Key Concepts*, 16.

6 Max Weber, *Economy and Society:An Outline of Interpretive Sociology*, eds. Guether Roth and Ckus Wittich (Berkeley, CA: University of California Press,1978), 53.

7 Ghassan Hage, 'Warring Societies and Intellectuals', *Transforming Cultures e-Journal* 1.1 (2006): 47. http://epress.lib.uts.edu.au/journals/TfC

who threaten to expose its true nature as an occupying force. Our Settler state allows freedom of speech so long as it is void of ethical content and denies it only in 'exceptional circumstances', which of late have come to characterize the usual state of affairs, by becoming as Giorgio Agamben would put it, a permanent 'state of exception'.[8] While this situation certainly makes it difficult to achieve speech acts that will engender the kind of thinking necessary for social transformation, it is perhaps now even more important to redouble our efforts to find ways to think and act creatively and this is why artists need to be involved.

If we consider speech acts to have the potential to be lenses of recognition, through which we see each other anew and with a common humanity it may become apparent that art has the potential to act as such a lens. The recognition that art brings, however, is not always comfortable and it often exposes the tensions or rifts that exist in our society. Adorno states that 'the unsolved antagonisms of reality return in artworks as immanent problems of form',[9] and it is with such problems of form that art concerns itself. Further to this, the artist duo Claire Fontaine argue, 'We are not providing a social service with our art, but giving shape to disturbing and painful things'.[10] Art is not merely an illustration of social realities but rather a response to them, a visual language of materials and processes by which artists conduct something of a contract with the viewer. Such affective art invokes a relationship with the viewer that is performative in that it slows the viewer down, engages them and draws a response from them. The viewer is pulled into the work and in becoming part of it, is implicated in the ideas it presents. When artists are dealing with traumatic events we are very often dealing with experiences owned by others and because it is important not to colonise those experiences by attempting to re-tell or illustrate such events we attempt to make work that responds to the trauma. In an acknowledgement of the inability of illustrative forms of art to represent the unrepresentable trauma of grossly violent acts, Tim Long explains in his chapter "Auroras: A Chorus of Witnesses" that artists such as Atom Egoyan imply violence but keep it deliberately out of frame. Affective works attempt to avoid didacticism in favour of self-reflexivity. In this sense one might understand such art as being engaged in a transaction with the viewer rather than communication to them. These works engage in relational ethics: ethics

---

8 Giorgio Agamben, *State of Exception* (Chicago: University of Chicago Press, 2005), 2–3.

9 Theodore Adorno, *Aesthetic Theory*, edited by Gretel Adorno and Rolf Tiedemann (London: Bloomsbury Academic, 2013), 7.

10 Andrew Culp and Ricky Crano, 'Giving Shape to Painful Things', *Radical Philosophy* 175 (2012): 45.

as opposed to morals because ethics are response-able and open to agonism whereas morals are static and encoded: anathema to our project.

Art is about decisions, about problem solving and relationships: relationships between maker and materials, art and viewer, artist and world. When artists work consciously with affect it is the realm of feelings and emotions with which we are concerned. We endeavour to create works that will cause an affective response in the viewer because we believe this acts as a catalyst for deep and critical thought. Artists who work with affect want their audience to become part of a process, to become engaged with the work in such a way that it triggers both an emotional and intellectual response in the viewer and in that moment transforms their perception. Invoking sensations in the viewer forces them to engage, it creates the conditions for awareness and profound thinking. It is these conditions, enabled through art, which Deleuze and Guattari describe as being necessary for the creation of what they term 'people-to-come'.[11] Art as a speech act can 'summon' these becoming-people through creating the conditions whereby they might create themselves, for a 'people-to-come' can only come about in an Australian context through recognition of shame, remorse and ultimately the de-colonising of the Occupier self. As it struggles to respond to the antagonisms of contemporary Australian reality, art can engage in transactions with viewers that create the conditions for fundamental shifts in being.

Affective art is about trying to create the conditions for making meaning and this is what makes it so useful to our thinking around remorse and its centrality to healing after events of great trauma. Thinking (meaning making) occurs in the present, it is an action rather than an object. The purpose of affective art is not to manifest a traumatic memory as an object like a monument, but rather to invite people to think, to make meaning, and in doing so to act. When artists make spaces for thinking we are inviting people to participate in the works as witnesses, viewers become instruments of witnessing by participating in the process of the work, by engaging with it. The importance of the creation of a 'thinking space' is also detailed by Elizabeth Matheson in her discussion in this volume, of the spatial dynamics present in the practices of contemporary installation artists. While acknowledging that it is not possible to represent the suffering of others in its particularity, it may be possible to bear witness to that suffering, because as Cathy Caruth says, 'to bear witness to the truth of suffering over a traumatic event is to bear witness to that event's

11 Gilles Deleuze and Felix Guattari, *What Is Philosophy?* Translaed by Hugh Tomlinson and Graham Burchell (New York: Colombia University Press, 1994), 218.

incomprehensibility'.[12] It's a difficult project, the attempt to make space for meaning making about incomprehensible events and to accept that there may be things that we can never know or understand. The important thing is not to be distracted towards ends but to stay with the process; not to look for the closure provided by a monument but to maintain interactions through art that facilitate thinking. As artists we will never speak that which cannot be spoken but we might make a space to listen and reflect. This is our gift; this is what art can do.

The link between thinking and acting needs to be rebuilt. Adorno and Arendt basically argue that the moral catastrophe of the Holocaust severed the link between thinking and acting;[13] for Arendt, Eichmann's thoughtless actions as part of the Nazi war machine are an illustration of this. I would argue that Settler colonial consciousness is a further illustration of such deadly thoughtlessness. A reconnection between thinking and acting can happen through art because the collaborative tryst which art requires of us is also transformative, in that during the affective moment of perception the viewer's sense of self and of the world transforms. The site for this transformation is art; art understood as a space or zone[14] as Deleuze and Guattari claim or perhaps as an 'event site' as Alain Badiou terms it.[15] Either way art itself is not so much an object as an occurrence or location where events come into being. Art is immanent, impermanent, it is always coming into being, it is about creating experiences that are outside the mundane consciousness and are in some sense performative. Art inhabits the realm of the virtual, that which is always becoming, in the Deleuzean sense, the realm of affects that allows it to open up a space somewhere between the virtual and the real whereby we might overcome our known selves to become something ontologically new. From the perspective of acting and art as a speech act, we can think about what an artwork can do through its employment of affect. It can make the invisible visible and allow us to perceive the imperceptible; art is almost magical in its transformative potential. In a world so absurd that it is perhaps beyond our abilities to make any sense of it,

---

12 Cathy Caruth, *Trauma: Explorations in Memory* (Baltimore: The Johns Hopkins University Press. 1995), 156.

13 For a more detailed discussion of these ideas see Adorno in his 1949 essay 'An Essay on Cultural Criticism and Society' in Theodore Adorno, *Prisms,* Cambridge MA: MIT Press, 1997 and Arendt in *The Human Condition* (Chicago: University of Chicago Press, 1958) and especially *Eichmann in Jerusalem. A Report on the Banality of Evil* (New York: Viking Press, 1968) and *The Life of the Mind* (New York: Harcourt, 1978).

14 Deleuze and Guattari, *What Is Philosophy?* 173.

15 Alain Badiou, *Deleuze: The Clamour of Being,* translated by Louise Burchill (Minneapolis: University of Minnesota Press, 1999), 84.

art offers a way to think and make meaning through the affective processes of being and becoming rather than through representation.

Thus it is important to speak of art as a work in progress or process, something open and shifting that allows for change and argument and disagreement. The object oriented perspective that demands premature foreclosure must be avoided if we are to build something that has integrity. Artists very often make strategic use of unanswered questions, as is the case put by Tim Long in his chapter concerning the Canadian film-maker Atom Egoyan, who leaves it up to the viewer to fill the space created. In this sense the viewer activates the artwork and the possible readings remain multiple. We must not try to build a Parthenon, as it were, but something response-able, reflexive that can change, and be adjusted as necessary. To focus on outcomes, on feeling comfortable and resolved will not bring about healing but rather leave so much unsaid and unacknowledged. In Australia we cannot reconcile because there never was an initial relationship of honesty and respect that was lost and to which we might return.[16] Yet we can try now to make a relationship of sincerity and trust between Occupier Australians and the First Peoples of this country but it will be a daily effort, a process, a dialogue, a stumbling, faulting attempt and we will probably fail, but if the process has integrity we will not give up, we will return to our task of becoming something better than we are.

Art has something special to offer this project because as artists we know what it is to take on a daunting, seemingly hopeless project and try to find a way to ask the questions that might reveal a new perspective. We work with rules and boundaries and we know when to push them and just how far, how much the materials will tolerate. We take risks, we fail, we ask what went wrong and what went right, we learn and we go back and we try again. We sometimes do this alone and at other times we collaborate with others, there is often a shifting between these positions of working alone and then in groups but even when seemingly working alone in our studios we are in dialogue with ourselves and with the world around us.

And so to practicalities: what does it look like when visual artists make art that is process and materially driven? What relationship can this have to the concerns of trauma studies and notions of justice? One example from my own practice involves a print making technique strategically employed because of the language it speaks, its grammatology, if you like. Viscosity printing, simultaneous colour etching or Hayter technique was developed in the 1930s by

16 For a discussion of ethical processes for reconciliation in an Australian context see Deborah Bird Rose, *Reports From a Wild Country: Ethics of Decolonisation* (Sydney: University of New South Wales, 2004).

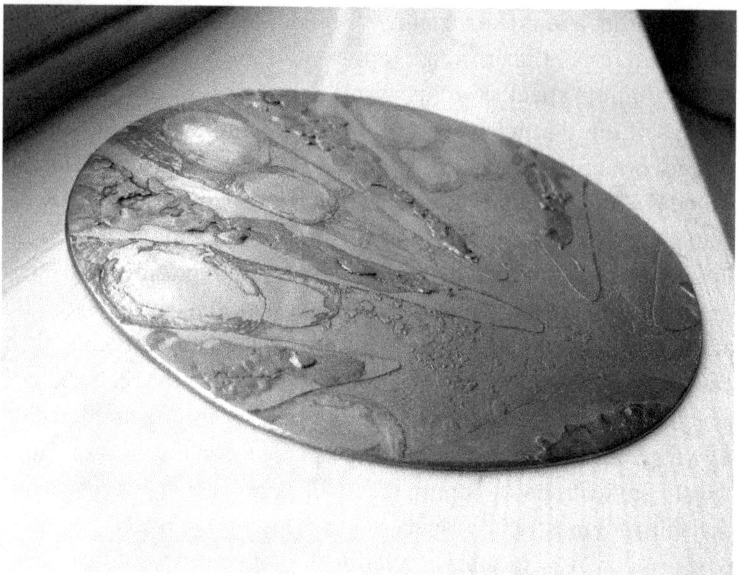

FIGURE 11.1 *Hayter etching plate*
© 2014. PHOTOGRAPHER RACHEL JOY. USED WITH PERMISSION.

chemist turned artist Stanley William Hayter. It is necessary here to explain something of the processes involved as understanding them will aid in appreciating their relationship to our theoretical concerns. The technique involves the simultaneous printing of many colours on one etching plate. Previous to this most etchings were either single colour, usually utilising dark ink and if colour was required it was painted in by hand or separate plates were employed for each colour. The Viscosity process involves the relationship of plate, inks, rollers and paper. The plate (figs 11.1 and 11.2), protected by a thin layer of bitumen, has a design scored into it, this is then *bitten* (placed in an acid bath) and the acid etches the surface area left uncovered.

The plate can be re-covered with bitumen and etched numerous times creating planes of different depths, rather like a three dimensional topographical map. Inks need to be prepared before being applied to the plate. These will have plate oil added to them in tiny amounts so as to create differences in viscosity. Thus if one has four different colours each will have a different viscosity. The final consideration before printing is the density of the rubber rollers, their softness or hardness. Each colour is rolled with a single roller and applied to the plate in a single pass so as not to muddy the inks. The interplay between the densities of each roller, the viscosity of the ink and the depth of each plane of the plate mean that each ink colour remains separate and is forced to a

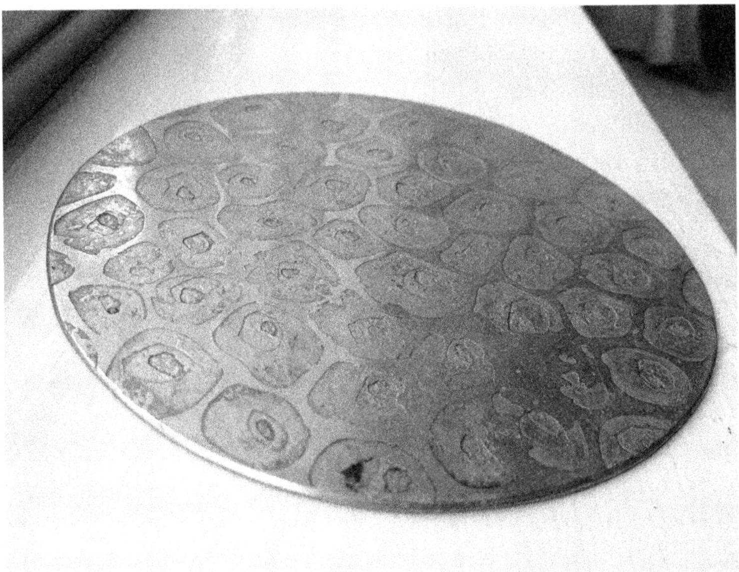

FIGURE 11.2 *Hayter etching plate*

particular level in the plate. The dampened paper can then be gently lowered onto the plate before it is run through the press and printed. Because of the number of variables involved and especially the difficulty in controlling the viscosity of the ink, multiples, known as editions, are rarely made using this technique; rather the unique state of each print is what is treasured.

For me the use of Hayter technique has many resonances with the processes that are necessary for healing in Australia and perhaps in other contexts also. Broadly, the conditions for the process involve the relationship between many seemingly oppositional or agonistic forces; these elements must firstly be understood in their specificities and then in terms of their relational aspects. The plate is the site that holds the event, most often it is made from copper or zinc (base metals cherished by alchemists) we cover it with bitumen (which also comes from the earth) and this is called a 'ground'. We scrape the ground and bite it; the process is visceral. We re-apply the ground and mark it with another story, another layer; it is now contested ground. The bitumen both masks and protects, where it is scraped back it opens to reveal the base metal of the plate or site and allows the acid to bite, to score and change it. As the acid etches the plate, tiny bubbles of hydrogen form on the corroded surface, the by-product (so much hot air) of all this activity. Etching takes time, we wait, we watch the bubbles form and we do not foreclose on the process. There comes a time when enough layers have been etched into the plate, when it holds all it will hold and we know the site must be made ready to receive the inks. It must be cleaned of bitumen; unmasked.

The inks have different colours and qualities, thicker or thinner, and will reside in different locations on the plate but there will sometimes be a little bleeding, overlapping, merging. Each new application of inks to the plate reveals a slightly different relationship of colour to space or place and when the print is finally pulled from the plate the result is unique. Although there are rules and each element has specific qualities, the relational aspects of which imply the outcomes most likely, in the end the results can be surprising. For me the time, repetitions of process, competing narratives and contested site involved in the practice of viscosity printmaking are important. These elements and the commitment to their honest employment to create an event, a method with an open outcome where the specificities of each element are respected but where they come together in unexpectedly beautiful ways offers so much promise and embodies a way to work together that offers hope for healing and for summoning a 'people-to-come'.

Healing is not a process that can occur alone. Cherokee scholar Daniel Justice reminds us that if First Nations people and Settlers are to move forward together 'collaboration is a necessity not an option'.[17] I have spoken of the need for artists to work both alone and at other times in collaboration. Although much of my practice is a very solitary pursuit and I admit that I often find working collaboratively a frustrating and at times frightening prospect, it is also a necessary one. And when it works it can be really beautiful. If my practice is truly to reflect the process I deem necessary to making a space for becoming better people and to moving towards achieving justice for all of us then I cannot work entirely alone. There are many ways to collaborate but in Australia collaboration between white Settler artists and Indigenous artists must involve a process in which Settlers acknowledge and relinquish our white privilege and Occupier status and listen. An example from my practice involved a project of which I was part on the country of the Ngaanyatjarra people of the Western Desert region of Western Australia. The project was initiated by the senior women of the community who were worried that the younger unmarried women (*Kungkas*), were not learning about and collecting *bush tucker*[18]

---

17 Daniel Justice, 'A Better World Becoming: Placing Critical Indigenous Studies' (paper presented at the Public Lecture Series, University of Melbourne, Australia, November 6, 2014).

18 Australian colloquialism denoting food (from both animal and plant sources) collected from the countryside as opposed to processed food purchased from shops.

and this meant a reliance on the unhealthy food available at the local shop. The senior women wanted to do a project where all the women would be involved in making a *wirra* (fig 11.3), a multipurpose digging implement and container, essentially an open-lipped elliptical bowl with sharp edges. When the women had made the wirras they could then use them for hunting and collecting bush tucker and any surplus ones could be painted for the tourist trade and sold at the art centre.

Why did they need to work with an outsider? The most senior female artist had experimented with making wirras from various materials and had hacked one from the body of a wrecked car using an axe. The sheet steel used in car panels is light, strong, can be easily shaped and keeps a relatively sharp true edge, especially when compared with the traditional material: Mulga[19] wood. Additionally, steel is a material that is free of cost and found locally in abundance because of the number of broken down abandoned cars in the rubbish tip outside the community. They had the materials and knew there had to be a better way to cut and shape the metal wirras but they didn't have the tools or the skills to use them. The elders requested the arts centre employ an artist with metal working skills to collaborate with the senior artists on the project and for reasons of cultural appropriateness the artist needed to be female. I was that artist.

Soon after arriving in the township I sat down in the red dust under a tree with the senior women who would work with me on the project. Facilitated by a young Ngaanyatjarra woman who worked for the land council, I listened as the women told me their ideas about what they wanted to do, identified the community members who would be involved and explained how things would run. Could I help them cut the cars? Could we make these shapes? Could they learn to use the tools to make more wirras whenever they wanted? Yes. The arts centre had bought the necessary tools and these would be available to the women whenever they needed them once we had completed the project.

There was a lot of hilarity over the safety boots, ear goggles and gloves we had to wear when handling the tools but everyone was very keen to wear the tinted 'sunglasses' provided for eye protection. Over the next few days we spent many hours scouring the tip for the most beautifully coloured cars to cut up. Then it was time to learn the difference between cutting and grinding disks, how to safely change them and how to operate both the generator and the angle grinder. Following a little practice the kungkas set to cutting the basic shapes from the cars and smoothing their edges, after which the wirras could

19 Acacia Aneura is a small tree native to Western Australia.

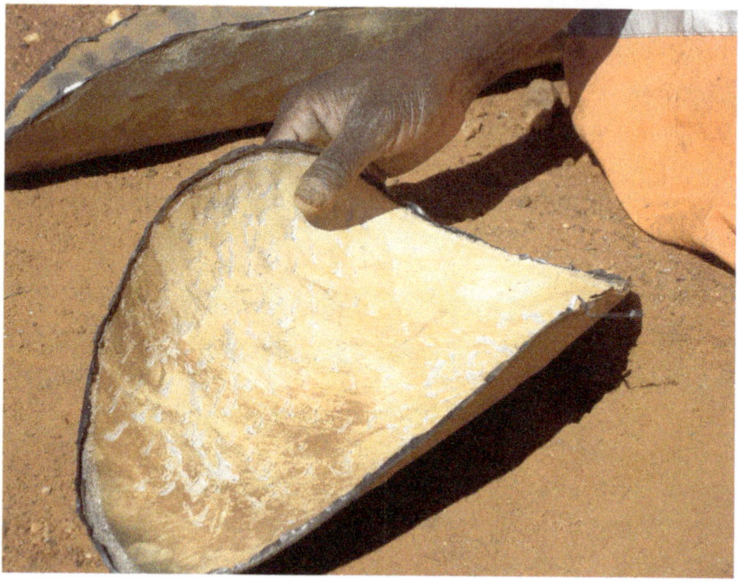

FIGURE 11.3 *Metal Wirra*, Ngaanyatjarra Lands

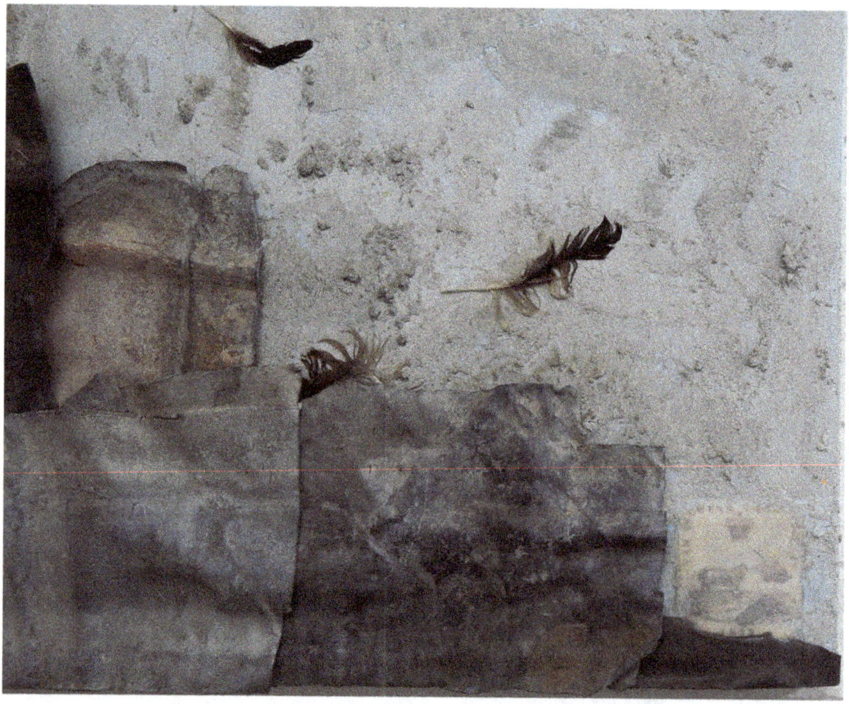

FIGURE 11.4 *Cape Grim 1828*, detail

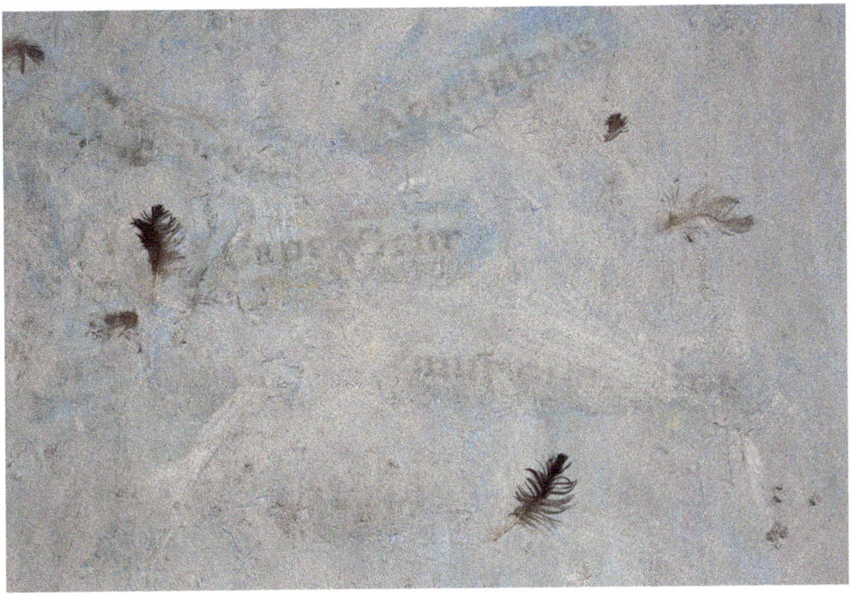

FIGURE 11.5 *Cape Grim 1828*, detail

be beaten into a curved dish shape using hammers or the back of an axe. We made lots of wirras and the following week we collected all the kungkas and their wirras and went out bush to dig for lizards, honey ants and other delicacies; everyone laughed a lot and we were very happy.

In this collaboration I did a lot of listening and learning. Because English is a second language in the Ngaanyatjarra lands, I taught primarily by showing and doing and the women learned through watching and copying. In the context of our collaboration, what I could contribute were my technical skills (I was considered a *ninti kungka* – clever unmarried woman) but by being open to the processes of the Ngaanyatjarra women and their elders I also helped to facilitate a cultural project that was devised by those women on their terms, on their country, that helped them to maintain a connection to their land and cultural practices and that would also lead to better health outcomes. During our collaboration we created a space where skills, stories and experiences were shared; skills in metal work, in locating and hunting or gathering bush tucker, stories about country and experiences in speaking, acting and listening. The space we made attempted to be creative and in a sense transformative, by utilising both the knowledge of the Ngaanyatjarra women and my own skill-set, and participating in a process by which each of us valued the other and the knowledge that we possessed and shared. For this project my role was to be a

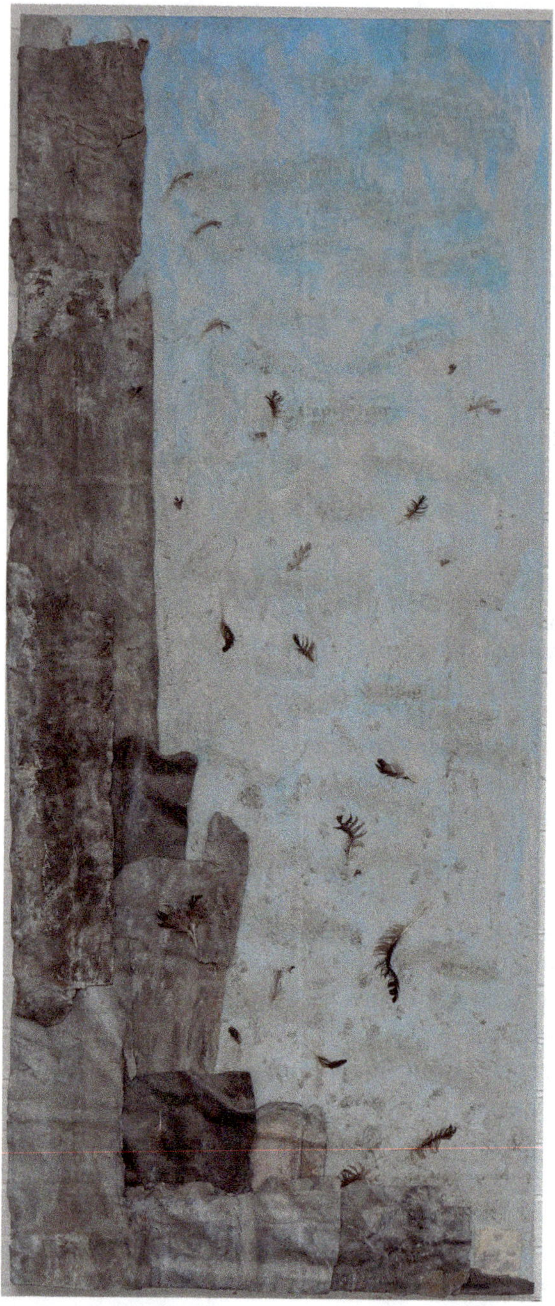

FIGURE 11.6 *Cape Grim 1828*
© 2010. PHOTOGRAPHER RACHEL JOY. USED WITH PERMISSION.

technician and a teacher but also to bear witness to the survival of Indigenous knowledge systems and ontological relationships to place.[20] My collaboration with the Ngaanyatjarra women allowed me to bear witness to their sovereignty.

My efforts to illustrate how art can make a space for identity transformation, and potentially for healing have so far touched on technical production processes, collaborative processes and finally I'd like to elucidate on the manner in which a language of materials and techniques can be employed to encourage emotionally informed critical thinking.

Time is an important element in making space for transformation as is the investment of self in an artwork and there is a significant relationship between the two. When works of art use materials in such a way as to obfuscate our first attempts to read them it causes frustration and discomfort, something that colonised people experience every time they encounter the forces of the Occupier, which for many Indigenous people, is most days. Will the viewer give up and think 'it's all too hard' or will they remain curious and continue to attempt a reading of the work? So as not to entirely alienate the viewer it is important that they invest something of themselves in their interaction with the artwork. In our world of sound bites and memes, art has a lot of competition for the limited attention spans of our audience, so once we have it, we need to keep it for long enough so that they make this necessary investment in the experience. We need to slow down their encounter and involve them in the work; techniques for this may involve using tiny detail, layering or partially obscuring elements of the work or revealing aspects of a work over time. These choices mean the viewer must make an effort to look in a different way. Destabilising linear notions of time or temporality changes the way we look at things including the way we understand the past. As such it may remind the viewer that the past is not cut off from the present. In the collision of past and present, exists a differentia of time and a dissonance that destabilises the established order, allowing a space for new understandings to be created. It is this crisis point from which something new might be born that offers so much promise to artists should they be able to evoke it in the minds of their audience. If we can open a space for the viewer to engage with the work they can be active participants in the art not merely passive recipients of a message that is already decided for them. In slowing the viewer down, the work obliges us to give something of

20 For further reading on Australian Indigenous knowledge systems and ontology begin by reading 'I Still Call Australia Home: Indigenous Belonging and Place in a White Postcolonizing Society' by Aileen Moreton-Robinson, in *Regroundings: Questions of Home and Migration*' edited by Sara Ahmed, C. Castameda, A.Marie Fortier and M. Sheller, (Oxford: Berg, Oxford University Press, 2003), 23–40.

ourselves to it, we allow ourselves to be moved, to ponder the title and perhaps to *feel* something. This is witnessing, it is acknowledging someone else's pain. The theorist Mieke Bal states 'The past is always out of our grasp. We always arrive too late. What can art do? It can *know*. To know is important'.[21]

Materials have a language that speaks to viewers in a visceral and direct way and with an immediacy unmatched by words. Materials and objects can speak of, or evoke pathos, misery, melancholy, absurdity, fear, rage, confusion, disgust or any number of emotional responses. The emotional *hook* engages the viewer and invites them to stay a little longer with the work, to look again, a little more deeply and perhaps to think about what the work makes them feel. Such artworks are hoping for some degree of self-reflexivity to be activated in the viewer so that while the thinking process might be initiated by the artwork it is internalised by the viewer and in so doing they are to some degree transformed. My work *Apologists* presents ox tongues cast in latex posed as oversized human tongues in a museum display-case. This collection of tongues belongs to the mythic species 'Homo Erectus Mendax' (sub-species Australis), mendax being Latin for liar. This work is initially disturbing as the tongues have a fleshy lifelike quality, but quickly becomes absurd when their size is taken into account and the collection is contextualised within its glass case (also referencing the collection of Indigenous people's body parts by European trophy hunters and scientists). The museum-style case also renders colonialist discourse a relic of the past and evokes the possibility of a future decolonised space. When the title is considered, the work perhaps becomes challenging for some, but if the viewer has stayed with the work this long and their curiosity has been aroused they may reflect on the long tradition of Settler justifications of colonialism and its continuation in contemporary forms of vacuous double-speak. Thus the work also alludes to issues of freedom of speech in Australia and who it is that most often gets to speak. While the work is intentionally provocative it is also silly, proving the power of absurdity to unmask truth and allowing the viewer the space to become part of this process through sharing the joke.

An example from my practice that utilises both the language of materials and obfuscating techniques is a work (fig 11.6) that concerns the 1828 massacre of Indigenous families conducted by shepherds, at what is now called Cape Grim, in northern Tasmania. The cliff, over which the people were driven, is represented by layers of lead sheet (fig 11.4) (a material with strong connections

---

21 Mieke Bal, *Of What One Cannot Speak: Doris Salcedo's Political Art* (Chicago: Chicago University Press, 2010), 225.

to death and the afterlife in Western culture). Text about the event is embedded in the work (fig 11.5) but largely obscured with paint and bees wax as it falls down the length of the canvas, the wax attempting to entomb the narrative and sever it from the present. Sand (a material found on the marginal shifting spaces of shorelines) is mixed in with the paint and wax at the bottom of the work, and delicate grey/black mutton-bird feathers drift among the text in reference to the birds the families were hunting when they were ambushed. In this part of Tasmania today, the traditional art form of threading shell necklaces is being revived and in acknowledgement that indigenous Tasmanian's have survived the terrible attempts to annihilate them I am in the initial stages of conversation with local women about the possibility of incorporating shell work, as an example of living culture, into this artwork. This work is for me, a reflection on a particular historic incident but not an attempt to illustrate or retell it; furthermore the intention is to reveal the connection between past and present and thus to express grief for the murder of these families while also acknowledging that the first Tasmanians continue to resist the invasion and occupation of their lands. Viewers' comments on this work have been various, ranging from horrified disbelief to melancholic reflection, to unease about a white artist tackling such subject matter. The content of the responses themselves are of less concern to me than the fact that the work succeeds in creating a space for conversations around this event and others like it.

The destabilising effects of the approaches used by artists may not provide the comfort and closure of answers. Indeed if art is doing its job it most certainly will not. What art can do is employ its visual language to evoke an emotionally informed thinking and reflection about the effects of colonialism. In doing so it creates a space where the burden of responsibility can be lifted from Indigenous Australians and offers an opportunity for Settlers to begin to transform their-selves as people-to-come. This space is perhaps something like the horizon: we don't know exactly what it looks like, in fact we just have to trust that it really exists, but in attempting to move towards it we make a journey of becoming and are changed by our efforts.

Bibliography

Adorno, Theodore. 'An Essay on Cultural Criticism and Society'. *Prisms*. Translated by Samuel and Shierry Weber, 19–32. Cambridge: MIT Press, 1967.

Adorno, Theodore. *Aesthetic Theory*, edited by Gretel Adorno and Rolf Tiedemann. London: Bloomsbury Academic, 2013.

Agamben, Giorgio. *State of Exception*. Chicago: University of Chicago Press, 2005.

Arendt, Hannah. *The Human Condition.* Chicago: University of Chicago Press, 1958.

Arendt, Hannah. *Eichmann in Jerusalem. A Report on the Banality of Evil.* New York: Viking Press, 1968

Arendt, Hannah. *The Life of the Mind.* New York: Harcourt, 1978.

Badiou, Alain. *Deleuze: The Clamour of Being.* Translated by Louise Burchill. Minneapolis: University of Minnesota Press, 1999.

Bal, Mieke. *Of What One Cannot Speak: Doris Salcedo's Political Art.* Chicago: Chicago University Press, 2010.

Caruth, Cathy. *Unclaimed Experience: Trauma, Narrative, and History.* Baltimore: The Johns Hopkins University Press, 1996.

Culp, Andrew and Ricky Crano. 'Giving Shape to Painful Things'. *Radical Philosophy* 175 (2012): 43–52.

Deleuze, Gilles and Felix Guattari. *What Is Philosophy?* Translated by Hugh Tomlinson and Graham Burchell. New York: Colombia University Press, 1994.

Hage, Ghassan. 'Warring Societies and Intellectuals'. *Transforming Cultures e-Journal* 1.1 (2006): 43–49.

Hayden, Patrick. ed. *Hannah Arendt Key Concepts.* Durham: Acumen Publishing, 2014.

Huyssen, Andreas. *Present Pasts: Urban Palimpsests and the Politics of Memory.* Stanford: Stanford University Press, 2003.

Justice, Daniel. 'A Better World Becoming: Placing Critical Indigenous Studies'. Paper presented at the Public Lecture Series, University of Melbourne, Australia, November 6, 2014.

Laub, Dori. 'Truth and Testimony: The Process and the Struggle'. *Explorations in Memory*, edited by Cathy Caruth, 61–75. Baltimore: The Johns Hopkins University Press, 1995.

Aileen Moreton-Robinson, Aileen. 'I Still Call Australia Home: Indigenous Belonging and Place in a White Postcolonizing Society'. *Regroundings: Questions of Home and Migration*, edited by Sara Ahmed, C. Castameda, A. Marie Fortier and M. Sheller, 23–40. Oxford: Berg, Oxford University Press, 2003.

Rose, Deborah Bird. *Reports From a Wild Country: Ethics of Decolonisation.* Sydney: University of New South Wales, 2004.

Weber, Max. *Economy and Society: An Outline of Interpretive Sociology*, eds. Guenther Roth and Ckus Wittich. Berkeley: University of California Press, 1978.

Young, James E. *Holocaust Memorials in History: The Art of Memory.* New York: Prestel-Verlag, and New York: The Jewish Museum, 1994.

PART 5

The Curatorial Turn: Objects, Space, and Frames of Testimony

CHAPTER 12

Haunted Geographies in Atom Egoyan's *Calendar* and *Return to the Flock*

Christine Ramsay

Abstract

Testimony and its witnessing grounded our collaborative curatorial project, *Atom Egoyan and the Place of the Witness*, a study of the lens-based installation work of internationally acclaimed Canadian-Armenian art filmmaker Atom Egoyan. The project considered Egoyan's migration between the art film and film installation art — the black box of the film theatre and the white cube of the gallery space — through his installation works, with a special focus on an exhibition of his masterpiece, *Steenbeckett*, at the MacKenzie Art Gallery (5 November, 2016-January 2, 2017, Regina, Canada). The exhibition, which was the North American premiere of this important work, was also Station 9 on the larger durational series of exhibitions entitled *Meet in the Middle: Stations of Migration and Memory between Art and Film* (*Regina 2014–2017*) (Regina, Canada, 2014–2017). Egoyan's relationship to the contexts and genres of testimonial production rests on his recurring thematic interest in memorializing the events of the Armenian Genocide, diasporic identities, and acts of witnessing; and his formal fascination with the analog/digital divide, the malleability of the moving image, 'screen subjectivity', and our immersion in the image. Often reworking dramatic narratives as installations, his work mobilizes the tensions between the two-dimensional cinematic screen and the three-dimensional gallery space. We are interested in the ways Egoyan uses the gallery as a space of 'decomposition' in which 'the single screen gives way', to quote Maeve Connolly, to new and different creative strategies of recomposing, expanding and immersing subjects in the moving image. This contribution to the section theme of 'Objects and Performance of Testimony' consists of a suite of three chapters which explore Egoyan's installations through questions of collective and personal trauma, memory and witnessing: Christine Ramsay on *Return to the Flock* (1996), Timothy Long on *Auroras/Testimony* (2007), and Elizabeth Matheson on *Steenbeckett* (2002).

 | DOI:10.1163/9789004391130_014

Keywords

testimony – trauma – memory – truth – Armenian Genocide – screen – subjectivity – film installation art – immersive media – expanded cinema – socially engaged – art

1 Armenia: a Haunted Geography

Acts of witnessing, the play of memory and forgetting, and the production of testimony are foundational themes in the narrative films and lens-based installation work of internationally acclaimed Canadian-Armenian art filmmaker Atom Egoyan. As he himself says apropos of Arshile Gorky, in the talk he delivered at *Arshile Gorky: A Retrospective*, a career exhibition of the renowned Armenian-American painter at the Tate Modern (London, February 10-May 3, 2010):

> This concept — of finding a way of recording and ascertaining experience, of proving and acknowledging, of translating the complexity of personal and collective memory — has found its way in much of my work.[1]

Egoyan goes on to relate the importance of his encounter with one of Gorky's most famous works, 'The Artist and His Mother', at London's Whitechapel Gallery in 1990. He speaks about how many of his own films and installations over the next twenty years would be profoundly influenced by Gorky's legacy and, like Gorky himself, the legacy of the Armenian Genocide — works such as *Calendar* (1993), *A Portrait of Arshile* (1995), *Return to the Flock* (1996), *Early Development* (1997), *America, America* (1997), *Diaspora* (2001), *Ararat* (2002), and *Auroras/Testimony* (2007). Gorky painted two versions of 'The Artist and His Mother' between 1926 and 1942, one now held at the National Gallery of Art in Washington — the one Egoyan saw — and the other at the Whitney Museum in New York. In 'Arshile Gorky and the Armenian Genocide', renowned American-Armenian poet, writer and translator Peter Balakian excavates the significance of the subject matter: the paintings were based on a photograph of Gorky and his mother taken in Van in 1912, when Gorky was nine, and 'three

1 Atom Egoyan, 'Gorky', Tate Modern, April 21, 2010, unpublished manuscript, 1.

years before the Turks would destroy his home village'[2] and attempt to annihilate his family and his people through abduction, torture, forced death marches, and outright slaughter. Gorky's mother died of starvation in his arms in 1919, and Balakian describes both portraits as profound works of grief and mourning, disclosing a 'single psychological process: the experience of a survivor confronting the nightmare of his past'.[3]

In his talk, Egoyan reminisces about picking up a poster depicting the painting in the gallery shop at the Whitechapel, and describes the importance of such 'fetish'[4] objects in the transmission of experiences in and across cultures, in his own life, and in the very form and content of his creative work. He ends on the keynote of the importance of such 'cultural artefacts' to his process of 'creating meaning and significance' through representations concerned ultimately with the 'complexity and precariousness of cultural transposition, especially the transposition and telling of trauma'.[5]

David Pike has written insightfully about Egoyan's and his characters' obsessions with the personal collections and public archives of things and images which house and mediate our individual and collective memories and enable their expression. In 'The Passing of Celluloid: The Endurance of the Image: Egoyan, *Steenbeckett*, and *Krapp's Last Tape*', Pike observes how 'bits and pieces of the real world' find their way into the great museum building projects of the 19th century, libraries, Hollywood movies and media representations of all kinds, including art such as Egoyan's, thus coming to bear great symbolic weight and ferry rich performative capacity on behalf of our cultural memory:

> Egoyan's oeuvre is packed with images of archives and collections, and there is often an unresolved tension between them — the father who tapes over the video archive of his family in *Family Viewing*, only to have the tapes erased by his son; the video mausoleum in *Speaking Parts*; the photographer's "collecting" of images of Armenian churches rather than making an archive of their history and meaning in *Calendar*. ... But Egoyan also shows the need of individuals to be freed from the compulsion to collect or archive. ... Consider Arianne, the first victim introduced in *The Adjuster*, who allowed an electrical fire to grow from a spark in her kitchen to consume her house and who is wholly uninterested in reclaiming

2 Peter Balakian, 'Arshile Gorky and the Armenian Genocide', *Art in America* 84.2 (1996): 66.

3 Balakian, 'Arshile Gorky', 66.

4 Egoyan, 'Gorky', 1.

5 Ibid., 8, 11.

> anything from it, apparently relieved to be rid of it all. ... Obsession with archiving may lead to depression in Egoyan's films, but failure to cathect one's things and one's memories leads instead to suicide.[6]

I am particularly interested in addressing the symbolic power of the cultural artefacts of the church, the sheep, and the Armenian countryside as Egoyan artfully deploys them in oblique yet moving testimony to the Armenian Genocide in his feature *Calendar* (1993) and again in his installation *Return to the Flock* (*The Event Horizon*, Irish Museum of Modern Art, Dublin, November 2, 1996-February 2, 1997). Together, these three artefacts work to cathect for the artist and the viewer the fraught mental and emotional energy of Armenia's 'haunted geography' — a situation caused by the Ottoman Turkish government's orchestrated slaughter of two million souls between 1895–1896 and 1915–1917, followed to this day by its abject denial of responsibility for such carnage.[7] As Balakian writes in *Black Dog of Fate: An Armenian Son Uncovers His Armenian Past*, in reflecting on the writing of his book of poems *Sad Days of Light*, his work also emerged out of a similar gesture of the unearthing of 'things I could lay claim to':

> Armenia had become an Atlantis to my imagination. Lost Armenia, where my family had lived only seventy years ago. Armenia, whose misfortune had helped to define modernity, as Michael Arlen noted, because the "harnessing of modern technology for mass murder began with the Genocide of the Armenians" and it was the source of "the bloody river linking the great murderous events of our century."[8]

I will analyse how these artefacts Egoyan mines, as 'bits and pieces of the real world', come to *mean* and *signify*, both formally *between Calendar* and *Return to*

6 David Pike, 'The Passing of Celluloid, the Endurance of the Image', *Image and Territory: Essays on Atom Egoyan*, edited by Monique Tschofen and Jennifer Burwell (Waterloo: Waterloo University Press, 2006), 115.

7 The definitive eye-witness account is Henry Morgenthau, *Ambassador Morgenthau's Story* (Detroit: Wayne State University Press, 2003 [1919]), and Peter Balakian has translated his uncle's account: Grigoris Balakian, *Armenian Golgotha: A Memoir of the Armenian Genocide*, translated by Peter Balakian with Aris Sevag (New York: Alfred A. Knopf, 2009). See also Akçam Taner, *A Shameful Act: Turkish Responsibility and the Armenian Genocide* (New York: Henry Holt, 2006).

8 Peter Balakian, *Black Dog of Fate: An American Son Uncovers His Armenian Past* (New York: Basic, 2009 [1997]), 274–275.

the Flock as dramatic narrative and lens-based installation, respectively, and thematically *among* them and the works of influential Armenian and Armenian-diasporic filmmakers that have gone before: Elia Kazan's *America America* (1963) and Artavazd Pelechian's *The Seasons* (1972). But before doing so, I will provide the contexts of this study, situating it, and Egoyan's oeuvre, in a larger collaborative curatorial project — entitled *Atom Egoyan and the Place of the Witness* — on the artist and the scope of his ongoing concern with the cultural transposition of testimony about personal and collective trauma, through strategies of immersive subjectivity, in the contemporary field of expanded cinema.

2 Atom Egoyan and the Place of the Witness

Renowned as an independent feature filmmaker, theatre and opera director, Atom Egoyan has also been at the center of expanded cinema practice as an internationally prize-winning and collected artist for his exemplary immersive lens-based installations on trauma, memory and witnessing as they frame historical events (the Armenian Genocide and diaspora) and more personal histories and identities (involving desire, lost love, and family relations). He has shown at the Venice and Istanbul biennales; is collected by prestigious institutions, such as Museo de Arte Contemporáneo de Castilla y Léon (Spain); and has received the El Pochote International Award for Digital Cinema (Mexico), among many other accolades. A recent prize is one of Canada's highest honours: the 2015 Governor General's Performing Arts Award for Lifetime Artistic Achievement in Film.

Atom Egoyan and the Place of the Witness was a collaborative curatorial research project investigating Egoyan's artistic achievement by surveying the depth and breadth of his career from the mid-1990s to the present through five key themes: 1) Diasporic identities; 2) Trauma and the place of the witness; 3) Installation art and the role of the archive; 4) Art/film and the place of artists' filmmaking; and 5) *Steenbeckett* and the spaces of memory. Inspired by the importance of marking the centenary of the Armenian Genocide, and by our interest in the complexities of personal and collective memory for Egoyan, the project's goal was to consider Egoyan's work as it variously makes place for witnesses and their transposition and telling of trauma, while migrating between the art film and film installation art (fig 12.1).

We simultaneously configured this interest in Egoyan as part of the larger Regina-based durational series of exhibitions, screenings and events entitled *Meet in the Middle: Stations of Migration and Memory Between Art and Film* (2014–2017). Conceived as a succession of fourteen way stations connected by

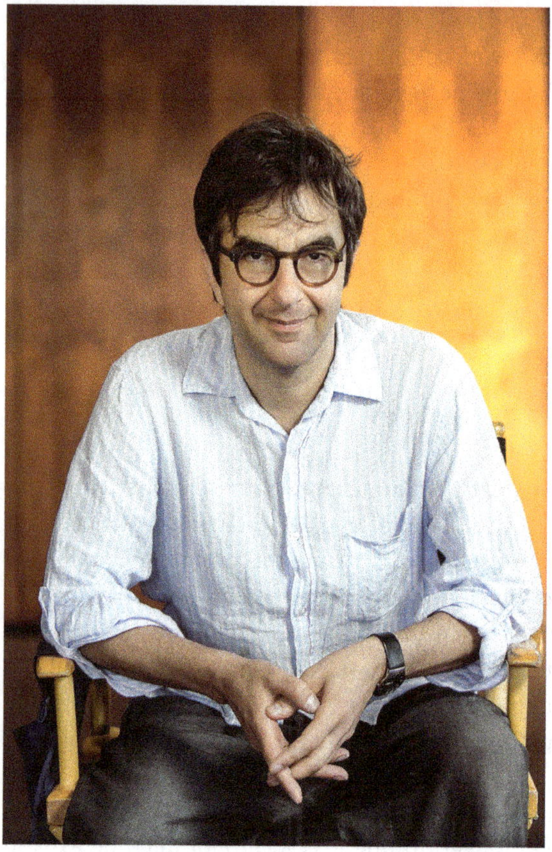

FIGURE 12.1 Atom Egoyan
PHOTOGRAPHER: TINA ROWDEN. © EGO FILM ARTS, 2015. PERMISSION GRANTED BY EGO FILM ARTS.

common concerns underlying global migration and unfolding over three years, *MITM* enabled artists, audiences, and curatorial researchers to stopover, encounter, intersect, reflect, locate and relocate themselves relative to the pressing questions of migration, memory and personal/political trauma, recalled and documented, imagined and represented, through the art/film practices of expanded cinema. As leading practitioners of 'art/film' in the gallery space, renowned Iranian-American artist Shirin Neshat, and Atom Egoyan, were the high-profile international artists chosen to bookend the project and frame the other stations, which included established Saskatchewan and Armenian artists, filmmakers and curators also working on themes of migration, memory and trauma in their work. *Meet in the Middle* began in winter 2014 with *Shirin Neshat: Soliloquy* (1999) at Regina's MacKenzie Art Gallery — the province of Saskatchewan's provincial museum[9] — and its capstone station was *Atom Egoyan: Steenbeckett* in fall 2016, including a critical catalogue of the same name on the contexts of *Steenbeckett* (Black Dog Publishing, 2018) and culminating in an international symposium (MacKenzie Art Gallery, November 2–5, 2016).

The *Meet in the Middle* concept emerged from the fact that new curatorial models are demanded to meet the transdisciplinary complexities of what is known, after the groundbreaking work of Gene Youngblood in the 1960s,[10] as the field of 'expanded cinema' — the explosion of the screen outward, 'toward immersive, interactive, and interconnected forms of culture'.[11] Jackie Hatfield has also been influential in redefining 'cinema' in the digital era to signify a 'wide-ranging historical and philosophical discourse', rather than 'film' per se: 'Importantly', she writes, the term 'cinema' is no longer

> yoked to the material conditions of a medium, and the cinematic experience can cross media boundaries and be achieved through a range of media combinations. A cinematic configuration could involve intermedia, performance, spectacle, video, art and technology in addition to film, and could be located within the "black box" of the theatre or the "white cube" of the gallery.[12]

---

9 The Regina-based curatorial collaborators on *Meet in the Middle* are Timothy Long (Head Curator, MacKenzie Art Gallery); Elizabeth Matheson (Curator and President, Strandline Curatorial Collective); Christine Ramsay (Associate Professor, Film and Media Studies, University of Regina); and Rachelle Viader Knowles (Senior Lecturer, School of Art and Design, Coventry University, UK). For further information, see the MITM website, viewed 20 December 2018, https://meetinthemiddle.squarespace.com

10 Gene Youngblood, *Expanded Cinema* (New York: Dutton, 1970). See also Stan Vanderbeek, 'Expanded Cinema: A Proposal and Manifesto', *Tulane Drama Review* 11 (1996).

11 Janine Marchessault and Susan Lord, 'Introduction', *Fluid Screens, Expanded Cinema*, eds. Janine Marchessault and Susan Lord (Toronto: University of Toronto Press, 2007), 7. See also: A. L. Rees, 'Expanded Cinema and Narrative: A Troubled History', *Expanded Cinema: Art, Performance, Film*, edited by A. L. Rees, et al. (London: Tate Publications, 2011); Gene Youngblood, 'Afterword: What We Must Do', *Fluid Screens, Expanded Cinema*, edited by Janine Marchessault and Susan Lord (Toronto: University of Toronto Press, 2007), 321–326; and Dork Zabunyan, 'The Dispersion of Cinema and Extension of the Domain of Film', *Art Press* 21 (2011): 68–77.

12 Jackie Hatfield, 'Expanded Cinema: Proto-, Photo and Post-Photo Cinema', *Expanded Cinema: Art, Performance, Film*, edited by A. L. Rees, et al. (London: Tate Publications, 2011), 262. See also Jackie Hatfield, 'Expanded Cinema and Its Relationship to the Avant-Garde', *Millennium Film Journal* 39/40 (2003): 51–65.

Accordingly, as the boundaries blur between the filmmaker as cinema artist (exhibiting images on the screen as large-scale narrative spectacle in the darkened theatre), and the lens-based visual artist (exhibiting them as more abstract, intermediated and interactive sculptural forms in the gallery, or other public settings), international curatorial attention has turned to examine the interconnections between art and film. Over the past two decades, great interest has evolved in presenting the work of filmmakers as gallery artists, alongside and in context with visual artists, who also use media/moving image technology in innovative and compelling ways. Thus, *Meet in the Middle* and its stations offered a model adequate to understanding and presenting the complexities of curating immersive art/film works as both three-dimensional sculptural forms in the gallery as architectural space, and two-dimensional forms on screen.

In the case of *Atom Egoyan and the Place of the Witness*, we were theoretically informed by three key disciplines: Film Studies, Curatorial Studies, and Trauma Studies. First, we engaged in the broad domain of current thinking in Film Studies on the increasing 'malleability of the image'[13] in what Zygmunt Bauman has termed our new era of 'liquid modernity'.[14] Modernity and globalized capitalism are now characterized by extreme flexibility in time and space, creating simultaneous convergences and fragmentation (economic, social, political, cultural, artistic) through transnational flows, fluid identities, and increasingly hybridized and networked mediascapes. Arts and culture generally, and media/moving image arts specifically, are important aspects of this state of 'remediation' described by Jay Bolter and Richard Grusin[15] — the flow of images across places, spaces, artforms, platforms, and screens — as they deconstruct traditional cinema into its component elements (light, sound, image, the apparatus) while reconfiguring the screen in the gallery and beyond (in urban public spaces, on heritage buildings, in landscapes, etc.). This is the terrain of 'expanded cinema' in which Kate Mondloch argues we are now increasingly immersed as 'screen subjects'.[16]

Accordingly, this project emerged in the context of what Jan Holmberg suggests has always been the pressing question of the 'ideal of immersion'

13 Marchessault and Lord, *Fluid Screens*, 4.

14 Zygmunt Bauman, *Liquid Modernity* (Cambridge: Polity, 2000), *passim*.

15 Jay David Bolter and Richard Grusin, *Remediation: Understanding New Media* (Cambridge, MA: MIT Press, 2000), 5.

16 Kate Mondloch, *Screens: Viewing Media Installation Art* (Minneapolis: University of Minnesota Press, 2010), ii.

and the realization and experience of the 'immersion effect'[17] so desired by cinema-makers and cinema-goers since the birth of film, but which clearly persists into the digital era even as cinematic technologies expand and change.[18] This strong sense of bodily immersion in, or 'presence with' the image that Holmberg describes as so 'radically different' than the sense of 'identification crucial to the later classical style'[19] of narrative cinema and its primary reliance on psychological suture of the viewer into a story through editing, is a key characteristic of installation art and its art/film, sculpture/screen dynamic. As Andrew Uroskie observes, as the moving image 'enters and transforms the space of contemporary art', its now 'heterogeneous and often ambivalent location'[20] in the gallery and beyond is an issue at the forefront for leading immersive installation artists (such as Janet Cardiff, Tacita Dean, Stan Douglas, Douglas Gordon, Anthony McCall, and, of course Atom Egoyan). As Timothy Long declares, so is the location of the viewer relative to the image and to the screen as a sculptural object within the gallery architecture or other public spaces. 'Installation art', Long writes, 'with its insistent engagement with the physical space of the viewer, enables film to leave the safe confines of the theatre and move into the space of the spectator',[21] creating a profound sense of physical, in addition to psychological, immersion in the work. The curators of such work must keep pace with these shifts in practice, which affect display and reception, and advance critical/theoretical concepts and methods.[22]

Hence, current thinking in Curatorial Studies advocates new, immersive configurations in our curatorial practice to present these new kinds of immersive

17 Jan Holmberg, 'Ideals of Immersion in Early Cinema', *Cinemas: Journal of Film Studies* 14.1 (2003): 129.

18 Essential works include: Jill Bennett, et al., *The Future of Cinema: Immersive and Interactive (Dis)Locations* (Berlin: Hatjie Cantz, 2002); Oliver Grau, *Virtual Art: From Illusion to Immersion* (Cambridge MA: MIT Press, 2003); and Laura Marks, *Touch: Sensuous Theory and Multisensory Media* (Minneapolis: Minnesota University Press, 2002).

19 Holmberg, 'Ideals of Immersion', 129.

20 Andrew Uroskie, 'Windows in the White Cube', *Screen/Space: The Projected Image in Contemporary Art*, edited by Tamara Trodd (Manchester: Manchester University Press, 2011), 145.

21 Timothy Long, 'Atom Egoyan's *Auroras*: A Chorus of Witnesses' in this volume.

22 See Claire Bishop, *Installation Art: A Critical History* (London: Tate, 2005) and Beryl Graham and Sarah Cook, *Rethinking Curating: Art after the New Media* (Cambridge, MA: MIT Press, 2010).

art/film installation works in the gallery space.[23] Internationally, curators and galleries have demonstrated a growing interest in collaborating with academics to reconceptualize and critically theorize the presentation of moving imagery, as it moves off the strictly two-dimensional screen and takes the form of three-dimensional sculptural installations which 'activate the space of reception' in new ways.[24] Recent major exhibitions include *Expanding the Frame 2011: Cinema on Stage* (Minneapolis, Walker Art Center, 2011), curated by Sheryl Mousley; *Projections: A Major Survey of Projection-Based Works in Canada, 1964–2007* (Toronto, Justina M. Barnicke Gallery, 2007), curated by Barbara Fischer; and *Into the Light: The Projected Image in American Art 1964–1977* (New York, Whitney Museum of Modern Arts, 2002), curated by Christine Iles. The MacKenzie has also participated further in this critical reassessment, hosting *Projections* in 2009 and mounting several exhibitions curated by Timothy Long, including *After Presence* (2012); *My Evil Twin* (2009); *Double Space* (2008) and *Wanda Koop: Sightlines* (2002). These are exhibitions which have begun to answer Regina-based curator and educator Sheila Petty's call for displays of contemporary Canadian artists who 'contest'[25] traditional uses of exhibition space (single channel display monitors; chairs and headsets, etc.); who lead us to re-think traditional curatorial models (taxonomic classification; didactics, etc.) in more immersive, interactive, and theoretically-informed ways; and who challenge us to program work that is not only aesthetically groundbreaking but also politically provocative and relevant to transnational global issues.

Egoyan's installation work was a perfect vehicle to explore and advance these theoretical concerns in Film and Curatorial Studies as it takes its place in this fluid terrain of expanded cinema and remediation through his formal innovations, entering and transforming the contemporary spaces of immersive art/film practice and exhibition. But we were also interested, *pace* Petty, in thematic concerns of how the work takes up crucial social and political

23 See Catherine Fowler, *Remembering Cinema: Artists' Filmmaking in the Gallery Since 1990* (Edinburgh: Edinburgh University Press, 2013); Louise Ismert, *Atom Egoyan: Hors d'usage* (Montreal: Musée d'art contemporain de Montréal, 2002); *Curating Subjects* edited by Paul O'Neill (Amsterdam: de Appel and Open Editions, 2007).

24 See "Expanded Cinema: Activating the Space of Reception", London, 17–19 April 2009, viewed 20 December 2018. http://www.tate.org.uk/context-comment/audio/expanded-cinema-activating-space-reception-day-1

25 Sheila Petty, 'Categorization and Curation Criteria: Contesting the Exhibition Space', (Terms of Address: A Symposium on the Pedagogy and Politics of Film and Video Programming and Curating, Centre for Media and Culture in Education, University of Toronto, 6–8 March 2003).

matters. Since 1996 and his first foray into installation with *Return to the Flock*, Egoyan's characteristic issues as a film director — trauma, historical memory, witnessing and testimony, diasporic identities, the technological mediation of time, and the physicality of the screen in space — have migrated from the 'black box' of his narrative films to the 'white cube' of the gallery, a journey that we argue is important to trace, analyze and celebrate as a signal example of expanded cinema.

Atom Egoyan and the Place of the Witness was also designed to put Egoyan, a leading figure working between art and film in Canada, on stage among notable national and international media/moving image artists, curators and theorists working in the important field of Trauma Studies.[26] As Antonio Traverso and Nick Broderick write:

> During the past 100 years or so, traumatic historical events and experiences have been re-imagined and re-enacted for us to witness over and over by constantly evolving media and art forms. Perhaps due to the ubiquity and multiplication of such images and narratives in modern and post-modern culture, questions about the impulse to behold and depict both the suffering of others and of the self, as well as more general questions about the ontological status of the representation of trauma, have increasingly been raised within intersecting, inter-disciplinary fields of study over the past two decades.[27]

Thus, our curatorial model for showcasing Egoyan's unique artistic vision in representing trauma emerged clearly from interdisciplinary insights at the intersection of Film, Curatorial and Trauma Studies.

In regard to leading currents in Film Studies, Egoyan's practice fits perfectly Youngblood's definition of expanded cinema:

---

26 One of the most influential works in the field is Jill Bennett's *Empathic Vision: Affect, Trauma and Contemporary Art* (Paolo Alto: Stanford University Press, 2005). See also Cathy Caruth, *Unclaimed Experience: Trauma, Narrative, Experience* (Baltimore: John Hopkins University Press, 1996) and Ana Douglas and Thomas A. Vogler, *Witness and Memory: The Discourse of Trauma* (New York: Routledge, 2003). For applications of trauma theory to modern visual culture, see Lisa Saltzman and Eric Rosenberg, editors, *Trauma and Visuality in Modernity* (Hanover: Dartmouth College and University Press of New England, 2006).

27 Antonio Traverso and Mick Broderick, 'Interrogating Trauma: Towards a Critical Trauma Studies', *Interrogating Trauma: Collective Suffering in Global Arts and Media*, edited by Mick Broderick and Antonio Traverso (London and New York: Routledge, 2011), 3.

> Cinema is the art of organizing a stream of audio-visual events in time. It is an event-stream, like music. There are at least four media through which we can practice cinema — film, video, holography and structured digital code — just as there are many instruments through which we can practice music.[28]

For David Pike, Egoyan directly addresses across his work the tension that has been evident between 'analogue and digital' as cinema expands, but without the usual 'deep-seated suspicion' of new technologies. In fact, Pike says, as mentioned above, Egoyan embraces celluloid, tape, digital and recording machines of all kinds like an 'archivist' using 'containers' to store experience — and these containers are as 'essential' to the meaning of the experience as 'the experience itself'.[29] Our 'dependence on and visceral need for such recording media', adds Marie-Aude Baronian, is one of Egoyan's 'favorite topics'.[30] Monique Tschofen and Jennifer Burwell also firmly locate Egoyan in this expanded and ubiquitous cinematic flow of the image and identities across platforms, screens and spaces, but they also note that as Egoyan 'displays our cultish and fetishistic reliance on images and screens' and their ever-changing technologies, he also 'constructs the screen as a meeting place where new, profound, and consciousness-altering forms of exchange take place'.[31] This understanding of screen and image as 'meeting place' in the era of digital cinema — a key characteristic of Egoyan's narrative features[32] — is also spatially realized with startling originality in his lens-based installations, beginning with *Return to the Flock*, and their common interest in staging stories of traumatized bodies and traumatic witnessing. Moreover, the relationship between screen and

---

28 Gene Youngblood, 'Cinema and the Code', *Future Cinema: The Cinematic Imaginary after Film*, edited by Jeffrey Shaw and Peter Weibel (Cambridge, MA: MIT Press, 2003), 157.

29 Pike, 'The Passing of Celluloid', 102, 107, 114, 117.

30 Marie-Aude Baronian, 'History and Memory, Repetition and Epistolarity', *Image and Territory: Essays on Atom Egoyan*, edited by Monique Tschofen and Jennifer Burwell (Waterloo: Wilfrid Laurier University Press, 2007), 161. And see Baronian's *Cinema et mémoire: Sur Atom Egoyan* (Seraing-le-Chateau, Belgium: Bebooks, 2013).

31 Monique Tschofen and Jennifer Burwell, 'Introduction: In Media Res: Atom Egoyan's Utopian Praxis', *Image and Territory: Essays on Atom Egoyan*, edited by Monique Tschofen and Jennifer Burwell (Waterloo: Wilfrid Laurier University Press, 2007), 1.

32 There exists a wealth of academic material addressing and contextualizing Egoyan's work. Particularly influential in addition to Tschofen and Burwell are: Hamid Naficy, *An Accented Cinema: Exilic and Diasporic Filmmaking* (Princeton: Princeton University Press, 2001), *passim*; Jonathan Romney, *Atom Egoyan* (World Directors Series. London: BFI, 2003); and Emma Wilson, *Atom Egoyan: Contemporary Film Directors* (Urbana and Chicago: University of Illinois Press, 2009).

image enables the witnessing of that trauma by the viewer in more immersive ways — ways that enhance our engagement, in both mind *and* body, in the subject's traumatic experience, creating an 'active spectator' who thus participates in 'meaning-making' with heightened consciousness and intent.[33] Our curatorial model asked and aimed to reveal how Egoyan's immersive strategy in representing trauma works and functions to such great effect.

The curatorial inquiry undertaken by this research and exhibition project can be summarized in the question: *'How, in the flow between screen, space, and audience, does Egoyan install his traumatic subject(s) and, so, move his viewers?'* Starting from the theoretical premise established above that the gallery is now a key mediator of the shifting relationships between 'art and film', 'space and screen', and 'object and viewer' in the era of digital cinema, the curatorial model examined Egoyan's 'immersive practice' in the context of his masterful and moving articulations of screen subjectivity through his recurrent themes of trauma, memory, witnessing and testimony (fig 12.2). The question of immersion of the screen subject has deep resonances for Egoyan: 'I've always felt that entrance into a screen is a physical act', he says.

> In *Speaking Parts*, there are these moments where I would almost like to think of the screen as an installation site that you are able to interact with. ... Likewise, in the recent installations I've tried to create ways in which people can physically manoeuver themselves into the private and communal memories that are being investigated. There is a physical sense that the person is activating a process with their very presence.[34]

Inspired by the installations of Canadian compatriot Janet Cardiff, whom he admires for her ability to take narratives off the screen and into physical space,[35] Egoyan sees the gallery as the kind of immersive spatial context necessary for his audiences to experience, in mind and body, as *embodied subjects*,

33 Baronian, 'History and Memory', 159. See also an account of the curatorial development of the satellite project conceiving the screen as a meeting place, of which the Egoyan exhibition is the capstone station: Christine Ramsay and Elizabeth Matheson, 'Meet in the Middle: Stations of Migration and Memory Between Art and Film', presented at the Curating Time- Based Media Curatorial Intensive, Independent Curators International, New York City, October 6–15, 2013, viewed 20 December 2018, http://curatorsintl.org/intensive/proposal/meet-in-the-middle

34 Atom Egoyan, Interview with Monique Tschofen, 'Ripple Effects', *Atom Egoyan Interviews*, edited by T. J. Morris (Jackson: University Press of Mississippi, 2010), 164.

35 Atom Egoyan, Interview with Janet Cardiff, 'The Whispering Room: Janet Cardiff', *Bomb Magazine* 79 (2002): 60–67; 62. See also Davina Quinlivan, 'The House that Egoyan

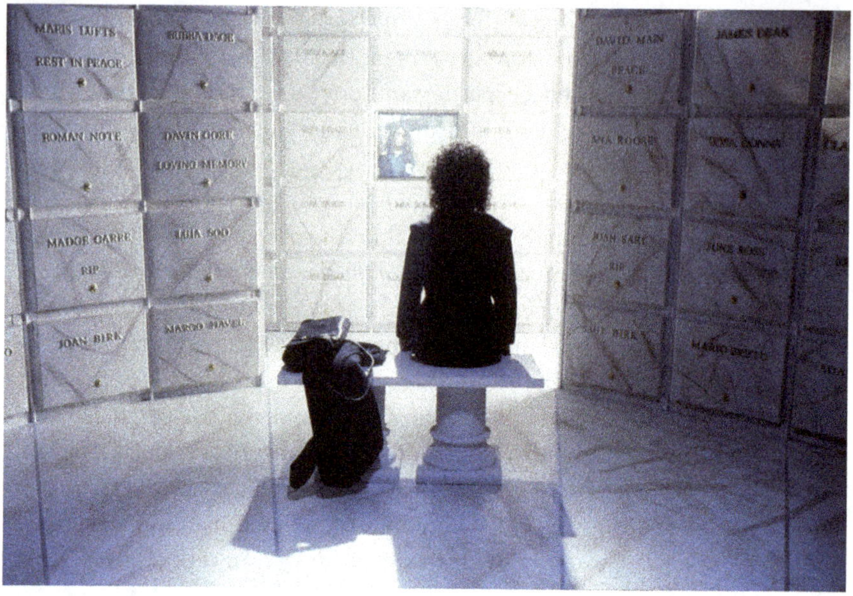

FIGURE 12.2 Still from *Speaking Parts*
COURTESY OF JOHNNIE EISEN.© EGO FILM ARTS. PERMISSION GRANTED BY EGO FILM ARTS.

his complex and challenging personal and political themes. He agrees with Cardiff that the body itself *is* the medium by which we mediate our current screen culture as screen subjects; the choice of technological platforms is obviously aesthetically important, but ultimately secondary to the primacy of the interactive subject who activates the screen in space. We contend that by variously reworking dramatic features (his own and others') as installations, Egoyan puts the cinema screen and the viewer in dialectic relationship to the space of the gallery, in effect immersing us as screen subjects in the productive tensions between *identifying* with the two-dimensional screen and *being closely present* with the screen in the three-dimensional gallery space. As Tschofen and Burwell describe Egoyan's strategy, 'in order to be *moved*, the viewer must *travel* into the image', exploring it, opening it to one's own subconscious: 'His own spatial metaphors point to a kinetic, embodied model of seeing that much resembles the phenomenological models of the cinema articulated by Vivian Sobchack (1992) and Laura Marks (2000)'.[36] For Marks, the place of the viewer

Built: Archives and Imagination in the Film of Atom Egoyan and the Art of Janet Cardiff', *The Place of Breath in Cinema* (Edinburgh: Edinburgh University Press, 2012).

36 Tschofen and Burwell, 'Introduction: In Media Res', 8.

in such works extends beyond the visual trope of the traditional cinematic 'gaze' onto the single screen to also encompass embodiment and the senses. Thus, the increased embodied proximity of the viewer to the image, the film, the tape, the screen, and ultimately, to the subject of the traumatic experience, in installations as opposed to narrative spectacles, enables the subject/image and the viewer a heightened co-being, mobilizing what Marks has provocatively called the art-screen's 'skin' as a 'multisensory' technology able to make bodies co-present in and through screen work and 'touch' the viewer in more expansive and moving ways.[37]

Atom Egoyan and the Place of the Witness took up these theoretical contexts that help explicate Egoyan's creative practice in order to engage his work responsively—in order to, in turn, help creatively facilitate, through curatorial practice and interpretation, the audience's relation to the work as a kind of 'kinetic, embodied model of *viewing*'. This Timothy Long calls 'theatroclasm' — literally 'the breaking of the place of the viewer', which happens whenever the anonymous cinematic voyeur is induced to 'question their place before the artwork and understand the controlling effect of the frame on collective experience'.[38] As Baronian notes, one of Egoyan's recurring tropes is to take the tension between objectivity and subjectivity, intimacy and distance, and make it an object of inquiry.[39] We argue that Egoyan has gravitated to installation in order to 'supplement' what traditional cinema and its distancing frame cannot achieve: 'bringing not just the voice and image' of the traumatized victims he represents to the consciousness of the spectator, but also the intimacy of the victims' 'aura or presence — a defining trait of visual art' — into the spectators' very space.[40] This implicates the history of 'the frame' in painting and film, which deconstructs and effaces itself, *pace* Jacques Derrida in *The Truth in Painting*, at the very moment it 'deploys its greatest energy'[41] in producing presence (or denying/manipulating it) for the viewer relative to the art object. Long's theory of theatroclasm underpinned *Atom Egoyan and the Place of the Witness* and provides a foundation for answering three key questions that the

37 Laura Marks, *Touch: Sensuous Theory and Multisensory Media* (Minneapolis: Minnesota University Press, 2002), 3.

38 Long, 'Chorus'. For an extended discussion of the concept, see also Timothy Long, *Theatroclasm: Mirrors, Mimesis and the Place of the Viewer* (Regina: MacKenzie Art Gallery, 2009).

39 Baronian, *Cinema et memoire*, 448–450.

40 Long, 'Chorus'.

41 Jacques Derrida, *The Truth in Painting*, trans. Geoff Bennington and Ian McLeod (Chicago: University of Chicago Press, 1987), 61.

artist's work raises: how traumatized bodies are made present in screen work; how gallery audiences become immersed in, identify with and respond to the experiences represented; and how witnessing functions for both the subjects in and the viewers of the work. By breaking the place of the viewer, Egoyan's installations variously restore bodily and sense memory to the viewer as they come into closer contact with the skin of the image and its power to mediate and memorialize experiences and testimonies of historical and personal trauma.

Therefore, *Atom Egoyan and the Place of the Witness* intended to capture, reflect, comment on and profile the ways Egoyan uses the museum/gallery as a fluid space of 'decomposition', in which 'the single screen gives way', as Maeve Connolly puts it,[42] to new and different creative strategies of recomposing, expanding, contracting, framing, and multiplying the image to immerse viewers and touch them in the deepest possible contemplation of his challenging themes. Accordingly, we researched, developed and executed a theoretically-based curatorial model coupling 'theatroclasm' with 'immersion' — the simultaneous immersion of the viewing subject within the space of the gallery on the one hand, and the world(s) represented within the screen on the other hand, inviting them to negotiate the content of the work and its spatial framing at one and the same time, and so to experience the juxtaposition of 'art/film' that the gallery site uniquely enables. Our theoretical thinking through the juxtaposition 'art/film' as Egoyan practices it is that the two-dimensional flat screen is matched, not only against, but within and through, its three-dimensional situation in space, becoming an object whose placement relative to the viewer (near or far, high or low, visible or obscured); size (large or small, square or rectangular); technological specifications (film or video, sound or silent, single or multiple channel); and content (collective and individual experiences of trauma) invoke the gallery as a truly active space of reception, which it is the curators' function and challenge to help the screen subject/audience notice, experience and navigate to the fullest.

As our contribution to this volume and its section theme of 'Objects, Spaces, and Frames of Testimony', my chapter touches on the representation of the historical memory of Armenia as a 'haunted geography' or 'spectral space' involving images of churches and sheep against the Armenian countryside as they migrate between Egoyan's feature film *Calendar* (1993)

---

42 Maeve Connolly, *The Place of Artists' Cinema: Space, Site, and Screen* (Bristol: Intellect, 2009), 64–65.

and *Return to the Flock* while paying homage to Elia Kazan's *America America* and Artavazd Pelechian's *The Seasons*. Timothy Long discusses *Auroras* (2007) through the lens of 'genre production' and 'historical memorialization'. *Auroras*, Egoyan's account of the traumatic experiences of Aurora Mardiganian, a survivor of the Armenian Genocide, is inspired by *Auction of Souls*, the lost 1919 Hollywood film about Mardiganian based on her autobiographical book *Ravished Armenia*, written in 1918. Elizabeth Matheson turns to *Steenbeckett* (2002) in the context of film installation art as an immersive 'thinking space' and 'theatre for memory' as it asks us to witness the reminiscences of Krapp, a haunted sexagenarian (played by William Hurt), as he reflects on the pain of hubris and lost love. Krapp was first introduced by Egoyan in his short dramatic film *Krapp's Last Tape* (2000), which was commissioned for the Irish-British co-production Beckett on Film, a project organized to film all of Samuel Beckett's nineteen plays, which screened at London's Barbican Centre in 2001. Working with and between the forms of narrative film and film installation art, how, we ask, has Egoyan made place for the witness as part of his navigation of the complexities of cultural transposition through his art, particularly the transposition and telling of trauma?

3 Cultural and Formal Transposition in the Telling of Trauma: *Calendar* and *Return to the Flock*

Churches, sheep and the Armenian countryside are sacred images in Armenian cultural consciousness. As mentioned above, I argue that they represent the kinds of 'cultural artifacts' of which Egoyan speaks as being key to his artistic process in the transposition and telling of Armenian cultural trauma. Indeed, given the iconic role they have played in Armenian and Armenian diasporic cinema, these artifacts can be seen to exemplify the kind of 'fetish' objects Egoyan describes: objects imbued with the spirit of the ways of life, architecture and predominantly Catholic traditions of the old country and of memories of the Genocide — Pike's 'bits and pieces of the real world' — part of the nation's collective and personal archive, if you will, in providing testimony to events that attempted to erase the national Armenian identity and that have, disgracefully, been denied by official history.

In 'An Archival Impulse', Hal Foster discusses the archival impulse in contemporary art as characterized not by a controlling 'will to totalize so much as a will to relate;' to probe a 'lost' or 'misplaced' past in order to make it physically reappear; to 'collate' its signs and fragments in order to create 'new orders of affective association' that can be useful to those in the present.[43] The recent turn to archival art, he suggests, emerges out of a 'failure in cultural memory', an obsession to connect a world that seems so 'frightfully disconnected'[44] in the digital age. Archival art takes its place in what Nicholas Bourriaud has called the era of 'postproduction' where we all mine and collage the fragmented image banks of globalized mass culture constantly, but where installation artists, invoking the modernist spirit of the 'readymade', are able to create new values by sampling, citing, collecting, combining, and tracing found images and objects in gestures that can produce important 'alternative knowledge' or 'countermemory' by remembering history, leaving space for the viewer, and calling out for 'human interpretation'[45] and thoughtful witnessing. Foster discusses many examples of works by artists who embrace this archival impulse, from Gerard Byrne, Tacita Dean, Stan Douglas, Sam Durant, Liam Gillick, Renée Greene, Douglas Gordon, Thomas Hirschhorn, Pierre Huyghe and Philippe Parreno to the incomparable writer Sebald. In the case of Dean, he describes how she plays with historical fact and its relationship to the present by recalling and recovering the *individual* 'lost souls' of history, such that her work 'functions as a possible portal between an unfinished past and a reopened future', while Durant's achievement lies in his ability to stage the archive as an associative terrain, creating a historical 'spatial unconscious'[46] that can conjoin the *collective* past with the desire to understand it in the present.

I suggest that Atom Egoyan works in similar ways in giving testimony to Armenia's lost souls and lost history across his oeuvre. Foster welcomes the way such artists variously turn those black holes of history — the 'excavation sites' of the modern world's genocidal violence and misery, such as Armenia — into 'construction sites' because 'it suggests a shift away from a melancholic culture that views the historical world as little more than the traumatic'.[47] The point Foster wishes to make is to testify to the value of installation art in *activating* the passive spectator as a *thinking subject* in relation to the screen as a deep site of cultural meaning: as Hirschhorn would say, in making productive 'spaces for the movement and endlessness of thinking;'[48] and, as Laura Marks puts it in 'Immigrant Semiosis', in making that thinking *embodied* — intimate,

43 Hal Foster, 'An Archival Impulse', *October* 110 (Autumn 2014): 21.

44 Ibid., 21–22.

45 Nicholas Bourriaud, *Postproduction: Culture as Screenplay: How Art Reprograms the World*, translated by Jeanine Herman (New York: Lukas & Sternberg, 2002), 4–5.

46 Foster, 'An Archival Impulse', 11, 15, 17.

47 Ibid., 22.

48 Ibid., 6.

experiential, emotional, personal, immersive — and, so, more significant, powerful and effective. As screen subjects, she reminds us, we are all semioticians, whether we are creating the images or contemplating them: 'Remember your body', she writes: 'remember how to think; keep learning how to communicate'.[49] This, I think, is how Atom Egoyan himself partakes in the archival impulse across *Calendar* and *Return to the Flock*, moving the unspeakable trauma of the Armenian Genocide into the realm of what he calls 'meaning and significance' for the deeply thinking, feeling and engaged gallery viewer, as I will now elaborate.

There is a 'spatial unconscious' running between Kazan's *America America*, Pelechian's *The Seasons*, and Egoyan's *Calendar* and *Return to the Flock*. Just as Gorky used the recovered photograph of him and his mother 'as a source for endless compositions',[50] likewise serial compositions can and have been drawn by Kazan, Pelechian and Egoyan from Armenian 'cultural artefacts' that have gripped, if not obsessed them and the Armenian people. In *Return to the Flock* Egoyan is of course borrowing and transposing the cultural artefacts of the sheep, the church and the Armenian countryside from his own narrative film *Calendar*, which in turn borrowed them from Elia Kazan's epic and Pelechian's poetic documentary. As Tschofen and Burwell suggested, Egoyan thus succeeds in constructing his screens as 'a meeting place' between artists, images, and viewers, where 'new, profound, and consciousness-altering forms of exchange take place'.[51]

In Kazan the church is an ambivalent site of collective belonging, as a church, which had been sheltering an Armenian community within the film's narrative about an immigrant youth's perilous journey from Turkish Anatolia to America in the early years of the 20th century, is intentionally set on fire by anarchists, evoking actual events of the Genocide and invoking traumatic witnessing in the youth and in the viewer, and traumatic memories for those Armenians and their families (like Gorky's, like Egoyan's, like Kazan's) who would have experienced such carnage. The film was directed and produced by Kazan from his 1962 book of the same name and won numerous prizes, including Best Picture, Best Director, and Best Screenplay at the 1964 Academy Awards. Kazan based the story of the immigrant youth, Stavros Topouzoglou (played by Stathis Giallelis), on the life of his own uncle. In 'The Immigrant Experience on Film: Kazan's *America America*', Brian Neve explains how

49 Laura Marks, 'Immigrant Semiosis', *Fluid Screens, Expanded Cinema*, edited by Janine Marchessault and Susan Lord (Toronto: University of Toronto Press, 2007), 45.

50 Atom Egoyan, 'Gorky', 4.

51 Tschofen and Burwell, 'Introduction: In Media Res', 1.

> Kazan's Uncle Joe, Avraam Elia Kazanjoglou, was one of thousands of Greeks who emigrated from Greece to Anatolia to the United States at the turn of the century. Most, like Kazan's uncle, made the journey alone and brought their families across later. Unlike mainland Greeks, whose chief motive was economic advancement, Anatolian Greeks were also influenced — as were the Armenians — by Turkish oppression, and they were more likely to view their journey to the United States as a permanent one.[52]

Within the narrative, Stavros helps and befriends Hohannes Gardashian (played by Gregory Rozakis) an Armenian youth seeking escape from Turkish persecution and passage to America as an immigrant labourer. After months of successive set-backs and harrowing trials in reaching Constantinople, told against the physical backdrop of the countryside of Turkish Anatolia and the history of the Genocide, the two embark on a ship to America, but in the end the tubercular and dying Hohannes sacrifices himself by exchanging his own passport with Stavros, so Stavros can 'legitimately' enter the country of his dreams. 'Yet', Neve writes, Kazan has made clear the fact that

> Stavros the human being, rather than Stavros the icon — the American Immigrant — has killed, lied and whored to get across. He has lost his innocence — including his innocence about America — and in the same process he has discovered the path to American success. ... Kazan has written that one of this hopes in the film was to show how Stavros, as he neared America, "became an American — in other words, someone who would do anything to reach his goal." Given that he has also revealed how in writing the script he came increasingly to be writing about himself, it is easy to recall Lillian Hellman's comments about the sons of immigrants. ... In one sense *America America* is an affirmation of an American ideal; in another it is an immigrant's attempt to understand his father's generation — and to come to terms with his own inheritance. Beyond its emblematic significance as a comment on American life and culture, the film remains a magnificent evocation of time and place.[53]

52 Brian Neve, 'The Immigrant Experience on Film: Kazan's *America America Film & History* 17.3 (September 1987): 63.

53 Ibid., 67.

Indeed, *America America* stands as a 'magnificent evocation' bringing to light not only early 20th century American immigrant life, but also testifying to the hidden and unspoken truths of the 'time and place' of *Armenia's* tragic experience, thus becoming an important touchstone for Egoyan as well. In first seeing the film's graphic scene of the Armenian church being burned, Egoyan relates how he thought he 'had found the first commercially distributed images of atrocities against the Turkish-Armenian population',[54] and how he thus came to 'fetishize' them, reprocessing and colourizing them for use in his own 1997 installation in the Armenian Pavillion at the Venice Biennale, entitled *America, America*. As mentioned above by Pike, this iconic image of the burning church is also invoked by Egoyan in the burning house in *The Adjuster* — another typically oblique, mediated and multivalent Egoyanesque reference, in portraying the traumatic destruction of *home*, to the traumatic destruction of *ravaged Armenia*. Similarly, in *Calendar*, the church is not literally represented aflame; rather, it is *translated* and *transposed*, and, in this instance, *multiplied* and *repeated*, marking its meaning as an explosive icon of the Turkish destruction of Catholic Armenia, as well as a sign of Armenia's power to endure.

Calendar stages a love triangle between a photographer from Toronto (played by Egoyan), his wife, who functions as his translator (played by Egoyan's wife, Arsinée Khanjian), and their Armenian driver and guide (played by Ashot Adamyan) as the obsessive, yet oddly distant and emotionally blank, photographer shoots multiple stills of Armenian churches for a calendar project. Cameras, video recorders, and answering machines self-reflexively intervene to tell — and show the telling — of this poignant story as we witness the end of a marriage set against the backdrop of the stunning Armenian landscape, its church architecture, and its ruins — the exact places where millions of people were marched and murdered, lambs to the slaughter.

Balakian describes these countryside 'death marches' in his trenchant account of the fate of Gorky and his family, quoting the eyewitness testimony of American Ambassador Henry Morgenthau, who wrote of the carnage in 1919 in *Ambassador Morgenthau's Story*:

> By the spring of 1915, Gorky's home was destroyed by the Turkish militia, local Turkish citizens and mercenary Kurds. On June 15, 1915, Shushanik and her children (Gorky, Vartoosh and their two half sisters), like nearly all the Armenians who weren't slaughtered outright, were sent off on a death march. Ambassador Morgenthau's memoir recalls that "from

54 Atom Egoyan, 'Gorky', 5.

> April to October, 1915, practically all the highways in Asia Minor were crowded with these unearthly bands of exiles. They could be seen winding in and out of every valley and climbing up the sides of nearly every mountain — moving on and on, they scarcely knew whither, except that every road led to death. Village after village and town after town was evacuated of its Armenian population. ... in these six months ... about 1,200,000 people started on this journey. ... 'Pray for us', they would say as they left their homes — the homes in which their ancestors had lived for 2,500 years."[55]

As Gorky himself explained in a letter to his nephew, Karlen Mooradian, which Balakian quotes, his painting, and the art and culture of Armenia itself, are imbued with the country's sense of *place* — its geographic and historical breadth of belonging across time and space. Again, Balakian merits quoting at length:

> Writing to his nephew, he explained that "though the Turks destroyed much of our art and killed our people we still struggled to express ourselves through art and many schools and styles of painting continued to flourish. But they have not received much publicity ... we are a small and humble people but in our time we have contributed our share to the advancement of art. ... The great art of our people lies hidden in ruins and amid the daily life of remote villages."

Gorky carried in his imagination an organic view of his Armenian culture. To him, it was a culture where architecture, technology, folk art, artisanry and high art were joined in one choral fugue, a Ruskian world where the energies of a society's imagination were entwined at all levels of creativity. Not unlike the Russian poet Osip Mandelstam, Gorky saw Armenia as an important nexus of civilization, part of a geographic and historical continuum.[56]

In both *Calendar* and *Return to the Flock*, Egoyan revisits these key Armenian cultural symbols of church ruins and remote village life, not unlike Gorky's 'choral fugue', creating a complex art/film/music metaphor for their significance to the Armenian landscape, the memory of a lost homeland and way of life, the catastrophic loss of life in the Genocide, and the endless peregrinations of the Armenian diaspora.[57] Taken together, *Calendar* and *Return to*

55 Balakian, 'Arshile Gorky', 62.

56 Ibid., 65.

57 See Katrin Kegel for an insightful analysis of the role and function of music in *Calendar* and across Egoyan's oeuvre: 'The Thirteenth Church: Musical Structures in Atom Egoyan's

the Flock are interesting because the pair instantiates Egoyan's self-proclaimed and self-reflexive immersive strategy throughout his work to show 'the frame as well as the picture'.[58] Moreover, they constitute his first gesture as an installation artist in decomposing/recomposing/reframing his images, and our experiences of them, as the immersive screen subjects whom he invites to migrate with him in new and surprising relationships to the screen, and between the cinema screen and the gallery space.

In *Calendar*, there is an arresting scene of the coldly intellectual photographer's pointing finger that literally and figuratively shows the frame, reaching around the camera as he tries to pose and control his exasperated subjects, his wife and the guide, breaking the diegesis, shattering the integrity of the film's narrative and its two-dimensional picture onto a closed cinematic world. It is Egoyan's highly original, symbolic and self-reflexive gesture regarding the power of the image-maker to construct, manipulate, and deconstruct the characters, the frame, and the story; and of the story and its characters to themselves escape that framing and, in an early gesture to Cardiff's work, come off the screen and into physical space. Within the diegesis, it is the image-maker's wife who seems to have the upper hand in her unmediated openness to her roots in Armenian historical reality, its traditions and way of life, its architecture, and its people. Of course, she begins to fall in love with their Armenian guide, leaving her husband truly outside the frame of the picture of the fraught history of Armenia that is emerging via the guide's knowledge, and also outside her capacity and desire to identify with and embrace their common traumatic heritage. The extreme low angle shot; the scaffolding intervening like a cross and seeming to protect the guide and the wife and sustain the building, while creating a barrier against the photographer; and the look of annoyed judgment toward the latter on the couple's faces — all work to emphasize the formation of a new, more vital couple against the backdrop of Armenia's rich and indestructible heritage. The church here, rather than succumbing to being burnt and destroyed, serves to support and privilege their relationship and its geo-political context, and the viewer is led to assume that, outside the diegesis, they go on to ignite their passion through their mutual sense of *belonging in and love for this ancient place*. While his wife remains with the guide, the photographer, who, as Pike observes above, has been obsessed with collecting pretty images of the churches rather than trying to understand their context

Calendar', *Image and Territory: Essays on Atom Egoyan*, edited by Monique Tschofen and Jennifer Burwell (Waterloo: Wilfrid Laurier University Press, 2007), 79–100.

58 Tschofen and Burwell, 'Introduction: In Media Res', 4.

in the Armenian landscape and for the Armenian people, returns to Toronto and helplessly tries to grasp both his personal loss and the political history of his ancestors by contemplating the fragmented document he has filmed of the dissolution of his marriage and his wife's decision to stay in Armenia and 'return to the flock'.

In addition to the symbology of the church, Egoyan litters *Calendar* strategically with a mesmerizing image of a flock of sheep streaming endlessly across the countryside and the screen like spectres of souls in passage, a multivalent reference to the victims of the Genocide, a flowing intertext with Artavazd Pelechian's *The Seasons*, and another clear marker of the power of this haunted geography to call its people home.

Daniel Fairfax describes *The Seasons* as a 'cosmological' film, and its imagery of sheep and shepherds, as 'one of the most sublime sequences in the history of the cinema'.[59] In Pelechian's famous meditation on the lives of shepherds in the harsh Armenian highlands, set to passages from Vivaldi's *Four Seasons*, the symbiotic relationship between the men and their animals is rendered in stunning black and white montage as the footage captures the men attempting to rescue the animals from torrential rivers, or from sliding down icy mountains into oblivion. As such, Fairfax writes, citing Pigoullié, Cioran and Matt, the film concerns itself with 'the little people', metaphorically presenting not only Armenia as 'a nation which has always been on the wrong side of history', but also larger 'epiphanies of the human condition in a permanent state of emergency'.[60]

Pelechian's work, as Baronian notes, owes its innovative formal structure and expressive power to the confluence between music and montage:

> Believing that music is movement itself and is therefore inevitably connected to image, Pelechian relies on a repetitive editing strategy comparable to musical composition in order to explore both infinite circularity and the tragic nature of movement that, for him, characterize life and existence. Egoyan borrows from Pelechian not only his Armenian ode to atemporal natural symbols, but also the fundamentally musical structural and editing techniques that convey the idea that everything in the world is moving, repeating, and reiterating.[61]

59 Daniel Fairfax, 'Artavazd Pelechian', *Senses of Cinema* 62 (March 2012): 14.

60 Ibid., 19.

61 Baronian, 'History and Memory', 166.

While Pelechian's theory of his editing strategy of 'distance montage' is notoriously complex, Fairfax explicates it well as the filmmaker's desire to have the viewer 'hear' his images and 'see' his sounds. Pelechian's goal is to edit film holistically, not simply by juxtaposing images in the Soviet style but by paying attention to the meaning generated by putting distance between images, and by joining them not only to each other but to sounds as well. Thus he intends to create a state of 'fugue' through the play of images with and against sounds, manipulating the screen's ability to produce an 'absent reality', so that, paradoxically, one can better feel reality's aura through the art form of cinema.[62] As François Niney has put it, and Pelechian relishes the description, the style achieves a 'dismantled reality'.[63] In 'Time Against Me, My Cinema Against Time', the director himself describes the essence of his unique approach as a gesture that installs absence between images to create '*an emotional field around the film*'[64] (his emphasis) — a gesture of *separation* that opens an immersive psychological space for the viewer's heightened absorption.

Indeed, Pelechian's strategy is clearly resonant with the contemporary forms of expanded cinema, film installation art and the archival impulse in which Egoyan situates himself — forms which value, as we have seen, theatroclastically breaking the place of the viewer and enabling them to travel around and into the image while the image, in turn, makes space for them to process and interpret its larger meaning. In *Calendar*, the image of the running sheep, while obviously narratively motivated as simply part of the terrain that the trio of characters are traversing in capturing images of churches for the calendar project, is again treated very self-reflexively. Held for an extreme duration, at least two minutes at the beginning of the film, and reappearing strategically at the end, as the wife tells the photographer she's leaving him for the guide, the sequence effectively bookends the film, its repetition rupturing the diegesis, much like Egoyan's pointed handling of the church within the frame, discussed above. In this breath-taking travelling shot, the sheep seem to run beyond the frame and time itself, now a blurred mass, now recognizable individuals, together symbolically taking on the extra-diegetic weight and aura of the scope of the Armenian Genocide, the lives of those killed, and the resulting diasporic condition of the survivors. This gesture recalls both Durant's desire to use installation strategies to conjoin the collective past to the present,

62 Fairfax, 'Artavazd Pelechian', 8–9.

63 François Niney, Interview with Artavazd Pelechian, 'Montage with Images that Don't Exist: Interview with Artavazd Pelechian', *Discourse* 22.1 (Winter 2000): 94–98; 97.

64 Artavazd Pelechian, 'Time against Me, My Cinema against Time', *Discourse* 22.1 (Winter 2002): 92.

and Dean's desire to recall history's individual lost souls, rendering the sheep Egoyan's living, breathing fetish objects culled from the archive of the Armenian experience.

Then, three years after filming *Calendar*, in a further gesture of decomposition, recomposition and reframing the subject of which Connolly speaks, Egoyan mines the church and the sheep to create *Return to the Flock*. As Egoyan's first work to migrate from narrative film to film installation art, *Return to the Flock* is a piece of record in his *oeuvre*. Twelve backlit still photos of Armenian churches are aligned horizontally above twelve video monitors showing looped footage of the flock of sheep from *Calendar* moving endlessly across the screen, and from screen to screen. In this light, Egoyan's work clearly bears comparison to that of Tacita Dean in terms of what Erika Balsom has called her thematic and formal articulation of a 'scattered cinema', and a 'cinema in ruins'. Balsom describes how, as analogue film becomes increasingly obsolete in the new screenscape of digitization and remediation, artists like Dean forego clinging to a 'purity of cinema' in favour of participating in the 'possibilities of its continuing metamorphosis'[65] by relocating it in the gallery space for us to witness — as art, as artifact, as relic, and as testimony to the traces of history and of time's passing.

The piece, as mounted at *The Event Horizon* exhibition at the Irish Museum of Modern Art, Dublin, in 1996 seems to extend to infinity, inviting us to flow bodily alongside, entering and leaving the frame(s) at our own pace. Thus, it offers the possibility for what Malcolm LeGrice has called the kind of enhanced 'spectator time'[66] that installation art provides for viewers to actively mobilize the work's meaning. With *Return to the Flock*, we experience Marks' and Hirschhorn's endless space for embodied thinking, for moving beyond the two-dimensional confines of the filmic space of *Calendar* and its tendency as dramatic narrative toward the singularity of 'one authorized, authoritative interpretation',[67] into the three-dimensional space of installation art's more immersive and interactive screen. Here, the rhythm of twelve — an ancient agrarian system for organizing and charting through the heavens the cycles of human social, religious and commercial life on earth, as well as a cross-cultural symbol of cosmic plenitude, completion, and integrity — is told in the multiple images of the stoically unmoving Armenian Catholic churches,

65 Erika Balsom, 'A Cinema in the Gallery: A Cinema in Ruins', *Screen* 50.4 (2009): 412.

66 Malcolm Le Grice, 'Time and the Spectator in the Experience of Expanded Cinema', *Expanded Cinema: Art Performance Film*, edited by A. L. Rees, et al. (London: Tate Publishing, 2011), 166.

67 Ibid., 169.

and underlined by the flowing energy of the Armenian sheep transposed from *Calendar*. With this gesture, Egoyan underwrites a formal metamorphosis, as the single channel screen of the film gives way, providing him with new possibilities for framing the picture and immersing the viewer in the gallery space while invoking Dean's notion of enacting 'a possible portal between an unfinished past and a reopened future'[68] as he artfully testifies to how the Genocide haunts the very fabric of Armenian national and diasporic identity. As Egoyan puts it, all of his 'post-genocidal stories are driven by a common anxiety: the anxiety of not being understood, of being ignored, of not being heard'.[69]

In this light, expanded cinema can be seen as a revitalized territory for the 'spiritualization of the image'[70] and the gallery space as a new environment of 'screen consciousness'[71] shared between artist, image, viewer and history for 'witnessing ourselves socially and politically'[72] – and, I would add, aesthetically. Between *Calendar* and *Return to the Flock*, his inaugural installation in 1996, we can see how Atom Egoyan began his fascinating and ongoing peregrination between the black box of cinema and the white cube of the gallery space, and how, as an artist and as a member of the Armenian diaspora, he began to migrate between the art film and film installation art, embracing new strategies to engage us in bearing witness to and making visible, seen and heard the fraught spaces of trauma, memory, and hard truths about home.

Bibliography

'America, America'. Atom Egoyan. *Armenian Pavilion*. Venice Biennale, Venice, Italy, June 15-November 9, 1997.

America, America. Directed by Elia Kazan. Los Angeles: Athena Enterprises, Warner Brothers, 1963. DVD.

Ararat. Dir. Atom Egoyan. Toronto: Alliance Atlantis Communications, Ego Film Arts, 2002. DVD.

Auction of Souls [original title: *Ravished Armenia*]. Dir. Oscar Apfel. Los Angeles: First National Pictures, 1919.

Auroras/Testimony. Atom Egoyan with Kutlug Ataman, *Luminato Festival*, Toronto, Canada, June 19–28, 2007.

68 Foster, 'An Archival Impulse', 15.

69 Atom Egoyan, 'Gorky', 11.

70 Rees, 'Expanded Cinema and Narrative', 13.

71 Marchessault and Lord, *Fluid Screens*, 7.

72 Connolly, *The Place of Artists' Cinema*, 10.

Balakian, Grigoris. *Armenian Golgotha: A Memoir of the Armenian Genocide*. Translated by Peter Balakian with Aris Sevag. New York: Alfred A. Knopf, 2009.

Balakian, Peter. 'Arshile Gorky and the Armenian Genocide'. *Art in America* 84.2 (1996): 58–67, 108–109.

Balakian, Peter. *Black Dog of Fate: An American Son Uncovers His Armenian Past*. New York: Basic, 2009 [1997].

Balakian, Peter. *Sad Days of Light*. Pittsburgh: Carnegie Mellon University Press, 1993.

Balsom, Erika. 'A Cinema in the Gallery: A Cinema in Ruins'. *Screen* 50.4 (2009): 411–427.

Baronian, Marie-Aude. *Cinema et mémoire: Sur Atom Egoyan*. Seraing-le-Chateau, Belgium: Bebooks, 2013.

Baronian, Marie-Aude. 'History and Memory, Repetition and Epistolarity'. *Image and Territory: Essays on Atom Egoyan*, edited by Monique Tschofen and Jennifer Burwell, 157–176. Waterloo: Wilfrid Laurier University Press, 2007.

Bauman, Zygmunt. *Liquid Modernity*. Cambridge: Polity, 2000.

Bennett, Jill. *Empathic Vision: Affect, Trauma and Contemporary Art*. Paolo Alto: Stanford University Press, 2005.

Bennett, Jill, James Donald, Ursula Frohne, Anna Munster and Peter Weibel *The Future of Cinema: Immersive and Interactive (Dis)Locations*. Berlin: Hatjie Cantz, 2002.

Bishop, Claire. *Installation Art: A Critical History*. London: Tate, 2005.

Bolter, Jay David and Richard Grusin. *Remediation: Understanding New Media*. Cambridge, MA: MIT Press, 2000.

Bourriaud, Nicholas. *Postproduction: Culture as Screenplay: How Art Reprograms the World*. Translated by Jeanine Herman. New York: Lukas & Sternberg, 2002.

Calendar. Dir. Atom Egoyan. Toronto: Ego Film Arts, 1993. DVD.

Caruth, Cathy. *Unclaimed Experience: Trauma, Narrative, Experience*. Baltimore: John Hopkins University Press, 1996.

Connolly, Maeve. *The Place of Artists' Cinema: Space, Site, and Screen*. Bristol: Intellect, 2009.

Derrida, Jacques. *The Truth in Painting*. Translated by Geoff Bennington and Ian McLeod. Chicago: University of Chicago Press, 1987.

Diaspora. Directed by Atom Egoyan. Toronto: Ego Film Arts, 2001. DVD.

Douglass, Ana and Thomas A. Vogler. *Witness and Memory: The Discourse of Trauma*. New York: Routledge, 2003.

'Early Development'. Atom Egoyan. *Les transports del l'image*. Le Fresnoy, Studio National des Arts Contemporains, Tourcoing, France, November 1997-January 1998.

Egoyan, Atom. 'Gorky'. *Arshile Gorky: A Retrospective*. Tate Modern, February 10-May 3, 2010. Unpublished manuscript. 1–11. Delivered 21 April, 2010. Viewed 16 May 2015. http://www.tate.org.uk/whats-on/tate-modern/exhibition/arshile-gorky.

Egoyan, Atom. Interview with Janet Cardiff, 'The Whispering Room: Janet Cardiff.' *Bomb Magazine* 79 (2002): 60–67.

Egoyan, Atom Interview with Monique Tschofen. 'Ripple Effects.' *Atom Egoyan Interviews*, edited by T. J. Morris. Jackson: University Press of Mississippi, 2010. 159–174.

Expanded Cinema: Activating the Space of Reception. Tate Modern, London, 17–19 April, 2009. Viewed 16 May 2015. http://www.tate.org.uk/context-comment/audio/expanded-cinema-activating-space-reception-day-1

Fairfax, Daniel. 'Artavazd Pelechian'. *Senses of Cinema* 62 (March 2012): 1–31.

Fischer, Barbara. *Projections: A Major Survey of Projection-Based Works in Canada, 1964–2007*. Toronto: Junstina M. Barnicke Gallery, April 8-June 17, 2007; Regina: MacKenzie Art Gallery, February 14-April 26, 2009.

Foster, Hal. 'An Archival Impulse'. *October* 110 (Autumn 2014): 3–22.

Fowler, Catherine. *Remembering Cinema: Artists' Filmmaking in the Gallery since 1990*. Edinburgh: Edinburgh University Press, 2013.

Graham, Beryl and Sarah Cook. *Rethinking Curating: Art after the New Media*. Cambridge, MA: MIT Press, 2010.

Grau. Oliver. 'Immersion and Interaction: From Circular Frescoes to Interactive Image Spaces'. *Media Art Net: A Survey of Media Art*, edited by Rudolf Frieling and Dieter Daniels, 292–313. Vienna: Springer, 2004.

Hatfield, Jackie. 'Expanded Cinema and Its Relationship to the Avant-Garde'. *Millennium Film Journal* 39/40 (2003): 51–65.

Hatfield, Jackie. 'Expanded Cinema: Proto-, Photo and Post-Photo Cinema'. *Expanded Cinema: Art, Performance, Film*, edited by A. L. Rees, Duncan White, Steven Ball and David Curtis, 262–266. London: Tate Publications, 2011.

Holmberg, Jan. 'Ideals of Immersion in Early Cinema'. *Cinemas: Journal of Film Studies* 14.1 (2003): 129–147.

Hors d'usage. Atom Egoyan, Musée d'art contemporain de Montréal, Quebec, August 29-October 20, 2002.

Iles, Christine. 'Between the Still and Moving Image'. *Into the Light: The Projected Image in American Art, 1964–1977*, 34–69. New York: Whitney Museum of American Art and Harry N. Abrams, Inc., 2001.

Iles, Christine. *Into the Light: The Projected Image in American Art, 1964–1977*. Whitney Museum of American Art, New York, 2002.

Iles, Christine. *Into the Light: The Projected Image in American Art, 1964–1977*. New York: Whitney Museum of Modern Art, 2002.

Ismert, Louise. *Atom Egoyan: Hors d'usage*. Montreal: Musée d'art contemporain de Montréal, 2002.

Kazan, Elia. Directed by *America, America*. New York: Popular Library, 1962.

Kegel, Katrin. 'The Thirteenth Church: Musical Structures in Atom Egoyan's *Calendar*'. *Image and Territory: Essays on Atom Egoyan*, edited by Monique Tschofen and Jennifer Burwell, 79–100. Waterloo: Wilfrid Laurier University Press, 2007.

Krapp's Last Tape. Dir. Atom Egoyan. UK: Blue Angels Films, 2000. DVD.

LeGrice, Malcolm. 'Time and the Spectator in the Experience of Expanded Cinema'. *Expanded Cinema: Art Performance Film*, edited by A.L. Rees, Duncan White, Steven Ball and David Curtis, 160–170. London: Tate Publishing, 2011.

Long, Timothy. *After Presence*. MacKenzie Art Gallery, Regina, Canada, February 4-April 15, 2012.

Long, Timothy. *Double Space*. MacKenzie Art Gallery, Regina, Canada, October 4, 2008-January 25, 2009.

Long, Timothy. *My Evil Twin*. Mackenzie Art Gallery, Regina, Canada, 2009.

Long, Timothy. *Theatroclasm: Mirrors, Mimesis and the Place of the Viewer*. Regina: MacKenzie Art Gallery, 2009.

Long, Timothy. *Wanda Koop: Sightlines*. MacKenzie Art Gallery, Regina, Canada, 2002.

Marchessault, Janine and Susan Lord. 'Introduction'. *Fluid Screens, Expanded Cinema*, eds. Janine Marchessault and Susan Lord, 3–28. Toronto: University of Toronto Press, 2007.

Mardiganian, Aurora. *Ravished Armenia: The Story of Aurora Mardiganian, the Christian Girl, Who Survived the Great Massacres*. [n.p]: IndoEuropean Publishing, 2014 [1918].

Marks, Laura. 'Immigrant Semiosis'. *Fluid Screens, Expanded Cinema*, eds. Janine Marchessault and Susan Lord, 284–303. Toronto: University of Toronto Press, 2007.

Marks, Laura. *Touch: Sensuous Theory and Multisensory Media*. Minneapolis: Minnesota University Press, 2002.

Meet in the Middle: Stations of Migration and Memory between Art and Film (Regina 2014–2016). Regina, Canada. Viewed 2 October 2015. https://meetinthemiddle.squarespace.com.

Mondloch, Kate. *Screens: Viewing Media Installation Art*. Minneapolis: University of Minnesota Press, 2010.

Morgenthau, Henry. *Ambassador Morgenthau's Story*. Detroit: Wayne State University Press, 2003 [1919].

Mousely, Sheryl. *Expanding the Frame 2011: Cinema on Stage*. Walker Art Centre. Minneapolis, 2011. Viewed 18 September 2014. http://blogs.walkerart.org/filmvideo/2011/01/20/expanding-the-frame-2011-cinema-on-stage/.

Naficy, Hamid. *An Accented Cinema: Exilic and Diasporic Filmmaking*. Princeton: Princeton University Press, 2001.

Neve, Brian. 'The Immigrant Experience on Film: Kazan's *America America*'. *Film & History* 17.3 (September 1987): 62–68.

Niney, François. 'Montage with Images that Don't Exist: Interview with Artavazd Pelechian.' *Discourse* 22.1 (Winter 2000): 94–98.

O'Neill, Paul, ed. *Curating Subjects*. Amsterdam: de Appel and Open Editions, 2007.

Pelechian, Artavazd. 'Time against Me, My Cinema against Time'. *Discourse* 22.1 (Winter 2002): 92–93.

Petty, Sheila. 'Categorization and Curation Criteria: Contesting the Exhibition Space'. Terms of Address: A Symposium on the Pedagogy and Politics of Film and Video Programming and Curating. Centre for Media and Culture in Education, University of Toronto, 6–8 March, 2003.

Pike, David. 'The Passing of Celluloid: The Endurance of the Image'. *Image and Territory: Essays on Atom Egoyan*, edited by Monique Tschofen and Jennifer Burwell, 101–122. Waterloo: Wilfrid Laurier University Press, 2007.

A Portrait of Arshile. Directed by Atom Egoyan. Toronto: Ego Film Arts, 1995.

Quinlivan, Davina. 'The House that Egoyan Built: Archives and Imagination in the Film of Atom Egoyan and the Art of Janet Cardiff'. *The Place of Breath in Cinema*. Edinburgh: Edinburgh University Press, 2012.

Ramsay, Christine and Elizabeth Matheson. 'Meet in the Middle: Stations of Migration and Memory Between Art and Film'. Presented at the Curating Time- Based Media Curatorial Intensive, Independent Curators International, New York City, 6–15 October, 2013. Viewed on 20 December 2018. http://curatorsintl.org/intensive/proposal/meet-in-the-middle.

Rees, A. L. 'Expanded Cinema and Narrative: A Troubled History'. *Expanded Cinema: Art, Performance, Film*, edited by A. L. Rees, Duncan White, Steven Ball and David Curtis, 12–21. London: Tate Publications, 2011.

Return to the Flock. *The Event Horizon*, Irish Museum of Modern Art, Dublin, 2 November 1996–2 February 1997.

Romney, Jonathan. *Atom Egoyan*. World Directors Series. London: BFI, 2003.

Saltzman, Lisa and Eric Rosenberg, editors. *Trauma and Visuality in Modernity*. Hanover and London: Dartmouth College and University Press of New England, 2006.

The Seasons. Dir. Artavazd Pelechian. Russia: Producer Unknown, 1972. Viewed 20 December 2018. https://www.youtube.com/watch?v=PNFTokKDPlk

Steenbeckett. *Atom Egoyan: Steenbeckett-An Installation*. (Former) Museum of Mankind, London, UK, February 15–March 17, 2002.

Taner, Akçam. *A Shameful Act: Turkish Responsibility and the Armenian Genocide*. New York: Henry Holt, 2006.

Traverso, Antonio and Mick Broderick. 'Interrogating Trauma: Towards a Critical Trauma Studies'. *Interrogating Trauma: Collective Suffering in Global Arts and Media*, edited by Mick Broderick and Antonio Traverso, 3–13. New York: Routledge, 2011.

Trodd, Tamara. 'Theorizing the Projected Image'. *Screen/Space: The Projected Image in Contemporary Art*, edited by Tamara Trodd, 1–22. Manchester: Manchester University Press, 2011.

Tschofen, Monique and Jennifer Burwell. 'Introduction: In Media Res: Atom Egoyan's Utopian Praxis'. *Image and Territory: Essays on Atom Egoyan*, edited by Monique Tschofen and Jennifer Burwell, 1–18. Waterloo: Wilfrid Laurier University Press, 2007.

Uroskie, Andrew. 'Windows in the White Cube', *Screen/Space: The Projected Image in Contemporary Art*, edited by Tamara Trodd, 61–106. Manchester: Manchester University Press, 2011.

Vanderbeek, Stan. 'Expanded Cinema: A Proposal and Manifesto'. *Tulane Drama Review* 11 (1996): np.

Wilson, Emma. *Atom Egoyan: Contemporary Film Directors*. Chicago: University of Illinois Press, 2009.

Youngblood, Gene. 'Afterword: What We Must Do'. *Fluid Screens, Expanded Cinema*, eds. Janine Marchessault and Susan Lord, 321–326. Toronto: University of Toronto Press, 2007.

Youngblood, Gene. 'Cinema and the Code'. *Future Cinema: The Cinematic Imaginary after Film*, edited by Jeffrey Shaw and Peter Weibel, 156–161. Cambridge, MA: MIT Press, 2003.

Youngblood, Gene. *Expanded Cinema*. New York: Dutton, 1970.

Zabunyan, Dork. 'The Dispersion of Cinema and Extension of the Domain of Film'. *Art Press* 21 (2011): 68–77.

This project has been generously funded by the Social Sciences and Humanities Research Council of Canada (2011–2017).

CHAPTER 13

Atom Egoyan's *Auroras*: a Chorus of Witnesses

Timothy Long

Abstract

In his lens-based installation *Auroras* (2007), Canadian filmmaker and artist Atom Egoyan re-presents the traumatic account of Aurora Mardiganian, a young woman who survived the Armenian genocide and whose story was published and then filmed in the United States under the titles *Ravished Armenia* and *Auction of Souls* (1919), in which she played herself. Egoyan's installation plays on the fact that Mardiganian, after collapsing during the film's promotional tour, was replaced by seven 'look-alikes'. Encountered as a series of projections or monitors, *Auroras* shows seven women retelling Aurora's harrowing story, which began as 15,000 Armenian women and children were ordered from their village. Their narrative culminates when Ottoman soldiers attack, raping a girl and killing her mother. Egoyan's staging of Mardiganian's testimony offers a startling reformulation of filmic witnessing. By multiplying the subjects who retell her traumatic story, and multiplying the screens on which they appear, Egoyan brings into question the filmic conventions by which victims are framed as sacred subjects and held at a safe remove from the viewer's world. Bringing the black box of cinema into the white cube of the art gallery or public space, Egoyan denies audiences the anonymity of the theatre and places them on an equal footing with the screens. The reversal of power is intensified through the encounter with seven culturally diverse actors portraying Mardiganian; the viewer is literally outnumbered and surrounded. In the place of a single witness there is a chorus, a resistant 'community of witnessing'.[1] Scapegoating logic is reversed, positioning viewer as victim with the goal of solidifying a sympathetic identification with the narrator-witnesses and engendering a physical experience of 'theatroclasm' or 'breaking the place of the viewer'.[2] Bodily memory is thereby restored to filmic memory, a key thematic of Egoyan's memorialisation of historical trauma.

1 See Shoshana Felman and Dori Laub, Testimony: Crises of Witnessing in Literature, Psychoanalysis and History (New York: Routledge, 1992), 211.

2 For a detailed explanation of this concept, see Timothy Long, *Theatroclasm: Mirrors, Mimesis and the Place of the Viewer* (Regina, Saskatchewan.: MacKenzie Art Gallery, 2009), 9–27.

 | DOI:10.1163/9789004391130_015

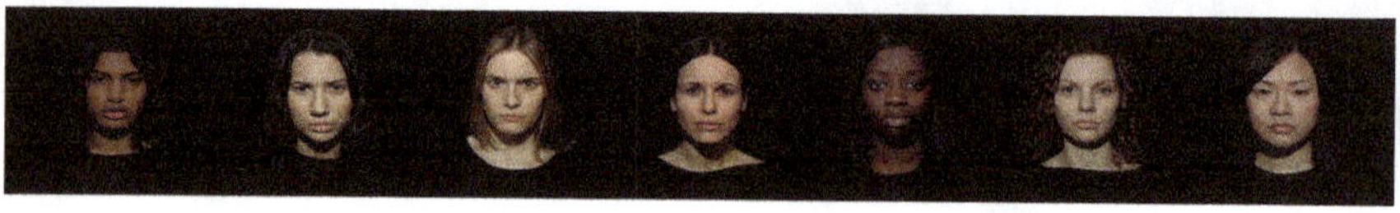

FIGURE 13.1 Atom Egoyan, Auroras, 2007, multi-channel video installation

Keywords

testimony – trauma – memory – Armenian genocide – film – installation art – immersive media – expanded cinema – socially engaged – art

1 Introduction

In his installation *Auroras* (2007), Canadian filmmaker and lens-based installation artist Atom Egoyan re-stages the traumatic testimony of Aurora Mardiganian, a young woman who survived the Armenian genocide of 1915–1917. Her first-hand account was published as a book and then filmed in the United States under the titles *Ravished Armenia* and *Auction of Souls* (1919), a cinematic production in which she played herself. Egoyan's installation plays on an unusual facet of this story. After collapsing during the promotional tour, Mardiganian was replaced by seven 'look-alikes' who carried on in her place. Encountered as a series of projections or monitors, *Auroras* shows seven women retelling Mardiganian's harrowing story, which began as 15,000 Armenian women and children were ordered from their village. Her narrative culminates when Ottoman Turkish soldiers attack, raping a girl and killing her mother.

As the world marks the 100th anniversary of the Armenian genocide, Mardiganian's testimony has continued relevance. Even today, the events of 1915–1917 are disputed. In 2014, Turkish Prime Minister Tayyip Erdogan expressed condolences to Armenians who suffered during the dying days of the Ottoman Empire, but his comments fell well short of a full apology and point to the ongoing importance of projects such as Egoyan's.[3] Significantly, the first presentation of *Auroras* was in the context of a two-person exhibition

3 'Turkey Offers Condolences to Armenia over WWI Killings', *BBC News*, 23 April 2014, viewed on 26 May 2015, http://www.bbc.com/news/world-europe-27131543.

with the Turkish artist Kutluğ Ataman at Artcore in Toronto as part of the Luminato Festival in 2007. Ataman's video *Testimony*, which appeared on a monitor in an adjacent room, featured an interview with an elderly woman who was nanny to the artist and his father; she was, in fact, an Armenian who had been taken in by the family after the genocide. Asked about this central event in her life, the woman is at a loss to remember, an amnesia which stands in stark contrast to the testimony which is at the heart of Egoyan's video installation. The two works were presented together at the 10th Istanbul Biennial later that same year. In 2015, Egoyan remounted *Auroras* as a solo installation in Berlin in the forecourt of the Maxim Gorki Theater, an emotionally charged setting which added new layers of historical resonance to the artwork.

As an artist of Armenian descent, Egoyan shares a deeply personal engagement with the question of genocide; both grandparents on his father's side lost most of their family during the massacres of Armenians which took place in Turkey around 1915.[4] Much of his work has dealt with, either directly or indirectly, the intergenerational effects of this genocidal violence.[5] These works range from his short films, such as *Open House* (1982), *Portrait of Arshile* (1995), and *Diaspora* (2001), to feature films, notably *Calendar* (1993) and *Ararat* (2002), to his lens-based installations, including *Return to the Flock* (1996), and *America, America* (1997), which was Armenia's official entry in the 1997 Venice Biennale. While these films and videos reference the events of 1915–1917, his work never offers a straightforward historical testimony. As Christine Ramsay points out, Egoyan's works, especially his feature film *Calendar* (1993) and his installation *Return to the Flock* (1996), offer an 'oblique yet moving testimony' to the Armenian genocide by invoking through symbol and cultural artifact Armenia's 'haunted geography'.[6] Egoyan underscores the need to bear witness to historical truth, all the while showing that the truth is inevitably, in his words, 'hidden, denied or simply forgotten'.[7]

4 Lisa Siraganian, 'Telling a Horror Story, Conscientiously: Representing the Armenian Genocide from *Open House* to *Ararat*', *Image and Territory: Essays on Atom Egoyan*, edited by Monique Tschofen and Jennifer Burwell (Waterloo, Ont.: Wilfrid Laurier University Press, 2007), 134.

5 Ibid., 133–156.

6 Christine Ramsay, 'Haunted Geographies in Atom Egoyan's *Calendar* and *Return to the Flock*', in this volume.

7 Atom Egoyan, 'Foreword' to *Ravished Armenia and the Story of Aurora Mardiganian*, edited by Anthony Slide (Jackson, Miss.: University of Mississippi Press, 2014), xi.

Against this backdrop, *Auroras* marks a striking departure. It offers what appears to be an unmediated, eyewitness account of the 1915–1917 genocide, as recorded by survivor Aurora Mardiganian. Within film history, the video shares characteristics with other examples of the genre, of which there are numerous examples related to the Holocaust.[8] However, this initial impression is incomplete and fails to take into account Egoyan's complex framing of Mardiganian's testimony, a staging which offers a startling reformulation of filmic witnessing.

2 Narrative

The script for *Auroras* was adapted by Egoyan with only a few changes from a section of *Ravished Armenia*, a book which remains one of the central texts in the archive of the Armenian genocide.[9] Thanks to the research of film historian Anthony Slide, we have an outline of the circumstances connected to the translation of Mardiganian's experiences into a book and film.[10] The book was based on an extended interview with Mardiganian by Harvey Gates and Eleanor Brown Gates, an American screenwriter and his wife who no doubt saw in Mardiganian's remarkable story an opportunity to capitalize on public interest in what was happening in Armenia. Mardiganian's harrowing ordeal had come to their attention after the *New York Sun* and the *New York Tribune* published stories based on interviews with the refugee – after arriving at Ellis Island on 5 November 1917, Mardiganian had placed ads in those same newspapers in a search for her brother whom she believed to be in the U.S.A. Mardiganian's story as told to Mr. and Mrs. Gates was serialized in fourteen instalments between August and November 1918 in the *New York American* and the *Los Angeles Examiner* under the titles 'My Two Years of Torture in Ravished, Martyred Armenia' and 'Ravished Armenia – My Two Years of Torture by the Turks', and subtitled 'The Diary of Arshalouys "Aurora" Mardiganian'. (By this time Mr. and Mrs. Gates had become Mardiganian's legal guardians and had anglicised her first

8 Notable examples include: *Shoah*, dir. Claude Lanzmann, BBC et al., 1985; *Nuit et Brouillard* (*Night and Fog*), dir. Alain Resnais, Argos Films, 1955; etc.

9 The book and film also appeared under the title *Auction of Souls* in the United Kingdom. For a comprehensive history of the book and film, including its use as an advocacy tool, see Anthony Slide, *Ravished Armenia*; and Leshu Torchin, '*Ravished Armenia*: Visual Media, Humanitarian Advocacy, and the Formation of Witnessing Publics', *American Anthropologist* 108.1 (March 2006): 214–220.

10 Slide, *Ravished Armenia*, 10–19. The following summary of details concerning Mardiganian's life and the development of the book and film are taken from this source.

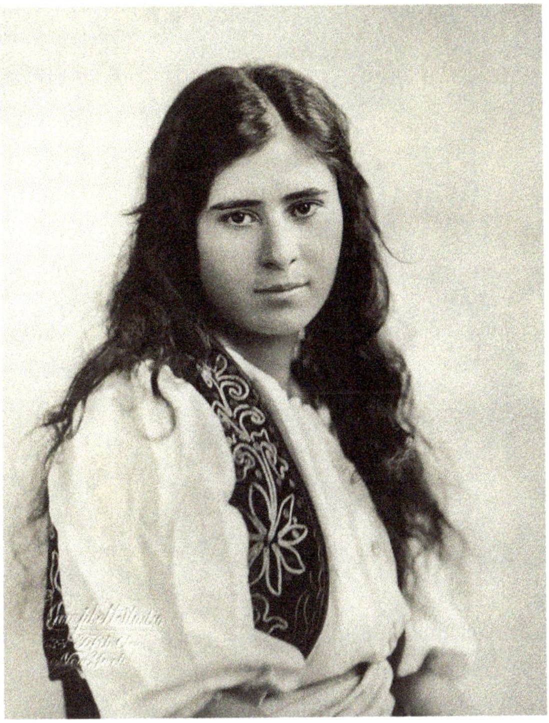

FIGURE 13.2 Aurora Mardiganian, publicity photo for *Auction of Souls*, 1919

name, changing it from Arshalouys to Aurora, and altered her last name, changing it from Mardigian to Mardiganian.) By the end of the year, the book was published in the U.S.A. as *Ravished Armenia* by Kingsfield Press in New York and in the U.K. as *The Auction of Souls* by Odhams Press in London.

Mardiganian begins her account on Easter morning, April 1915, in the home of her father, a wealthy businessman in the town of Tchemesh-Gedzak (present day Çemişgezek) in eastern Anatolia.[11] There the fourteen year old witnesses the beginning of the Ottoman purge of Armenian Christians, starting with the imprisonment and massacre of the town's men, including her father and brother. Rounded up along with the remaining women and children in her family, she is forced to join an unrelenting death march that will take her on a journey of over one thousand kilometres. Along the way, she is abducted by Kurdish raiders and sold into the harem of a Turkish official, but manages to escape and rejoin her family only to watch the death of her sister at the hands of the Ottoman police.

11 For the complete original text of *Ravished Armenia*, see ibid., 42–191.

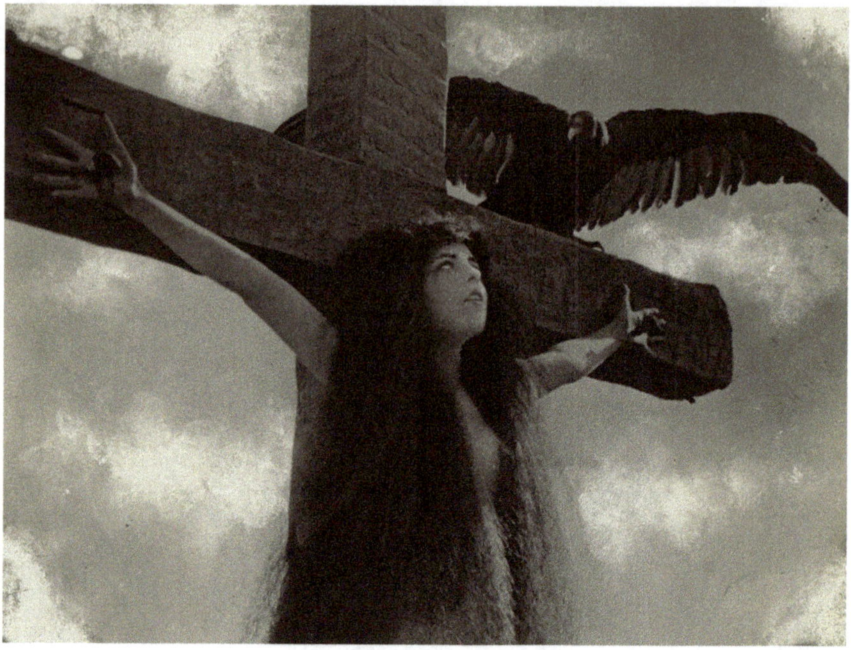

FIGURE 13.3 A vulture hovers over the crucifixion of an Armenian woman in a scene from *Auction of Souls*, 1919
© PUBLIC DOMAIN. COURTESY OF THE ACADEMY OF MOTION PICTURE ARTS AND SCIENCES.

Among the many atrocities she witnesses is the gruesome roadside spectacle of vultures gathered around the bodies of sixteen girls who had been nailed to makeshift crosses – a sight which greeted deportees upon their arrival at the city of Malatia (Malatya). (Mardiganian later corrected this somewhat sanitized version of events, noting that the crosses were in fact wooden stakes upon which the women had been forced to impale themselves through their vaginas.)[12]

The events recounted in *Auroras* take place shortly after their departure from Malatia, when a band of two hundred Kurdish horsemen descend on the column of deportees and commence to ravage, torture and kill several women.[13] Inspired by this violent spectacle, the Ottoman soldiers guarding the deportees attempt to drag off a young woman of their own, only to reject her because she is no longer 'a maid'.[14] When each woman that they

12 Ibid., 10.

13 The text used for *Auroras* appears in Chapter 8, 'In the Harem of Hadji Ghafour'. See ibid., 128–131.

14 In the script for *Auroras*, the word 'virgin' is consistently substituted for 'maid'.

subsequently accost also claims to be no longer a virgin, the soldiers suspect that they are being 'cheated'. They retaliate by threatening to put out the eyes of one of the older women unless a virgin comes forward. At this point, the daughter of the unfortunate woman breaks down, crying, 'My mother! My mother! Spare her – here I am – I am still a maid!' As the soldiers carry her away, she begs one last favour. 'I will go – I will go, and be willing – but let me kiss my mother!' The soldiers ignore her pleas and carry her away. Soon afterwards the mother collapses and dies. Upon her return the daughter buries her face in her shawl and remains with her mother until they are forced to resume their march the next day. The account ends with Mardiganian's terse summary:

> Every night such things happened. Other parties along that road had fared the same. Sometimes I counted the bodies of exiles who had preceded us until I could count no longer.[15]

For the remainder of the book, Mardiganian continues to recount a litany of horrors as she passes through the hands of a number of captors, including Turks, Chechens, Kurds, and Germans. Her final escape, which comes only after witnessing the death of her mother and younger sister, arrives at the hands of an elderly Armenian shepherd who rescues her from prison. A desperate flight across the open highlands leads her to the advancing Russian forces where she meets General Andranik, the leader of the Armenian volunteer regiments. Provided with money and a passport, she is sent to St. Petersburg – by now in the throes of the Russian Revolution – and from there to Oslo and the United States.

Mardiganian's vivid account of violent attacks and sexual depredations offered ample material for a film adaptation, which was clearly Harvey Gates interest from the start, a project endorsed by the American Committee for Armenian and Syrian Relief, who saw in Mardiganian's story a powerful tool for raising public awareness and financial support. Indeed, the front matter of *Ravished Armenia* includes a notice for the film that states the Committee's involvement with both the book and film.[16] Nora Waln is formally credited with the scenario, although Slide notes that it is Frederic Chapin's name that appears on extant copies of the script.[17] Waln was closely connected to Mardiganian in her role as publicity secretary of the American Committee for

15 Ibid., 131.

16 For a reproduction of the notice for the film, see ibid., 48.

17 Ibid., 12.

Armenian and Syrian Relief and had charge of Mardiganian at the time of her initial meetings with Gates. Production of the film was left to Colonel William N. Selig, who engaged Oscar Apfel to direct the film. Mardiganian travelled to Los Angeles in November 1918 for shooting, which was completed in less than a month. Playing herself in the film had its traumatic moments. Her first encounter with actors in Turkish costume aroused fears of renewed attack; only when they spoke to her in English was she reassured. Later she broke her ankle while filming a scene in which she was required to jump between rooftops. Despite the injury, she continued to act without a break. The film received its initial screening in January 1919 at the Alexandria Hotel in Los Angeles. Over the course of the next two years, it created a sensation in cities across Canada and the United States, breaking box office records in a number of centres.

The Armenian genocide, unlike many subsequent genocides of the twentieth century, is marked by a lack of documentary motion-picture records, a fact noted by Egoyan.[18] Film historian Marie-Aude Baronian points out

> the complex relationship which Armenians have with images in general: the lack of images – the destruction of the archives being an organised pursuit and the result of a policy of genocide – gives rise to a constant desire to reconstruct the past by whatever visual means possible.[19]

In the absence of a visual archive, Armenians have felt it necessary to create one, or, as in Egoyan's case, to recreate one of the early attempts to witness to the event. Of course, one might have expected Egoyan to use the 1919 Hollywood film rather than the book as his starting point. Unfortunately, this film is all but lost; what remains today is a ten minute segment which was preserved by the Armenian diaspora as an educational tool in their battle to have the atrocities recognised. Interestingly, subsequent to creating *Auroras*, Egoyan visited the archives of the Academy of Motion Picture Arts and Sciences in Hollywood and discovered a score of production stills and promotional images from the film, material which gives a sense of the account rendered by the Hollywood production.

The passage which Egoyan chose for his narrative offers a moment of high drama which conveys the brutality of the treatment suffered by Armenians at the hands of Ottoman troops and their allies. Many similar passages

---

18 Egoyan, 'Foreword', xiii.

19 Marie-Aude Baronian, *Cinéma et mémoire. Sur Atom Egoyan* (Seraing-le-Château, Belgium: Bebooks, 2013), Kindle edition. Author's translation.

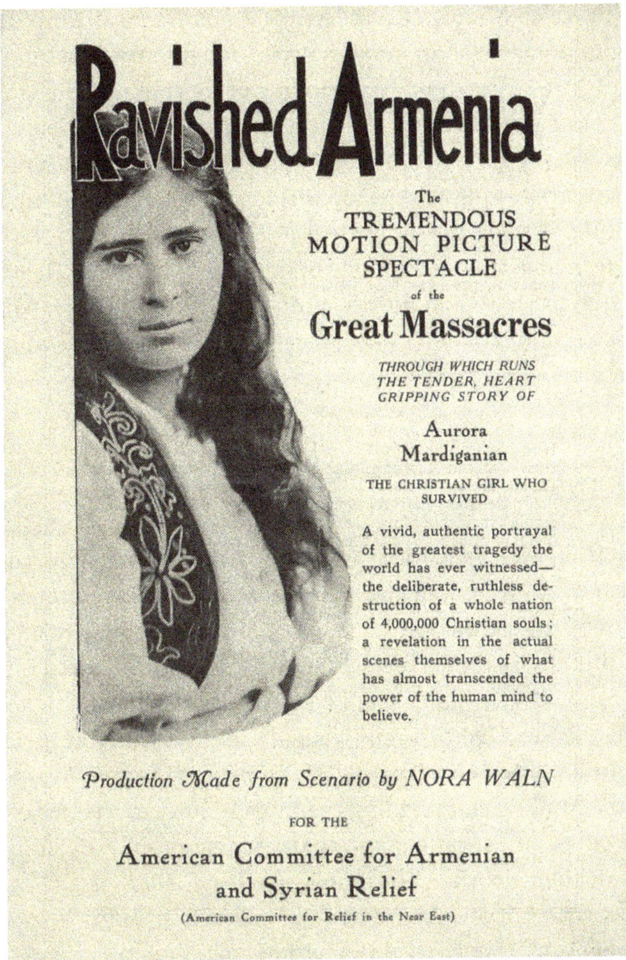

FIGURE 13.4 Advertising flyer for *Ravished Armenia*, 1919

could have been chosen, but this particular passage has three aspects which particularly suit Egoyan's purposes. First, it contains a parental relationship in which a young woman loses her mother. The transmission of testimonials through parental relationships is a theme which deeply interests Egoyan. In the short film *Portrait of Arshile*, for example, Egoyan explains to his son that he is named after the Armenian-American artist Arshile Gorky, a painter who conveyed the profound sense of anguish at the loss of his mother in a refugee camp in canvases such as *The Artist and His Mother* (c. 1926–36, Whitney Museum of American Art). Second, while the narrative is a first-person testimonial, it relates an incident in which Mardiganian herself was not directly involved. The act of witnessing trauma, of seeing an atrocity, is brought into focus and then further intensified by the account of the blinding of the mother, a loss of sight that makes the act of witnessing all the more unbearable. A consistent theme throughout Egoyan's work is his interest in how people react to traumatic events, as opposed to showing the violence itself, which is almost always out-of-frame in his films.[20] Finally, the narrative is a story of self-sacrifice, but one that fails to liberate or alleviate the suffering of the victims involved. There is no redemption offered to viewers in the uncomfortable encounter created by this work. It is about trauma and its effects on survivors and those who receive their testimony.

3 Performers/Performance

While the testimony itself follows certain well-worn conventions, Egoyan makes a distinctive contribution in the staging of the testimony. As already noted, in conceiving this installation, Egoyan responded to a peculiar circumstance related to the promotional tour for the 1919 Hollywood film based on Mardiganian's book. After over a year of appearances, Mardiganian broke down and threatened suicide. One can only imagine the toll which it took on the seventeen-year-old, after dictating her story, playing herself in the film recreation, and then telling and retelling her horrific story in a series of unfamiliar American cities. In Egoyan's assessment, she is not only a victim of genocide, but also of the celebrity culture that was then emerging.[21] The decision to replace her with not one, but seven look-alikes is a stunning fact which is the basis for Egoyan's restaging. This decision has a number of ramifications. First, the actors which Egoyan cast for *Auroras* are not playing Mardiganian per se, but rather they represent the actors hired to play the young Armenian. Thus, it is not Mardiganian's presence and personality that is recreated by Egoyan, but rather the process of substitution by which testimony is transmitted and kept alive. This missing presence is in effect the frame of the piece, a displacement which animates the testimony with the question of who is speaking for whom.

Egoyan's decisions around casting further broaden the question of who bears witness to genocide. By choosing actors of Asian, African, and European descent,

20 See Sirangian, 'Telling a Horror Story', 140–141.

21 Egoyan, 'Foreword', xii.

he moves the question beyond the concern of a single nationality or ethnic group, be it Armenians, Bosnians, Tutsis, or Jews, and makes it a broadly human question.[22] The collective witness implies a collective audience, a mirror of humanity. In choosing this approach, Egoyan recognises his position as an assimilated subject, a Canadian citizen first and foremost, despite his ties to the Armenian community. *Auroras* accepts this position, not as a disadvantage, but as a launching point for the translation and transmission of the Armenian genocide as a global phenomenon in the modern era.[23]

From a dramaturgical perspective, the staging of a monologue with seven actors poses an obvious challenge. Egoyan's solution is to distribute Mardiganian's narrative evenly among the seven actors. The effect is akin to a reading or rehearsal in an actor's workshop. The tone is sombre and dispassionate; the actors, set against a black background, deliver their lines looking straight at the camera without facial expression or gesture. However, as the narrative progresses to its violent climax, the centrally positioned actor, played by Sarah Casselman, emerges from this colourless delivery, her voice breaking with emotion as she recounts the plea of the young woman to the soldiers. Grief-stricken, she extends her hands toward the camera in supplication and then, with a loud cry, buries her face in a green shawl. The contrast of passion and dispassion among the actors embodies the tension which is often found in testimonial accounts: between a need for objectivity that risks emotional flatness, and a desire for subjective engagement that risks accusations of emotional manipulation. *Toronto Globe and Mail* critic Liam Lacey poses this very question in his review of the Artcore presentation:

> Is it wrong to wring emotions out of horrors? Or, on the contrary, is it legitimate to remain dispassionate about them? … Egoyan's films are filled with questions of the legitimacy of different kinds of testimony, and how the legacy of loss is passed on.[24]

Egoyan does not answer this question, but leaves it for the viewer to decide. Consistent with his other films and videos, Egoyan takes the tension between

22 The actors cast were Sarah Casselman, Tammi Chau, Robyn Thaler Hickey, Isabella Lauretano, Mina James, Assumpta Michaels and Amelia Sirianni. Liam Lacey, 'Painful Stories, Powerful Work from Egoyan and Ataman', *Toronto Globe and Mail*, June 5, 2007.

23 For a discussion of the role of translation in Egoyan's work in general, see Monique Tschofen, 'Speaking a/part: Modalities of Translation in Atom Egoyan's Work', *London Journal of Canadian Studies* 21 (2005–6): 29–48.

24 Lacey, 'Painful Stories'.

objectivity and subjectivity, between intimacy and distance, and makes it an object of inquiry.[25]

4 Spectator

The two most fully realized presentations *Auroras*, at Artcore (2007) and at the Maxim Gorki Theater (2015), offer one final layer of complexity to this inquiry. Both created a multipart engagement with the spectator: one through a seven projector video installation that surrounded the viewer, the other through a linear configuration of monitors which allowed viewers to encounter the individual performers in sequence.

In considering the implications of these divergent approaches to the installation, it is important to note that Egoyan's decision to branch out from film into lens-based installation began in 1996 with *Return to the Flock*, a work that reflected on the contradictions of post-genocide Armenian identity. I would argue, along with Christine Ramsay and Elizabeth Matheson, my fellow collaborators in the curatorial research project *Atom Egoyan and the Place of the Witness*, that Egoyan was attracted to installation art for its ability to supplement what cannot be achieved in cinema alone.[26] Installation art, with its insistent engagement with the physical space of the viewer, enables film to leave the safe confines of the theatre and move into the space of the spectator, bringing not just the voice and image of the victim, but a sense of the person's aura or presence – a defining trait of visual art. This is a key element for considering how art and trauma are intertwined. My contention is that the artwork, in its basic structure, is analogous to a surrogate victim, and that the frame both controls and obscures the viewer's knowledge of this fact. *Auroras* plays on this truth and uses it to create a new relationship between artwork and spectator by inverting the traditional frame of art, so that the places of spectator and art object are reversed – what I would describe as a kind of 'theatroclasm'.[27] Theatroclasm – literally 'the breaking of the place of the viewer' – is a term which I developed to describe a type of mirroring-effect which induces viewers to question their place before the artwork and understand the controlling effect

25 See Baronian, *Cinéma et mémoire*.

26 For a full description of the project *Atom Egoyan and the Place of the Witness*, see Ramsay, in this volume. For an analysis of Egoyan's move from the black box of cinema to broader architectural frames of reference, see Elizabeth Matheson, 'Immersive Space and the Place of the Witness', in this volume.

27 See Long, *Theatroclasm*, 9–27.

of the frame on collective experience. Originally developed in relation to the historical artwork, I have extended it to describe lens-based practices, which mirror and destabilise the spaces that define the relationships between the moving image and its audiences within the museum.

'Theatroclasm' is a concept which takes as its starting point the history of the frame which both painting and film share. From the religious icon, to the Renaissance picture window, to the cubist breakdown of one-point perspective, to the modernist monochrome, the frame has been essential for producing presence. Jacques Derrida, in his essay on the nature of frames identifies a crucial point. He writes,

> the *parergon* [or frame] is a form which has as its traditional determination not that it stands out but that it disappears, buries itself, effaces itself, melts away at the moment when it deploys its greatest energy.[28]

In other words, the presence produced by the frame is created at a cost through a disappearance or expulsion. The cinematic image shares this essential condition.

Following the cultural anthropology of René Girard, I would argue that the frame is essentially a sacrificial mechanism; the presence it produces derives from the same violent exclusionary logic which drives other religious and cultural forms.[29] Just as scapegoating yields a sacred presence through the forcible expulsion of a single victim from the midst of the collective, so the frame yields aesthetic presence, what Walter Benjamin calls 'the aura', through the segregation of the image from the mundane world around it. In the process, the role of the image as a controller of collective behaviour is transformed. The redirection of the rivalrous desires of the collective through sacrificial expulsion is subsumed under the sign of the aesthetic, through which potential sources of conflicting desire – sexual, political, or economic – are now are mediated by the auratic function of the frame.

As an inheritor of the western image tradition, film also participates in this auratic regime. Just as the frame disappears in order to create the presence of the painted image, so the cinema screen must darken in order to bear the

28 Jacques Derrida, *The Truth in Painting*, translated by Geoff Bennington and Ian McLeod (Chicago: University of Chicago Press, 1987), 61.

29 See René Girard, *The Scapegoat*, translated by Yvonne Freccero (Baltimore: Johns Hopkins University Press, 1986). For an analysis of Girard's theory of the scapegoat as it pertains to visual art, see Long, *Theatroclasm*, 9–27.

projected image – a process which facilitates the passive identification of cinema-goers with the camera-eye's perspective.

Since the advent of modernism, theatroclastic artworks have subverted this paradigm in a number of ways, challenging the convention of the solitary, omnipotent viewer, and his or her imaginative occupation of the same virtual position as the video/filmmaker. While cinematic precedents can be found as far back as Andy Warhol's *Chelsea Girls* (1966), it is only with the development of film and video installation art that new possibilities for engagement with the physical space of the viewer are introduced, such as Douglas Gordon's *Play Dead: Real Time* (2003). In this work, unanimous violence is thematised in the endless circling of the camera around a central figure, in this case, a circus elephant. However, the viewer's illusion of being in a position of control is disrupted by the offset arrangement of freestanding and semi-opaque screens. Thus Gordon effectively undermines video's perspective system, all the while systematically exposing the projection's participation in a sacrificial mode of viewing.

Egoyan, who in his own words has 'always felt that entrance into a screen is a physical act',[30] has exploited the potential of the physical engagement of the viewer in a number of ways throughout his career as a lens-based installation artist. As he explains, he has

> tried to create ways in which people can physically manoeuvre themselves into the private and communal memories that are being investigated. There is a physical sense that the person is activating or initiating a process with their very presence.[31]

Two earlier lens-based installations provide examples of Egoyan's active engagement with the screen. In *Evidence* (1999), which is based on a video clip from his Hitchcockian thriller *Felicia's Journey* (1999), Egoyan forces the viewer to the confront the screen at extreme proximity while sitting in a corner just inches away from the video monitor. This claustrophobic viewing situation echoes the sense of entrapment captured in the surveillance video taken in the car of serial killer Joseph Hilditch (Bob Hoskins) as he speaks to one of his young female victims. The confrontation with the screen is pushed even further in *Close* (2001), which Egoyan created for the Venice Biennale with visual

30 Atom Egoyan, 'Ripple Effects: Atom Egoyan Speaks with Monique Tschofen', *Image and Territory*, 348.

31 Ibid.

artist Julião Sarmento. In this installation, close-up video of freshly clipped toenails being dropped one-by-one onto a woman's tongue is rear-projected onto a monumental screen that is suspended just a few feet from the wall. The narrow viewing corridor thereby created forces viewers into an unbearable intimacy with the screen. In both installations, spectators are manoeuvred into a physical relationship to the screen as a means of challenging their voyeuristic relationship to the screen subjects.[32]

While *Evidence* and *Close* demonstrate Egoyan's theatroclastic use of both projection screens and monitors, *Auroras* complicates this engagement by multiplying the screens involved. The installation at Artcore featured seven over-life size projections of the heads and shoulders of the seven 'Auroras'. The projections appeared on three walls of a large rectangular-shaped room. By creating an installation which hems in the viewer on three sides Egoyan induced viewers to recall the encirclement of the Armenian women by the Ottoman troops.[33] More broadly, by multiplying the subjects who retell Mardiganian's traumatic story, and multiplying the screens on which they appear, Egoyan, a filmmaker himself, brings into question the filmic conventions by which victims are framed as sacred subjects and held at a safe remove from the viewer's life world. By bringing the black box of cinema into the white cube of the art gallery, Egoyan denies audiences the anonymity of the theatre and places them on an equal footing with life-sized screens. The reversal of power is intensified through the encounter with seven culturally diverse actors portraying Mardiganian; the viewer is literally outnumbered and surrounded. In the place of a single witness there is a chorus, a resistant 'community of witnessing', to borrow Shoshana Felman's term.[34] Scapegoating logic is thereby reversed, positioning the viewer as victim with the goal of both solidifying a sympathetic identification with the narrator-witnesses, and engendering a physical experience of theatroclasm.

This physical engagement with the witness is given a public articulation in the installation of *Auroras* that took place in the forecourt of the Maxim Gorki Theater, a building which originally housed the Singakademie. The invitation from the theatre to reconfigure *Auroras* for this location came in response to a suggestion made by Egoyan's wife, the actor Arsinée Khanjian, who had been engaged to perform as part of 'Es schneit im April (It Snows in April)', a

32 See William F. Van Wert, '*Close*: Voyeurism and the Idea of the Baroque', *Image and Territory*, 295–305.

33 See Baronian, *Cinéma et Mémoire*.

34 See Felman and Laub, *Testimony*, 211.

multi-disciplinary project dedicated to the 100th anniversary of the Armenian genocide.[35] Included among the plays, film series, concerts, lectures and exhibitions which made up the program were a screening by Fred Kelemen of the remaining fragments of *Ravished Armenia* and *Auction of Souls*, a lecture-performance by Khanjian that used the film script to reconstruct Mardiganian's story and connect it to reports from other survivors.

Formally included as part of 'It Snows in April', *Auroras* was sited outdoors in a long plaza which connects the theatre to a number of historical buildings in central Berlin, including the Neue Wache, home of the memorial to the 'Victims of War and Tyranny', and the Palais am Festungsgraben, which houses the Saarländische Galerie and Theater in Palais. For this installation, Egoyan installed monitors in the four advertising kiosks which visitors pass on their way to the Maxim Gorki Theater. The first three kiosks held side-by-side monitors on the front and back, each monitor featuring one of the actors portraying Aurora, while the fourth kiosk, nearest to the theatre, held a monitor beside an informational text about the historical figure of Aurora Mardiganian. Each of the seven actors appeared twice: as visitors passed a kiosk, they encountered the same pair of actors located on both sides. The viewer thus had an experience of being followed by a Janus-like gaze that looked both forward and backward. For those familiar with Mardiganian's story, the linear arrangement recalls the death march which the deportees were forced to take. In passing by, the viewer unwittingly assumes the position of the Ottoman guards in their surveillance of the column of deportees, or the position of the onlookers who witnessed the march. If viewers choose to stop and take a closer look, upon entering the space between kiosks, they find themselves momentarily hemmed in, a position akin to that created by the Artcore presentation in which viewers provisionally assume the position of the victim. The movement between the position of victim and victimizer which this artwork allows offers a sophisticated reading of genocide, one that acknowledges that any individual has the potential to be either a victim or a victimizer depending on their historical circumstances. This reading is especially pointed in light of the polarity of circumstances occupied by the citizens of Berlin over the course of the twentieth century.

By chance, the resonance with German history was further intensified in the nearby Neue Wache, where the soundtrack for *Auroras* could be overheard

35 Atom Egoyan, personal communication to the author, 6 July 2015. For a full listing of the events connected with 'It Snows in April', see Maxim Gorki Theater, 'Es schneit im April', viewed on 29 January 2016, http://english.gorki.de/programme/special-events/it-snows-in-april.

in the interior of this former guard house for the Prussian royal family. In the centre of the unadorned, stone-faced interior stands Käthe Kollwitz's bronze sculpture, *Mother with her Dead Son* (1937), a work recalling a traditional Christian pietà. For Kollwitz, who lost one of her sons during World War One, the work had a deeply personal significance. It was created at a time when she found herself increasingly marginalized by Germany's Nazi government, which had by this time forced her to resign from the faculty of the Akademie der Künste in Berlin and had banned the exhibition of her work in response to her vocal opposition to the Nazi Party. Placed under the open oculus which is the building's only source of light, it is exposed to the elements, and gives a personal focus to the memorialisation of victims of war and despotic governments.

The installation is the most recent example of what Elizabeth Matheson describes as Egoyan's use of immersive spatial contexts for 'confronting the moral challenges' of genocide and for helping audiences 'cope with traumatic pasts'.[36] By inserting the memory of the Armenian genocide into the heart of Berlin, Egoyan reminds viewers of the history of atrocities which have followed in the wake of this event over the course of the past century. Indeed, it was on the eve of the invasion of Poland that Adolph Hitler cited the 'annihilation of the Armenians' as a precedent for his project of ethnic cleansing.[37] In this context, Egoyan's selective edits to the text of *Ravished Armenia* for the script of *Auroras* take on special significance. While retaining Mardiganian's identification of herself and her fellow deportees as Armenian, Egoyan deliberately leaves out any mention of the identity of the attackers, whether Kurdish or Turkish. Furthermore, he omits the reference to 'Allah' which is included in one of the soldier's taunts. Egoyan's focus is on the identification with the victims, rather than on the identification of the victimizers; empathy, not demonization, is the goal. Although unplanned, the spillover of the *Auroras* soundtrack into the Neue Wache offered another opportunity to contemplate this message. For visitors overhearing Mardiganian's heart-wrenching tale as retold by a chorus of seven distinct voices, a felt connection to Kollwitz's sculpture is spontaneously produced. This connection is all the more intense given the absence of the images of the speaking subjects. Kollwitz's expressive modelling of a mother's embrace of her dead son fills the void, giving physical expression to Aurora's story and embodying anew the suffering caused by the inhumanity of genocidal regimes across time and geography.

---

36 Matheson, in this volume.

37 Siraganian, 'Telling a Horror Story', 133.

As a lens-based installation, *Auroras* restores bodily memory to filmic memory, a key thematic of Egoyan's memorialisation of historical trauma through a filmic investigation of testimony. Whether in the context of an installation in an art gallery or an intervention in public space, *Auroras* destabilizes the place of the viewer by implicating them in a dramatic restaging of historical testimony. The theatroclastic impetus of Egoyan's work gives Mardiganian's witness account renewed power and a wider relevance a century after the events which devastated her family and the Armenian people.

Bibliography

Baronian, Marie-Aude. *Cinema et mémoire. Sur Atom Egoyan*. Seraing-le-Château, Belgium: Bebooks, 2013. Kindle Edition.

Derrida, Jacques. *The Truth in Painting*. Translated by Geoff Bennington and Ian McLeod. Chicago: University of Chicago Press, 1987.

Egoyan, Atom. 'Foreword', *Ravished Armenia and the Story of Aurora Mardiganian*, edited by Anthony Slide, xi–xiv. Jackson, Mississippi: University of Mississippi Press, 2014.

Egoyan, Atom. 'Ripple Effects: Atom Egoyan Speaks with Monique Tschofen'. *Image and Territory: Essays on Atom Egoyan*, edited by Monique Tschofen and Jennifer Burwell, 343–357. Waterloo, Ont.: Wilfrid Laurier University Press, 2007.

Felman, Shoshana and Dori Laub. *Testimony: Crises of Witnessing in Literature, Psychoanalysis and History*. New York: Routledge, 1992.

Girard, René. *The Scapegoat*. Translated by Yvonne Freccero. Baltimore: Johns Hopkins University Press, 1986.

Lacey, Liam. 'Painful Stories, Powerful Work from Egoyan and Ataman'. *Toronto Globe and Mail*, June 5, 2007.

Long, Timothy. *Theatroclasm: Mirrors, Mimesis and the Place of the Viewer.* Regina, Sask.: MacKenzie Art Gallery, 2009.

Siraganian, Lisa. 'Telling a Horror Story, Conscientiously: Representing the Armenian Genocide from *Open House* to *Ararat*'. *Image and Territory: Essays on Atom Egoyan*, edited by Monique Tschofen and Jennifer Burwell, 133–56. Waterloo, Ont.: Wilfrid Laurier University Press, 2007.

Slide, Anthony, ed. *Ravished Armenia and the Story of Aurora Mardiganian*. Jackson, Miss.: University of Mississippi Press, 2014.

Torchin, Leshu. '*Ravished Armenia*: Visual Media, Humanitarian Advocacy, and the Formation of Witnessing Publics'. *American Anthropologist* 108.1 (March 2006): 214–20.

Tschofen, Monique. 'Speaking a/part: Modalities of Translation in Atom Egoyan's Work'. *London Journal of Canadian Studies* 21 (2005–6): 29–48.

'Turkey Offers Condolences to Armenia over WWI Killings'. *BBC News*, 23 April 2014. Viewed on 26 May 2015. http://www.bbc.com/news/world-europe-27131543.

Van Wert, William F. '*Close*: Voyeurism and the Idea of the Baroque'. *Image and Territory: Essays on Atom Egoyan*, edited by Monique Tschofen and Jennifer Burwell, 295–305. Waterloo, Ont.: Wilfrid Laurier University Press, 2007.

CHAPTER 14

Immersive Space and the Place of the Witness

Elizabeth Matheson

Abstract

This chapter considers testimony situating moving imagery and filmic installation as an immersive form of 'life writing genres' through *Steenbeckett* (2002). Egoyan uses excerpts from his film of Samuel Beckett's *Krapp's Last Tape*, in which a haunted sexagenarian reviews self-important reel-to-reel tape recordings he made in his prime, to reflect on the pain of hubris and memories of lost love. The viewer is immersed in Krapp's reverie through a dense aesthetic layering of technologies in space. Two thousand feet of celluloid travels around the darkened gallery on a system of pulley suspended sprockets, propelled through the Steenbeck editing table, whose small screen also serves as our fittingly obscure and distanced window onto Krapp. In her theory of 'the kiss' within architectural space as it relates to film projection, Lavin sees a 'coming together of two similar but not identical surfaces that soften, flex, and deform when in contact[1].' Caruth analyzes this 'coming together' in filmic architectural encounters through the lens of bearing witness to history and memory. Pérez-Gómez sees the gallery as, in fact, 'a theatre for memory'[2] capable of uncovering truths, while Agamben shows that the ways of seeing experience in filmic installations are akin to the position of the witness. Alongside these developments, Grau advocates that this witnessing in moving image installations is by its very nature an immersive 'thinking space.' Steenbeckett is such a 'thinking space.' Its structural and compositional features channel and inform the body's resonance with and immersion in its immediate surroundings. Consequently, I propose that the reciprocal relationship between the bodily gesture, Egoyan's installation art and the gallery is best described through the notion of 'dialectical immersion': a temporary embodied spatial encounter that can only be fully understood from within.

1 Sylvia Lavin, *Kissing Architecture* (Princeton, N.J.: Princeton University Press, 2011), 5.

2 Alberto Pérez-Gómez, 'The Architecture of Richard Henriquez: A Praxis of Personal Memory,' *Richard Henriquez: Memory Theatre*, edited by Howard Shubert (Montreal/Vancouver: Canadian Centre for Architecture and Vancouver Art Gallery, 1993), 9.

 | DOI:10.1163/9789004391130_016

Keywords

testimony – genre and production in – installation – dialectical immersion – witnessing – Atom Egoyan

1 Witnessing and Immersive Space

We live in an age of failing states with unprecedented abuses of human rights. Partitions, wars, calamities and ceaseless conflict have eclipsed what was thought possible after the extreme cruelties of World War II and the Holocaust. In the midst of these sinister planetary transformations we all have unwittingly become witnesses to these catastrophic events. It has left us dumb with fear. How are we to make meaning out of this? In this rapid unravelling of the world, cultural spaces have begun to play an increasingly important role in understanding the harshness of this reality. In the first few pages of *Kissing Architecture* critic Sylvia Lavin reflects upon a theory of formal purity proposed at the height of the Cold War and internal politics in the USA by influential art critic Clement Greenberg (1909–1994). It is the idea that our only possible relation to representation is one of Kantian detachment. For Kant, an aesthetic response was characterized by detachment.[3] For Greenberg and his fellow American modernist colleagues, to react to say, a representation of trauma, with feelings of grief or other sensations was in their mind no less than the obliteration of the aesthetic dimension.[4] Lavin points out that this has been radically transformed whereby people are increasingly using the possibilities of built spaces to re-engage with modernity—both as it relates to historical and personal narratives, alternative histories and to space and time.

This re-engagement with built space comes at a time when it is becoming increasingly hard to ignore the reshaping of the visible world with the presence of moving imagery and undoubtedly many of these cultural gestures mirror contemporary society dominated by watching a screen, be it a computer,

3 Immanuel Kant, *The Moral Law: Kant's Groundwork of the Metaphysics of Morals*, translated by H. J. Paton (London: Hutchinson, 1972), 98.

4 Clement Greenberg, 'Modernist Painting,' *Clement Greenberg: The Collected Essays and Criticism*, vol. 4 of *Modernism with a Vengeance 1957–1969*, edited by John O'Brian (Chicago: University of Chicago Press, 1993), 86.

cell phone, movie, or television. Discussions around how moving imagery remediate our worldview, have become especially pitched of late. So much so, in fact, well-established theoretical discourses around moving imagery, initially developed in relation to cinematic apparatus and its language, have begun to turn to the experience of immersion itself. Perhaps this development is not all that surprising given the elastic category of moving imagery and the fact that it seems—in both the minds of artists and viewers—to be an important point of engagement. Unlike a public space dotted with advertising screens, marked by the temporal and transitory, Lavin suggests that moving image installations in built spaces, such as art galleries, permit the momentary generation of new affects that in turn form the basis of alternative possibilities in the social aesthetic world. What is perfectly clear is that the enlightened ideal of the social contract that extended to built space and social attention rooted in a sense of hierarchy, autonomy, and legibility—has been breached by the inclusion of an infinite range of interlopers including moving image installation art. Critics like Sylvia Lavin liken this to a kiss, a 'coming together' like a centrifugal force of attraction between two exquisitely similar but yet distinct things of multiplicity produces a new form of eidetic experience.[5]

Scholars have frequently turned to spatial turning points to explain the intimate link between ourselves and the re-shaping of the visual world. Cathy Caruth, for instance, analyses this 'coming together' in filmic architectural encounters though the lens of bearing witness to World War II history and memory. Architectural historian Alberto Pérez-Gómez sees this rise in architectural space interest in the latter part of the twentieth-first century as, the inherent role of cultural space to serve as 'theatres of memory' capable of uncovering truths. Philosopher Giorgio Agamben also speaks to this in a more radical sense that the ways of seeing in built spaces is akin to the position of witnessing in which viewers are confronted with the difficulties of imagining not only atrocity, but one's own ability to see oneself as a witness to that atrocity.[6]

None of this of course is news. Anyone, with a glancing familiarity with the twentieth-first, century knows that the intimate relation between the dynamics of seeing and representation as acts of reckoning with loss and trauma has been continuous in shaping cultural spaces. Within the history of galleries themselves there is a long tradition of the exhibition space being important as the work itself, dating back to the beginnings of the 1955 Documenta

5 Sylvia Lavin, *Kissing Architecture* (Princeton, N.J.: Princeton University Press, 2011), 5.

6 Alberto Pérez-Gómez, 'The Architecture of Richard Henriquez: A Praxis of Personal Memory,' *Richard Henriquez: Memory Theatre*, edited by Howard Shubert (Montreal/Vancouver: Canadian Centre for Architecture and Vancouver Art Gallery, 1993), 9.

exhibition initiated by architect Arnold Bode. Dramatically hanging giant white curtains across the bombed-out shell of Kassel's neoclassical Fridericianum, one of Germany's oldest museums, Bode brought together a number of previously banned 'Entartete Kunst' (Degenerate Art), in an attempt to create something moving, dynamic and extremely modern in the midst of post-war rubble, where 'the exhibition space itself represented a kind of manifesto.'[7] This was born precisely out of the terror of a split society and out of the desire to heal it. For that reason, Bode's conception of space was immensely relevant in post-war Europe, when the ideas of reconstruction were tied to addressing the hidden history of National Socialism and its war of aggression. In some ways, this manifesto of exhibition space was prefigured by Germany's post-war cinema's fascination with rubble and the still standing steel frame remnants of bombed out buildings to visualize time and history in modernity. Windows, screens and other openings in ruined buildings became symbolic of the conflicted spaces of European history—allowing spectators to come to terms with loss by offering access to events and experiences that seemed to defy representation.[8]

This is a feeling that appears elsewhere in post-war culture and seems to extend from an inability of language to convey the great sense of irrevocable loss. After World War II, the ethnic makeup of the continent changed dramatically. Within its depopulated European cityscapes, Jewish neighbourhoods and homes stood empty, synagogues had been reduced to ashes, along with the irreplaceable loss of Jewish colleagues, friends and family. The unspeakable had happened. By the 1950s, after the programme of American 'de-Nazification,' the motto of the new civic, industrial and media infrastructure across Europe was to 'forget the past' and not to look back.[9] The post-war period, both for perpetrators and survivors, was one that left a gaping hole in the consciousness that one could neither acknowledge nor discuss.

The Holocaust, with its disappearances and remains, as a symbol of the failure of Western life, became the foundational trauma for post-war art and politics. Standing at the crossroads of all the arts, post-war theatres were characterized by a noticeable emptiness with a great loss of the artistic and cultural community. During reconstruction, theatres were either stripped barewith minimal props, or immense stages were created that dwarfed actors

7 Lorenzo Benedetti, 'Arnold Bode and the Perfect Combination of History, Environment and Contemporary,' *Cura* 11 (2012): 40.

8 Hester Baer, *Dismantling the Dream Factory: Gender, German Cinema, and the Postwar Quest for a New Film Language* (New York: Berghanon Books, 2012), 12.

9 Tony Judt, *Post War: A History of Europe since 1945* (New York: Penguin, 2005), 13.

and audiences who wanted to consummate their experiences.[10] The empty theatre and the bare stage became a symbolic gesture to subvert the visual legacy of jubilant crowds at Nazi parades, rallies and the red and black fervour of fascism. It created an undeniable stir in post-war Europe.

These reverberations were keenly felt at the epicentre of the Holocaust—Poland. The list of Polish thinkers who have explored this territory is long from Tadeusz Borowski and Jerry Ficowski to Jerzy Grotowski and Tadeusz Kantor.[11] This kind of work spurred ground-breaking projects by theatre artists such as Jan Klata. For his recent play on post-war relations between Germany and Poland titled *Transfer!* Klata created an intensely affective environment of sound, light into an architectural volume that itself was barely rising to the generic black box. Reflecting on current debates about the relations between the Polish state and Polish Jews, this play brought together people who had witnessed the war. One of the most striking features of the work is the bareness of the stage with the exception of a skeletal frame. The audience cannot help but pay notice to this skeletal scaffolding, and the witnesses who present themselves asking to be read, understood, pleading for the audience to understand them. They are presented as corrective to the historical amnesia that surrounds the tragic history of occupied Poland and offer the theatre's walls as compensatory transparency: you may not be aware of the complicated circumstances of Polish-Jewish relations during the Holocaust but you can understand on some level the significance of this violent rupture that fundamentally altered Poland's concept of itself as a nation and the world. Here Klata's kiss is neither an assault on the space nor a reinforcement of the space but a heightened experience—of intense affect. And despite its theatrical insistence on narrative and its demand that the audience respond as readers, the play's material effects on the building opens up other modes of perception and experiences. That is to say, unlike German post-war rubble films, contemporary theatrical examples such as this operate outside the framework of total collective redemption and reconciliation. With this performance and for most of his work, Klata takes his place in a long line of thinkers who have proposed at one time or another that space offers something more rewarding than lamentation—the possibility of thinking, particularly in its quest to address historical amnesia and oblivion.

10 Magda Romanska, *The Post-Traumatic Theatre of Grotowski and Kantor: History and Holocaust in 'Akropolis' and 'Dead Class'* (New York: Anthem Press, 2014), 115.

11 Magda Romanska, *The Post-Traumatic Theatre of Grotowski and Kantor*, 5.

Within the annals of European cinema itself there is a history of space (perceived and real) being important in this regard, dating back to the revolutionary Soviet cinema with the publication of 'Montage and Architecture' written by Russian filmmaker Sergei Mikhailovich Eisenstein, who experienced first-hand one of the greatest transformations of space in which centuries old palaces and government buildings were upturned and re-visioned. Considered to be pivotal in understanding the interplay between architecture, film and movement through space, Eisenstein created a fundamental link between built space and film. A multiplicity of practices, a montage of viewpoints and dialectical immersion not only guide the cinema but architecture itself—so said Eisenstein. Changes in height, size, angle and scale of the view, as well as space are embedded in the very language of architectural as well as filmic shots, editing and movement. And by walking around cultural and built spaces one could experience '… the perfect example of one of the most ancient film …'.[12] And indeed, she who wanders through a building or a site acts precisely like a film spectator absorbing and connecting visual spaces. For Eisenstein grasping reality or in his words 'the external events of the world' could only come through this dialectical understanding of the world.[13] In this immersive condition, in which space is varied and dynamic, one is allowed to withdraw into self, to a place of bodily sensation.

Visitors to contemporary cultural spaces, who also engage the anatomy of the building as they transverse, travel to specific areas, who go from work to work, room to room, floor to floor, similarly draw the itinerary of such a walking practice. And as filmic installation demonstrates, immersive space in contemporary cultural settings remains fundamentally an experiential space. It succeeds in disconnecting spectators from their everyday surroundings and transporting them to a place of contemplation. Although it is safe to say that moving imagery is seen as an emerging practice in galleries, it seems installation has become the default of contemporary art and we are still dealing with the theoretical implications of this transformation. In the current period, the phenomenon of a projector at one end of the room and a projected image on the other wall has been called into question and once again we are seeing a rise in experimentation as once again our way of images is being radically transformed. And the work of Atom Egoyan and others testifies to the desire of current installation practice to intensify the link between moving imagery and

12 Sergei Eisenstein, 'Montage and Architecture,' *Assemblage* 10 (1989): 116.

13 Sergei Eisenstein, 'A Dialectical Approach to Film Form,' *Film Form*, edited by Jay Leda (New York: Harcourt, 1977), 45.

built space, refashioning the strong connection that, in theory and in practice came into place in the 1930s around the notions of montage, immersion and the dialectic. This space has become even more crucial in the rapid unravelling of the visible world. As Lavin writes:

> Today we need the aesthetic to produce new experiences rather than to evacuate them and more forms of interestedness rather than less. Today, affect should be defined as the internalization of perception and not as feelings over determined by cultural codes. We no longer need to equate detachment and distance with intellection and abstraction nor feeling with crude sentimentality and so we can return to experience with new theoretical vigour.[14]

It should be mentioned that this is a much-neglected space in curatorial studies. Even where the studies explore space, they are very content-focused with a division between built space as real and medium space as imaginary. And yet the effects of immersion are very real. This project *Atom Egoyan and the Place of the Witness* requires forms of thinking about immersion that consciously go beyond inquiring into that which can be only understood as packaging of environments (such as didactics, text panels) or an experience of totality (designed and lush environments offering sensory or narcissistic pleasure) to a more dynamic way of seeing. For these reasons, it is difficult to think about that connection, that relationship between our viewing experiences in installation and a material sense of installation within curation alone. One reason for that really is the naïve ontologies of built space and moving imagery, essentially the culturally constructed body of the screen which might correspond to the imaginary anatomy of the gallery or theatre where the screen becomes the placeholder for the painting or operating like a technological fetish. But it is perhaps not surprising that naïve ontologies such as these do not recognize the built space itself in terms of its structure, massing, spatial organization and circulation. It could be said that if the latter is attended to, then questions of participation and how viewers make these spaces meaningful becomes possible. And for me that is why for curatorial studies these articulations of space and a deeper understanding of immersion is so very necessary and without this we cannot properly grasp the effects

14 Clement Greenberg, 'Modernist Painting,' *Clement Greenberg: The Collected Essays and Criticism*, vol. 4 of *Modernism with a Vengeance 1957–1969*, edited by John O'Brian (Chicago: University of Chicago Press, 1993), 86.

of the 'immersive condition' of cultural spaces, what it does to us or, to go back to Eisenstein again, we need to be able to see how built space determines our situation.

In the field of gallery curation in Canada, the mention of Atom Egoyan as an installation artist (rather than as a filmmaker of such epoch defining films as the 1990's *Exotica* and *The Sweet Hereafter*) often produces a flicker of bodily unease. This rather nervous reaction from curators is understandable, perhaps. Of course, there is still an uneasy relationship between the moving image and cultural spaces in Canada—and it is still not unusual to hear 'Why should a filmmaker place a work in a cultural space other than a cinema?' The answer is why not? And really the deeply conservative assumption underlying this question echoes the continuing internalization that began under modernism, for not only an attempt with other groups for cultural authority but also a protective attitude towards cultural spaces as institutional spheres rather than sites of experimentation.

The fact that this question is being asked is also part of the deeply rooted investment in the object merged with the suspicion based on the reading of film and video as separate disciplines to that of visual art—each possessing its own discreet history, theoretical framework and models. And this suspicion is the result of what many art historians see as the failure of a brief wave of cinephilia amongst artists such as Duchamp, Man Ray etcetera in Europe in the teens and early 1920s especially in Paris which came and went before the radical fulfilment was washed away by the realities of the art market and also the political events of the 1930s.

So in a sense this question that is still asked is the ultimate legacy of this failure, which produced a hardening between art and film, which really has taken a long time to soften. Part of this softening has been credited to a wave of artists who have turned to cinematic techniques to envelop the viewer. However, for some cultural theorists such as Claire Bishop, the issue really is that visual arts are looking in the wrong way at the wrong place. In her text on installation and what she has termed 'the immersive condition,' Bishop has argued that in fact the built space of the cinema set up all the parameters for installation of the late twentieth century and produced particular forms of installation.[15] Along with cinema, media technologies have not only ordered the world, but do so at speeds and time too fast for us to perceive. Despite this escalation, the cinematic experience continues to dominate the public language of visual cultures and along with it—an ongoing desire for immersion in a communal

15 Claire Bishop, *Installation Art: A Critical History* (London: Tate, 2005), 13.

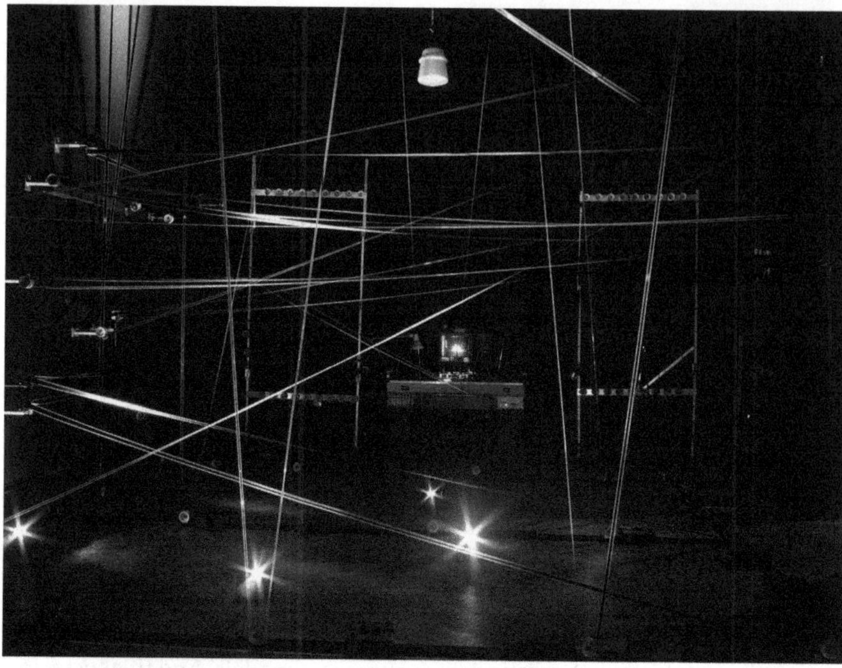

FIGURE 14.1 View of Atom Egoyan's *Steenbeckett*

activity. All the more reason, says Bishop, not to look at the screen alone, the questions of immersion through cinematic apparatuses, nor indeed through cinematic language since in none of these dimensions can we grasp the essentials of what is ordering our world. What we should do, she says, is to look closer at the viewing experience in built space and to consider spatial concepts. The point that art historian and media theorist Oliver Grau advocates is that the viewing experience in moving image installations is no longer singular and by its very nature has created an immersive 'thinking space' for viewers that is very well taken here.[16] The call then is for a moment of perception; that is, to find the patterns of culture we should explore the spatial practices and structures of cultural spaces. It seems to me that to understand the patterns of culture we should explore space through participation or in the geometries of the actual architecture. It is there that we should find what we might term the immersive dialectic.

16 Oliver Grau, *Virtual Art: From Illusion to Immersion* (Cambridge: MIT Press, 2004), 254.

2 Atom Egoyan's *Steenbeckett*

One place then where these ideas of immersion and dialectics have appeared in my work is around Atom Egoyan and his installation work *Steenbeckett* (2002). What I want to do with the rest of this chapter is to make some observations about that work and also to connect very specifically to some of the things that give rise to immersion in cultural spaces. The installation *Steenbeckett*, shown recently at the Whitworth Gallery in Manchester, visualizes and traces Samuel Beckett's well-known play *Krapp's Last Tape* (1958) into a visual field, but does so in a totally encompassing way. As a centrepiece of this installation Egoyan uses his own directed film of *Krapp's Last Tape* (2000), in which a haunted sexagenarian played by John Hurt reviews self-important reel-to-reel tapes he made in his prime, to reflect on the pain of hubris and memories of loss.

The viewer is immersed in Krapp's reverie through a dense aesthetic layering of technologies in space. Two thousand feet of 35 mm celluloid travels around the darkened gallery on a system of pulley-suspended sprockets attached to the gallery walls, propelled through a Steenbeck editing table, whose small screen also serves as our fittingly obscure and distance window onto Krapp. In traditional film, the position of the viewer is physically passive—the process of spectatorship is physically still. The film becomes the point of spectatorship and the body is largely left behind. Here the viewer experiences greater eye mobility, shifting points of view, and an uncanny sense of architectural closeness. This experiential dimension—a sense of closeness—was recognized by Walter Benjamin when he related cinema's new mode of spectatorship to the way we respond to buildings. In his view the spectatorial practice established by architecture is based on collective use:

> The distracted mass absorbs the work of art. This is most obvious with regard to buildings. Architecture has always represented the prototype of a work of art the reception of which is consummated by a collective in a state of distraction.[17]

In this hybrid of a white cube and black box, each model informs and modifies the characteristics of each other. And while the potency of this work lies in the transgression of the surface of the wall, it shapes experience by nudging the

17 Walter Benjamin, 'The Work of Art in the Age of Mechanical Reproduction,' *Illuminations*, translated by Harry Zohn (New York: Harcourt Brace Jovanovich, 1968), 572.

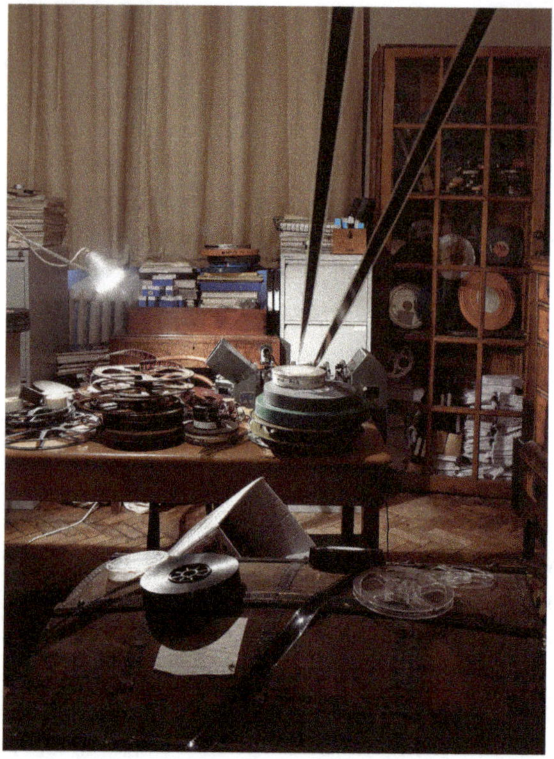

FIGURE 14.2 View of Atom Egoyan's *Steenbeckett* (2002) in *Projections: Works from The Artangel Collection* (2011).
© ATOM EGOYAN, 2002. PHOTO CREDIT: COURTESY THE ARTIST AND THE WHITWORTH ART GALLERY, THE UNIVERSITY OF MANCHESTER. USED WITH PERMISSION.

viewer into new forms of experience. And as Sylvia Lavin points out 'Kissing is a means of extending and identifying architectural effects.'[18]

These extending and identifying effects are visible in the rest of the exhibition space. Off in the corner of the darkened installation through a doorway is another visual field of an illuminated room arranged like Krapp's den packed with objects. Its structural and compositional features channel the body's resonance with and immersion in its immediate surroundings. The intimate detail provided by the space (spools, canisters, etc.) gives the viewer a sense of familiarity, however its attraction resides in the fact that the viewer is confronted with simultaneous sites: the visible simulation and its real counterpart. It is well known that Beckett was deeply involved in the resistance against fascism

18 Lavin, *Kissing Architecture*, 33.

choosing to join the Resistance and remain in Nazi-occupied France during World War II. Less well known is Beckett's writing on the ruined spaces and reconstructed buildings in war-torn France as emblematic of the timelessness of suffering.[19] At first glance, it may seem curious that Beckett considered built space in the midst of genocide. There is a very good reason for this. Although, people were repeatedly told to move forward and forget the past in the name of reconstruction and progress, for most, the Holocaust was arguably a present absence.

What one learns from Beckett's writing applies to the self, and to everyone, it is a commentary on selective forgetting rather than memory itself. Beckett seems to be showing that it is not enough to simply think of memory, but also by time, action and importantly space. It is not enough to simply remember an individual, as that person may be entirely different depending on the space and time of reference. If one was to talk about the past, the question arises: what and how does one remember? What and how does one forget? Only through careful consideration can this be resolved.

This becomes clearer with recent re-evaluations of Beckett's work that reveal how his writing was irrevocably changed by the events of World War II and in particular France's deathly indifference to the mass deportation and murder of thousands of its Jewish citizens.[20] In order to heal the state, one was asked to forget terrible experiences undergone by its Jewish citizenry under the war-time French government. While it is interesting to understand that historical and social crisis became the impetus and inspiration for Beckett, the decisive thing is to understand that this selective forgetting around the Holocaust led him to see space not as simple, nor as something without meaning. One may ask why? The answer lies in post-war spatial turn in cultural practices across Europe described earlier. Like many of his post-war generation, Beckett understood that language was not enough to describe the devastating effects of World War II and its genocidal legacy. Beckett's plays manifest these anxieties not only in the words and in the rhythm of their dialogue, but importantly in the mood-inducing environment of space itself. His ensuing struggle

19 Samuel Beckett, 'The Capital of Ruins' *The Complete Short Prose 1929–1989*, ed. S.E. Gontarski (New York: Grove Press, 1995), 275.

20 Recent research on Beckett's war years include, Jackie Blackman 'Beckett Judaizing Beckett: "A Jew from Greenland" in Paris,' *Samuel Beckett Today/Aujourd'hui* 18 (2007): 325–340; James McNaughton 'Beckett, German Fascism and History: The Futility and Protest,' *Samuel Beckett Today/Aujourd'hui* 15 (2005): 101–116; Jackie Blackman, 'Beckett's Theatre "After Auscwitz",' *Samuel Beckett: History, Memory, Archive*, edited by Sean Kennedy and Katherine Weiss (New York; Palgrave Macmillan 2009), 71–87.

to make meaning out of this dark period of European history led to the placement of audiences in front of empty stages in which the bare walls of theatre left audiences to grapple with lingering ghosts and hold-over ideologies of an accelerated war-time modernity. And this brings us to the heart of the matter.

The likes of Bode, Beckett and other post-war thinkers did not have the slightest intention of creating empty formalism: they interpreted space in a manner to elicit emotive responses. By shaping space, Beckett's work created affective environments in post-war visual expression in which bearing witness to the Holocaust was complicated by the fact that so many who witnessed these atrocities were murdered in the gas chambers.

In *Remnants of Auschwitz*, Giorgio Agamben writes:

> The witness usually testifies in the name of justice and truth and as such his or her speech draws consistency and fullness. Yet here the value of testimony lies essentially in what it lacks: at its centre it contains something that cannot be borne witness to and that discharges the survivors of authority. The 'true witnesses,' the 'complete witnesses' are those who did not bear witness and could not bear witness. The survivors speak in their stead, by proxy, as pseudo-witnesses: they bear witness to a missing testimony.[21]

This becomes clearer if we go back once again to *Steenbeckett*. Missing testimony is signalled in *Steenbeckett* installation, encountered again and completed by another screen situated in a separate room where one can watch the entirety of the film *Krapp's Last Tape*. Krapp sits in his den—as he does every year to record his impressions of the past year—but instead is drawn to recordings from his past. The endless repetitive movement of 35mm celluloid throughout the gallery space, in its iconic movement, offers a visual parallel to Krapp's listening to the narrated episodes of his life that pass from spool to spool. While sitting watching *Krapp's Last Tape*, one can consider Krapp's reverie of his career and sexual prowess and his own present self's amusement and anger at his youthful folly:

> Hard to believe I was ever that young whelp. The voice! Jesus! And the aspirations! (*Brief laugh Krapp in which Krapp joins.*) And the resolutions! (*Brief laugh in which Krapp joins.*) To drink less, in particular. (*Brief laugh of Krapp alone.*) Statistics. Seventeen hundred hours, out of the preceding eight thousand odd, consumed on licensed premises alone.

21 Giorgio Agamben, *Remnants of Auschwitz: The Witness and the Archive* (New York: MIT Press, 2007), 34.

> More than 20%, say 40% of his waking life. (*Pause*). Plans for a less ... (*hesitates*) ... engrossing sexual life. Last illness of his father. Flagging pursuit of happiness. Unattainable laxation. Sneers at what he calls his youth and thanks to God that it's over. (*Pause.*) False ring there. (*Pause.*) Shadows of the opus ... magnum. Closing with a—(*brief laugh*)—yelp to Providence. (*Prolonged laugh in which Krapp joins.*) What remains of all that misery?[22]

Amidst this dialectic of apotheosis and self-deprecation, Krapp moves into the darkness of the stage only to return to the lit desk to stare out to the audience and listen to the remains of his life. The image of John Hurt's return into the light is seared into the mind of many theatregoers as the centrepiece of *Krapp's Last Tape*. The sudden weariness of his expression, the failed writer, the human being bearing witness to the depth of his own lack of compassion—leaves a deep impression and prefaces the retelling of his collective memory. The individuality of each memory is preserved and at the same time its negative aspect remains—doubt. Here on this stage, there is no general view, no official version of events. Krapp's monologue builds this little by little with the audience, simultaneously acknowledges and challenges memory through the act of re-telling. Krapp's world becomes our own: its pettiness, its lost visions—and through all that, something untouchable, yet inescapable—the interconnectedness of all things. Rather than being auto-biographical, *Krapp's Last Tape*, looks at how regret is universal. The dominant element of Beckett's work is not about splitting memory into opposing poles, but its symbolic reunification lies within the character Krapp. This is the immersive dialectic, in which the opposites, instead of separating and entering into conflict, exist in function of one another, reinforcing one other. Such for Beckett, is the relation between loss and possibility. Such for Egoyan, is the mixed feelings between looking and not looking. Such for Lavin is the kiss between ephemeral images and affective constitutive environments. Such is the relationship that binds the walls in the gallery to other forms of visual practices temporarily shifting contexts while generating material closeness. Such finally, is the momentary generation of alternative possibilities between the audience and the work. The more immersive and affective, the more these elements shape experience, perception and understanding.

22 Samuel Beckett, *Krapp's Last Tape and Other Dramatic Pieces* (New York: Grove Press, Inc., 1957), 16.

Much like Beckett himself, Egoyan does not consider memory to be a mechanistic storehouse in which everything is preserved, according to a category and marked. Rather, Egoyan has argued that learning to embrace ambiguity and allowing a viewer to move through space in a meaningful ways provides a way to cope with traumatic pasts because it pushes people to keep confronting the moral challenges the events pose, rather than storing them away neatly as over and done with.[23] In this way, dialectical immersion is a central achievement of both these men—who both work to enact the voices of those who cannot speak. Therefore amongst such a thinking space, one can say the unsayable, witnessing as a proxy-witness so that to bear testimony, as Agamben suggests,

> ... is to place oneself in one's own language in the position of those who have lost it, to establish oneself in the living language as if it were dead, or in a dead language as if it were living ... It is not surprising that the witness' gesture is also that of the poet, the *auctor* par excellence ... Poets—witnesses—found language as what remains, as what actually survives the possibility, or impossibility, of speaking.[24]

When one returns to the darkened gallery to watch the ceaseless spinning celluloid it comes to mind that *Steenbeckett* raises another issue: that of endless tension without any apparent ending, reflecting a key problem for life in the visually mediated 21st century. Much like the windows in bombed out buildings and empty stages, we can only come to recognize this through the shaping of space for us in the promise of its meaning. In this sense, the immersion found in cultural spaces offers us something by subtly revealing something about our own anxiety in the midst of a period dominated by the politics of fear; a time when our expectations have been raised and lowered and we are exhausted from never knowing if the moment is at hand or still to come. While the end is what we all seek to avoid, *Steenbeckett* and other immersive installations demonstrate that in spite of the emitted sense of weariness and finality—an ending is not all and reminds us that the spaces placed in front of us often serve as thresholds to the possible, and that in spite of our individual limitations, one can move back into the light and something transformative can still occur.

23 Quoted in David Pike, 'The Passing of Celluloid, the Endurance of the Image: Egoyan, Steenbeckett and Krapp's Last Tape,' *Image and Territory: Essays on Atom Egoyan*, edited by Monique Tschofen and Jennifer Burwell (Waterloo: Wilfrid Laurier University Press, 2007), 101.

24 Agamben, *Remnants of Auschwitz: The Witness and the Archive*, 161.

Bibliography

Agamben, Giorgio. *Remnants of Auschwitz: The Witness and the Archive*. New York: MIT Press, 2007.

Baer, Hester. *Dismantling the Dream Factory: Gender, German Cinema, and the Postwar Quest for a New Film Language*. New York: Berghanon Books, 2012.

Benedetti, Lorenzo. 'Arnold Bode and the Perfect Combination of History, Environment and Contemporary.' *Cura* 11 (2012): 34–44.

Beckett, Samuel. *Krapp's Last Tape and Other Dramatic Pieces*. New York: Grove Press, Inc. 1957.

Beckett, Samuel. 'The Capital of Ruins.' *The Complete Short Prose 1929–1989*, edited by S.E. Gontarski, 275–278. New York: Grove Press, 1995.

Benjamin, Walter. 'The Work of Art in the Age of Mechanical Reproduction.' *Illuminations*. Translated by Harry Zohn. New York: Harcourt Brace Jovanovich, 1968.

Bishop, Claire. *Installation Art: A Critical History*. London: Tate, 2005.

Blackman, Jackie. 'Beckett Judaizing Beckett: "A Jew from Greenland" in Paris.' *Samuel Beckett Today/Aujourd'hui* 18 (2007): 325–340.

Blackman, Jackie. 'Beckett's Theatre "After Auscwitz." ' *Samuel Beckett: History, Memory, Archive*, edited by Sean Kennedy and Katherine Weiss, 71–87. New York: Palgrave Macmillan, 2009.

Caruth, Cathy. *Unclaimed Experience, Trauma, Narrative and History*. Baltimore: Johns Hopkins University Press, 1996.

Eisenstein, Sergei. 'A Dialectical Approach to Film Form.' *Film Form*, edited by Jay Leda, 45–63. New York: Harcourt, 1977.

Eisenstein, Sergei. 'Montage and Architecture.' *Assemblage* 10 (1989): 110–131.

Exotica. Directed by Atom Egoyan. Canada: Alliance Entertainment, Ego Film Arts, Miramax, Ontario Film Development Corporation and Téléfilm, 1994. DVD.

Grau, Oliver. *Virtual Art: From Illusion to Immersion*. Cambridge: MIT Press, 2004.

Greenberg, Clement. 'Modernist Painting.' *Clement Greenberg: The Collected Essays and Criticism*, vol. 4 of *Modernism with a Vengeance 1957–1969*, edited by John O'Brian, 85–93. Chicago: University of Chicago Press, 1993.

Judt, Tony. *Post War: A History of Europe since 1945*. New York: Penguin, 2005.

Kant, Immanuel. *The Moral Law: Kant's Groundwork of the Metaphysics of Morals*. Translated by H.J. Paton. London: Hutchinson, 1972.

Lavin, Sylvia. *Kissing Architecture*. Princeton, NJ: Princeton University Press, 2011.

McNaughton, James 'Beckett, German Fascism and History: The Futility and Protest.' *Samuel Beckett Today/Aujourd'hui* 15 (2005): 101–116.

Pérez-Gómez, Alberto. 'The Architecture of Richard Henriquez: A Praxis of Personal Memory.' *Richard Henriquez: Memory Theatre*, edited by Howard Shubert, 9–29. Montreal/Vancouver: Canadian Centre for Architecture and Vancouver Art Gallery, 1993.

Pike, David L. 'The Passing of Celluloid, the Endurance of the Image: Egoyan, Steenbeckett and Krapp's Last Tape.' *Image and Territory: Essays on Atom Egoyan*, edited by Monique Tschofen and Jennifer Burwell, 101–122. Waterloo: Wilfrid Laurier University Press, 2007.

Romanska, Magda. *The Post-Traumatic Theatre of Grotowski and Kantor: History and Holocaust in 'Akropolis' and 'Dead Class.'* New York: Anthem Press, 2014.

The Sweet Hereafter. Directed by Atom Egoyan. Canada: Alliance Communications Corporation, Ego Film Arts, Téléfilm Canada, Harold Greenberg Fund, The Movie Network, Canadian Film or Video Production Tax Credit. DVD.

Index

www.ingramcontent.com/pod-product-compliance
Lightning Source LLC
Chambersburg PA
CBHW071425230926
51846CB00001B/119
9789004376748